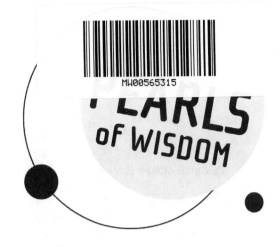

Pediatric
BOARD REVIEW

Third Edition

Peter Emblad
Scott H. Plantz
Robert M. Levin
Huiquan Zhao

McGraw-Hill
Medical Publishing Division

New York Chicago San Francisco Lisbon London
Madrid Mexico City Milan New Delhi
San Juan Seoul Singapore
Sydney Toronto

Pediatric Board Review, Third Edition

Copyright © 2006 by The McGraw-Hill Companies, Inc. All rights reserved. Printed in the United States of America. Except as permitted under the United States Copyright Act of 1976, no part of this publication may be reproduced or distributed in any form or by any means, or stored in a data base or retrieval system, without the prior written permission of the publisher.

1 2 3 4 5 6 7 8 9 0   CUS/CUS   0 9 8 7 6 5

ISBN 0-07-146444-1

The editors were Catherine A. Johnson and Marsha Loeb.
The production supervisor was Phil Galea.
The cover designer was Handel Low.
Von Hoffmann Graphics was printer and binder.

This book is printed on acid-free paper.

Cataloging-in-Publication data for this title is on file at the Library of Congress.

INTERNATIONAL EDITION ISBN: 0-07-110883-1

Copyright © 2006. Exclusive rights by The McGraw-Hill Companies, Inc. for manufacture and export. This book cannot be re-exported from the country to which it is consigned by McGraw-Hill. The International Edition is not available in North America.

DEDICATION

To my daughter, Annika, a source of endless amusement and amazement.
I look forward to watching you grow into the extraordinary woman
you are destined to become.

Peter Emblad

To my wife Cynna, thank you for picking me!

Scott H. Plantz

To my wife, Lisa A. Solinar, M.D., and to my children, Max, George, and Ana.

Robert M. Levin

To my parents and family, especially my son, he (at age 11) typed the first draft of my
mnemonics. To Drs. Farrell and Grabowski, and everyone in the Combined
Peds/Genetics Residency.

Huiquan Zhao

EDITORS:

Peter Emblad, M.D.
Department of Emergency Medicine
San Franscisco Kaiser Hospital
San Francisco, CA

Robert M. Levin, M.D.
Health Officer
Ventura County Public Health
Ventura, CA

Huiquan Zhao, M.D., Ph.D.
Divison of Human Genetics
Department of Pediatrics
Children's Hospital
Cincinnati, OH

Scott H. Plantz, M.D.
Associate Professor
Chicago Medical School
Mt. Sinai Medical Center
Chicago, IL

CONTRIBUTING AUTHORS:

Bobby Abrams, M.D.
Attending Physician
Macomb Hospital
Macomb, MI

Jonathan Adler, M.D.
Instructor
Harvard Medical School
Boston, MA

Raymond C. Baker, M.D.
Professor of Clinical Pediatrics
University of Cincinnati College of Medicine
Associate Director
Division of General & Community Pediatrics
Children's Hospital
Cincinnati, OH

Kristen Bechtel, M.D., MCP
Assistant Professor of Emergency Medicine
Allegheny University of Health Sciences
Attending Physician
Department of Pediatric Emergency
St. Christopher's Hospital for Children
Philadelphia, PA

Michelle L. Bez, D.O.
Newcomb Medical Center
Vineland, NJ

Frank M. Biro, M.D.
Professor of Clinical Pediatrics
University of Cincinnati College of Medicine
Associate Director
Division of Adolescent Medicine
Children's Hospital
Cincinnati, OH

David F.M. Brown, M.D.
Instructor in Medicine
Harvard Medical School
Massachusetts General Hospital
Boston, MA

Eduardo Castro, M.D.
Instructor in Medicine
Harvard Medical School
Massachusetts General Hospital
Boston, MA

Leslie S. Carroll, M.D.
Assistant Professor
Chicago Medical School
Toxocology Director
Mt. Sinai Medical Center
Chicago, IL

Marjorie Chaparro, M.D.
Department of Pediatrics
Mount Sinai Hospital
Chicago, IL

Deandra Clark, M.D.
Department of Pediatrics
University of South Florida
Tampa, FL

David Cone, M.D.
Assistant Professor of Emergency Medicine
Chief, Division of Emergency Medical Services
Department of Emergency Medicine
Allegheny University of Health Sciences
Philadelphia, PA

James Corrall, M.D., MPH
Clinical Associate Professor of Pediatrics and
Emergency Medicine
Indiana University School of Medicine
Indianapolis, IN

Judith A. Dattaro, M.D.
Attending, Emergency Department
The New York Hospital
Instructor, Department of Surgery
Cornell V.A. Medical Center
New York, NY

Carl W. Decker, M.D.
Madigan Army Medical Center
Fort Lewis, WA

Phillip G. Fairweather, M.D.
Clinical Assistant Professor
Mt. Sinai School of Medicine
New York, NY
Department of Emergency Medicine
Elmhurst Hospital Center
Elmhurst, NY

Craig Feied, M.D.
Associate Professor
Washington Hospital Center
George Washington University
Washington, D.C.

David Neal Franz, M.D.
Associate Professor of Pediatrics and Neurology
University of Cincinnati College of Medicine
Director
Tuberous Sclerosis Clinic
Children's Hospital
Cincinnati, OH

Anne Freter, RN, BSN
Intensive Care Unit
Hope Children's Hospital
Oak Lawn, IL

Lynn Garfunkel, M.D.
Assistant Professor of Pediatrics
Associate Director
Pediatrics Residency Training Program
Director
Combined Internal Medicine and Pediatric
Residency Training Program
University of Rochester School of Medicine and
Dentistry
Rochester, NY

Jay Gold, M.D.
MediStar
Madison, WI

Javier A. Gonzalez del Rey, M.D.
Associate Professor
University of Cincinnati College of Medicine
Associate Director
Division of Emergency Medicine and
Pediatrics Residency Training Program
Director
Pediatric Emergency Medicine Fellowship
Program
Children's Hospital
Cincinnati, OH

William Gossman, M.D.
Mt. Sinai Medical Center
Chicago Medical School
Chicago, IL

John Graneto, D.O.
Director, Pediatric Emergency Medicine
Lutheran General Children's Hospital
Park Ridge, IL

Ned Hayes, M.D.
Chief, Epidemiology Section
Bacterial Zoonoses Branch
Division of Vector-Borne Infectious Diseases
Centers for Disease Control and Prevention
Fort Collins, CO

James F. Holmes, M.D.
University of California, Davis-School of
Medicine
Sacramento, CA

Eddie Hooker, M.D.
Assistant Professor
University of Louisville
Louisville, KY

Ira Horowitz, M.D.
Director, Intermediate Intensive Care Unit
Department of Pediatrics
Division of Critical Care Medicine
Hope Children's Hospital
Christ Hospital and Medical Center
Oak Lawn, IL

Matt Kopp, M.D.
Department of Emergency Medicine
Rhode Island Hospital
Brown University School of Medicine
Providence, RI

Lance W. Kreplick, M.D.
Assistant Professor
University of Illinois
EHS Christ Hospital
Oak Lawn, IL

Deborah A. Lee, M.D., Ph.D.
Assistant Professor
Department of Psychiatry
Clinical Assistant Professor
Department of Pediatrics
Director
Child Neurology TP
Tulane University
New Orleans, LA

Gillian Lewke, P.A., CMA
Boston City Hospital
Boston, MA

Bernard Lopez, M.D.
Assistant Professor
Thomas Jefferson Medical College
Thomas Jefferson University Hospital
Philadelphia, PA

Mary Nan S. Mallory, M.D.
Instructor
University of Louisville
Louisville, KY

Bridget A. Martell, M.D.
Yale New Haven Hospital
Huguenot, NY

David Morgan, M.D.
Jules Stein Eye Institute
Los Angeles, CA

James J. Nordlund, M.D.
Professor
Department of Dermatology
University of Cincinnati College of Medicine
Children's Hospital
Cincinnati, OH

Peter Noronha, M.D.
Associate Professor of Clinical Pediatrics
Associate Program Director of Pediatrics
University of Illinois College of Medicine
Chicago, IL

Scott E. Olitsky, M.D.
Assistant Professor
Residency Program Director
Department of Ophthalmology

State University of New York at Buffalo and the
Children's Hospital of Buffalo
Buffalo, NY

Edward A. Panacek, M.D.
Associate Professor
University of California, Davis - School of
Medicine
Sacramento, CA

Geraldo Reyes, M.D.
Director
Critical Care Training
Hope Children's Hospital
Oak Lawn, IL

Karen Rhodes, M.D.
University of Chicago Medical Center
Chicago, IL

Luis R. Rodriquez, M.D., F.A.A.P.
Assistant Professor
Department of Pediatrics
Mt. Sinai School of Medicine
New York, NY
Elmhurst Hospital Center
Elmhurst, NY

Carlo Rosen, M.D.
Instructor
Harvard Medical School
Massachusetts General Hospital
Boston, MA

Bruce K. Rubin, M.D.
Professor of Pediatrics, Physiology and
Pharmacology
Brenner Children's Hospital
Winston-Salem, NC

Howard M. Saal, M.D.
Professor of Clinical Pediatrics
University of Cincinnati College of Medicine
Head, Clinical Genetics
Director, Medical Genetics Residency Program
Children's Hospital
Cincinnati, OH

Alan Schooley, M.D.
Children's Hospital
Boston, MA

Girish D. Sharma, M.D., FCCP
Assistant Professor
Section of Pediatric Pulmonology
The University of Chicago Children's Hospital
Chicago, IL

Rejesh Shenoy, M.D.
Department of Pediatrics
University of Illinois College of Medicine
Chicago, IL

Clifford S. Spanierman, M.D., FAAP
Pediatric Emergency Physician
Department of Emergency Medicine
Lutheran General Children's Hospital
Park Ridge, IL

Dana Stearns, M.D.
Instructor
Harvard Medical School
Massachusetts General Hospital
Boston, MA

Jack Stump, M.D.
Attending Physician
Rogue Valley Medical Center
Medford, OR

Joan Surdukowski, M.D.
Assistant Professor
Mt. Sinai Medical Center
Chicago Medical School
Chicago, IL

Loice Swischer, M.D.
Medical College of Pennsylvania
Philadelphia, PA

Nicholas Tapas, M.D.
General Pediatrician
Lutheran General Children's Hospital
Park Ridge, IL

Hector Trujillo, M.D.
General Pediatrician
Miami Children's Hospital
Miami, FL

Michael Zevitz, M.D.
Assistant Professor
Chicago Medical School
Chicago, IL

Stan Zuba, M.D.
Assistant Professor of Pediatrics
RUSH/The Chicago Medical School
Chicago, IL

INTRODUCTION

Congratulations! *Pediatric Board Review: Pearls of Wisdom*, will help you learn some medicine. Originally designed as a study aid to improve performance on the Pediatric Written Board exams or Pediatric In-service exam, this book is full of useful information. A few words are appropriate discussing intent, format, limitations, and use.

Since *Pediatric Board Review* is primarily intended as a study aid, the text is written in rapid-fire question/answer format. This way, readers receive immediate gratification. Moreover, misleading or confusing "foils" are not provided. This eliminates the risk of erroneously assimilating an incorrect piece of information that makes a big impression. Questions themselves often contain a "pearl" intended to reinforce the answer. Additional "hooks" may be attached to the answer in various forms, including mnemonics, visual imagery, repetition, and humor. Additional information not requested in the question may be included in the answer. Emphasis has been placed on distilling trivia and key facts that are easily overlooked, that are quickly forgotten, and that somehow seem to be needed on board examinations.

Many questions have answers without explanations. This enhances ease of reading and rate of learning. Explanations often occur in a later question/answer. Upon reading an answer, the reader may think, "Hm, why is that?" or, "Are you sure?" If this happens to you, go check! Truly assimilating these disparate facts into a framework of knowledge absolutely requires further reading of the surrounding concepts. Information learned in response to seeking an answer to a particular question is retained much better than information that is passively observed. Take advantage of this! Use *Pediatric Board Review* with your preferred source texts handy and open.

Pediatric Board Review has limitations. We have found many conflicts between sources of information. We have tried to verify in several references the most accurate information. Some texts have internal discrepancies further confounding clarification.

Pediatric Board Review risks accuracy by aggressively pruning complex concepts down to the simplest kernel—the dynamic knowledge base and clinical practice of medicine is not like that! Furthermore, new research and practice occasionally deviates from that which likely represents the right answer for test purposes. This text is designed to maximize your score on a test. Refer to your most current sources of information and mentors for direction.

Pediatric Board Review is designed to be used, not just read. It is an *interactive* text. Use a 3 x 5 card and cover the answers; attempt all questions. A study method we recommend is oral, group study, preferably over an extended meal or pitchers. The mechanics of this method are simple and no one ever appears stupid. One person holds the book, with answers covered, and reads the question. Each person, including the reader, says "Check!" when he or she has an answer in mind. After everyone has "checked" in, someone states his/her answer. If this answer is correct, on to the next one; if not, another person says their answer or the answer can be read. Usually the person who "checks" in first receives the first shot at stating the answer. If this person is being a smarty-pants answer-hog, then others can take turns. Try it, it's almost fun!

Pediatric Board Review is also designed to be re-used several times to allow, dare we use the word, memorization. A hollow bullet is provided for any scheme of keeping track of questions answered correctly or incorrectly.

We welcome your comments, suggestions and criticism. Great effort has been made to verify these questions and answers. Some answers may not be the answer you would prefer. Most often this is attributable to variance between original sources. Please make us aware of any errors you find. We hope to make continuous improvements and would greatly appreciate any input with regard to format, organization, content, presentation, or about specific questions. We also are interested in recruiting new contributing authors and publishing new textbooks. We look forward to hearing from you!

Study hard and good luck!

P.E., R.M.L., H.Z. & S.P.

TABLE OF CONTENTS

INFECTIOUS DISEASES

O **How quickly do patients infected with HIV become symptomatic?**

Five to ten percent develop symptoms within three years of seroconversion. Predictive characteristics include a low T4 count and a hematocrit less than 40. The mean incubation time is about 8.23 years for adults and 1.97 years for children less than 5 years old. When AIDS develops, the survival duration is about 9 months. However, new treatments often prolong this time period.

O **An HIV+ patient presents with a history of weight loss, diarrhea, fever, anorexia, and malaise. She is also dyspneic. Lab studies reveal abnormal LFTs and anemia. What is the most likely diagnosis?**

Mycobacterium avium-intracellular. Lab confirmation is made by an acid-fast stain of body fluids or by a blood culture.

O **Which drugs are used to treat CNS toxoplasmosis in AIDS patients?**

Pyrimethamine plus sulfadiazine.

O **What is the most common cause of focal encephalitis in AIDS patients?**

Toxoplasmosis. Symptoms include focal neurologic deficits, headache, fever, altered mental status, and seizures. Ring enhancing-lesions are evident on CT.

O **The differential diagnosis of ring-enhancing lesions in AIDS patients is what?**

Lymphoma, cerebral tuberculosis, fungal infection, CMV, Kaposi's sarcoma, toxoplasmosis, and hemorrhage.

O **What is the presentation of an AIDS patient with tuberculous meningitis?**

Fever, meningismus, headache, seizures, focal neurologic deficits, and altered mental status.

O **On physical exam, what is the most common eye finding in AIDS patients?**

Cotton-wool spots. It has been proposed that the cotton-wool spots are associated with PCP. These finding may be hard to differentiate from fluffy-white, often perivascular retinal lesions that are associated with CMV.

O **What is the most common opportunistic infection in AIDS patients?**

PCP. Symptoms may include a non-productive cough and dyspnea. A chest x-ray may reveal diffuse interstitial infiltrates or it may be negative. Although, Gallium scanning is more sensitive, false positives occur. Initial treatment includes TMP-SMX. Pentamidine is an alternative.

O **How is Candida of the esophagus diagnosed in the ED?**

An air-contrast barium swallow shows ulcerations with plaques. In contrast, herpes esophagitis produces punched-out ulcerations with no plaques.

○   **What is the risk of contracting HIV infection after an occupational exposure?**

0.32%. Eighty percent of the occupational exposure-related infections are from needle sticks.

○   **A patient is infected with *Treponema pallidum*; what is the treatment?**

The type of treatment depends upon the stage (1°, 2°, 3°) of the infection. Stages 1° and 2° syphilis are treated with benzathine penicillin G (2.4 million units IM X 1 dose) or doxycycline (100 mg bid po for 14 day). Stage 3° syphilis is treated with benzathine penicillin G, 2.4 million units IM X 3 doses 3 weeks apart.

○   **What is the cause of chancroid?**

Hemophilus ducreyi. Patients with this condition present with one or more painful necrotic lesions. Suppurating inguinal lymphadenopathy may also be present.

○   **What is the cause of granuloma inguinale?**

Calymmatobacterium granulomatis. Typically the onset occurs with small papular, nodular, or vesicular lesions that develop slowly into ulcerative or granulomatous lesions. Lesions are painless and are located on mucous membranes of the genital, inguinal, and anal areas.

○   **What is the causative agent in tetanus?**

Clostridium tetani. This organism is a Gram-positive rod, vegetative, and a spore former. *C. tetani* produces tetanospasmin, an endotoxin, which induces the disinhibition of the motor and autonomic nervous systems and thus the exhibition of tetanus clinical symptoms.

○   **What is the incubation period of tetanus?**

Hours to over 1 month. The shorter the incubation period, the more severe the disease.

○   **What is the <u>most</u> <u>common</u> presentation of tetanus?**

"Generalized tetanus" with pain and stiffness in the trunk and jaw muscles. Trismus develops and results in risus sardonicus (i.e., a sardonic smile).

○   **A patient presents with fever, dyspnea, cough, hemoptysis, and eosinophilia What parasite might cause this?**

Ascaris lumbricoides. This helminth is a roundworm. Serologic tests include an ELISA, a bentonite flocculation, and an indirect hemagglutination. Treat with pyrantel pamoate (pyrimidine pamoate) or mebendazole. An obstruction of the intestine may require surgery.

○   **How is hookworm, *Necator americanus*, infection acquired?**

In areas where human fertilizer is used and people don't wear shoes. Patients present with chronic anemia, cough, low-grade fever, diarrhea, abdominal pain, weakness, weight loss, eosinophilia, and guaiac positive stools. A diagnosis is confirmed if ova is present in the stool. Treatment includes mebendazole or pyrantel pamoate.

○   **What are the signs and symptoms of *Trichuris trichiura*?**

This hookworm lives in the cecum. Complaints include anorexia, abdominal pain especially RUQ, insomnia, fever, diarrhea, flatulence, weight loss, pruritus, eosinophilia, and microcytic hypochromic anemia. A diagnosis is made by examining for ova in the stool. Mebendazole is the treatment of choice.

○ **List 3 common protozoa that can cause diarrhea.**

1. *Entamoeba histolytica.* Occurs worldwide. Although half of the infected patients are asymptomatic, the usual symptoms consist of N/V/D/F, anorexia, abdominal pain, and leukocytosis. Determine the presence of this organism by ordering stool tests and performing an ELISA for extraintestinal infections. Treatment is with metronidazole or tinidazole followed by chloroquine phosphate.

2. *Giardia lamblia.* Occurs worldwide. This organism is one of the most common intestinal parasites in the U. S.. Symptoms include explosive watery diarrhea, flatus, abdominal distention, fatigue, and fever. The diagnosis is confirmed via a stool examination. Treatment is with metronidazole.

3. *Cryptosporidium parvum.* Occurs worldwide. Symptoms are profuse watery diarrhea, cramps, N/V/F, and weight loss. Treatment is supportive care. Medications may be needed for immunocompromised patients.

○ **Explain the pathophysiology of rabies.**

Infection occurs within the myocytes for the first 48 to 96 hours. It then spreads across the motor endplate and ascends and replicates along the peripheral nervous system, axoplasm, and into the dorsal root ganglia, spinal cord, and CNS. From the gray matter, the virus spreads by peripheral nerves back to tissues and organ systems.

○ **What is the characteristic histologic finding associated with rabies?**

Eosinophilic intracellular lesions found within the cerebral neurons called Negri bodies are the sites of CNS viral replication. Although these lesions occur in 75% of rabies cases and are pathognomonic for rabies, their absence does not eliminate the possibility of rabies.

○ **What are the signs and symptoms of rabies?**

Incubation period of 12 to 700 days with an average of 20 to 90 days. The initial signs and systems begin with fevers, headache, malaise, anorexia, sore throat, nausea, cough, and pain or paresthesias at the bite site.

During the CNS stage, agitation, restlessness, altered mental status, painful bulbar and peripheral muscular spasms, bulbar or focal motor paresis, and opisthotonos are exhibited. 20% develop ascending, symmetric flaccid and areflexic paralysis. In addition, hypersensitivity to water and sensory stimuli to light, touch, and noise may occur.

The progressive stage includes lucid and confused intervals with hyperpyrexia, lacrimation, salivation, and mydriasis along with brainstem dysfunction, hyperreflexia, and extensor planter response.

In the final stages, coma, convulsions, and apnea occur, followed by death between the fourth and seventh day for the untreated patient. The treated patient may survive for 14 days.

○ **What is the diagnostic procedure of choice in rabies?**

Fluorescent antibody testing (FAT).

○ **How is rabies treated?**

Prevention is the most effective treatment. Wound care of a suspected rabies bite should include debridement and aggressive irrigation. The wound must not be sutured; it should remain open. This will decrease the rabies infection by 90%. RIG 20 IU/kg, as much as possible at wound site and the remainer in the deltoid muscle, should be administered along with HDCV, 1-mL doses IM on days 0, 3, 7, 14, and 28, also in the deltoid muscle.

○ **What is the second <u>most</u> <u>common</u> tick borne disease?**

Rocky Mountain spotted fever (RMSF). The causative agent is *Rickettsia rickettsii* and the vectors are the female Ixodi ticks, *Dermacentor andersoni* (wood tick) and *D. variabilis* (American dog tick). Lyme disease is the most common tick borne disease.

○ **Which test should be performed to confirm RMSF?**

Immunofluorescent antibody staining of a skin biopsy or a serologic fluorescent antibody titer. The Weil-Felix reaction and complement fixation tests are no longer recommended.

○ **Which antibiotics are prescribed for the treatment of RMSF?**

Tetracycline or chloramphenicol. Antibiotic therapy should not be withheld pending serologic confirmation.

○ **Which is the most deadly form of malaria?**

Plasmodium falciparum.

○ **What is the vector for malaria?**

The female Anopheline mosquito.

○ **What lab findings are expected for a patient with malaria?**

Normochromic normocytic anemia, a normal or depressed leukocyte count, thrombocytopenia, an elevated sed rate, abnormal kidney and LFTs, hyponatremia, hypoglycemia, and a false-positive VDRL.

○ **How is the definitive diagnosis of malaria established?**

Visualization of parasites on Giemsa-stained blood smears. In early infection, especially with *P. falciparum*, parasitized erythrocytes may be sequestered and undetectable.

○ **What is the drug of choice for treating *P. vivax*, *ovale*, and *malariae*?**

Chloroquine.

○ **How is uncomplicated chloroquine-resistant *P. falciparum* treated?**

Quinine plus pyrimethamine-sulfadoxine plus doxycycline or mefloquine.

○ **How is complicated chloroquine-resistant *P. falciparum* treated?**

Quinidine gluconate IV plus doxycycline IV.

○ **Which type of parasite infections do not typically result in eosinophilia?**

Protozoa infections, such as amebas, Giardia, Trypanosoma, and Babesia.

○ **Which is the <u>most</u> <u>common</u> intestinal parasite in the US?**

Giardia. Cysts are obtained from contaminated water or passed by hand-to-mouth transmission. Symptoms include explosive foul-smelling diarrhea, abdominal distention, fever, fatigue, and weight loss. Cysts reside in the duodenum and upper jejunum.

○ **How is Chagas disease transmitted?**

The blood-sucking Reduviid "kissing" bug, blood transfusion, or breast feeding. A nodule or chagoma develops at the site of the bite. Symptoms include fever, headache, conjunctivitis, anorexia, and myocarditis. CHF and ventricular aneurysms can occur. The myenteric plexus is involved and may result in megacolon. Lab findings include anemia, leukocytosis, elevated sed rate, and ECG changes, such as PR interval, heart block, T-wave changes, and arrhythmias.

○ **What are two diseases that the deer tick, *Ixodes dammini*, transmits?**

Lyme disease and Babesia.

○ **How do patients present with Babesia infection?**

Intermittent fever, splenomegaly, jaundice, and hemolysis. The disease may be fatal in patients without spleens. Treatment is with clindamycin and quinine.

○ **When are patients most likely to acquire Lyme disease?**

Late spring to late summer with the highest incidence in July.

○ **How is Lyme disease diagnosed?**

Immunofluorescent and immunoabsorbent assays identify the antibodies to the spirochete. Treatment includes doxycycline or tetracycline, amoxicillin, IV penicillin (V in pregnant patients), or erythromycin.

○ **Which type of paralysis does tick paralysis cause?**

Ascending paralysis. The venom that causes the paralysis is probably a neurotoxin. A conduction block is induced at the peripheral motor nerve branches and thereby prevents the release of acetylcholine at the neuromuscular junction. Forty-three species of ticks have been implicated as causative agents.

○ **What is the <u>most</u> <u>common</u> sign of tularemia?**

Lymphadenopathy, usually cervical in children and inguinal in adults. It is caused by *Francisella tularensis* and is transmitted by the vectors *Dermacentor variabilis* and *Amblyomma americanum*.

○ **A patient presents with a sudden onset of fever, lethargy, headache, myalgias, anorexia, nausea, and vomiting. She describes the headache as retro-orbital and is extremely photophobic. The patient has been on a camping trip in Wyoming. What tick-borne disease might cause these symptoms?**

A virus of the genus Orbivirus, of the family, Reoviridae, causes Colorado tick fever. The vector is the tick *D. andersoni*. The disease is self-limited and treatment is supportive.

○ **What is the <u>most</u> <u>common</u> cause of cellulitis?**

Streptococcus pyogenes. *Staphylococcus aureus* can also cause cellulitis though it is generally less severe and more often associated with an open wound.

○ **What is the <u>most</u> <u>common</u> cause of cutaneous abscesses?**

Staphylococcus aureus is the most common aerobe in cutaneous abscesses; two-thirds are found in the upper torso, 97% are resistant to penicillin G.

○ **What is the probable cause of an infection arising from an animal bite that develops in less than 24 hours? More than 48 hours?**

Less than 24 hours is typically *P. multocida* or Streptococci. More than 48 hours is usually *Staphylococcus aureus*.

O   **A patient who was involved in a work-related crush injury to his foot is brought to your office a day after the injury in shock. The patient has a fever, severe pain, and a horrible smell coming from his foot. On palpation you feel crepitus. Diagnosis?**

Gas gangrene. Gas from the infection quickly invades the fascial planes accounting for the crepitus. Treatment is with wound debridement and systemic antibiotics. The drug of choice is penicillin G; an alternative is chloramphenicol.

O   **What is the <u>most</u> <u>common</u> cause of gas gangrene?**

Clostridium perfringens.

O   **What is the <u>most</u> <u>common</u> site of herpes simplex I virus infection?**

The lower lip. First the lip itches and burns. Then the small vesicle with the red base appears. These lesions are painful and can frequently recur since the virus remains in the sensory ganglia. Recurrences are generally triggered by stress, sun, and illness.

O   **What are the most common causes of otitis media?**

S. pneumoniae, non typeable *H. influenza, and M. catarrhalis.*

O   **An infant is brought to your office with fever and lethargy. On physical exam, you notice purulent rhinitis and an adherent membrane. The pt also has some shallow ulcers on the upper lip. What is your diagnosis?**

Diptheria in nares. This is more common in infants.

O   **What are the 3 stages of pertussis? How long does each last?**

Catarrhal, paroxysmal, and convalescent. Each stage lasts about 2 weeks.

O   **How do you calculate dosages for antibiotics in obese children?**

Calculate their ideal weight from height and use that.

O   **What are the most common viral causes of pneumonia in the otherwise healthy child?**

RSV, influenza, parainfluenza, and adenovirus.

O   **What viral cause of pneumonia can lead to acute fulminant pneumonia?**

Adenovirus.

O   **What is the treatment of choice for gastroenteritis caused by Shigella in an 8-year-old child?**

TMP/SMX or cefixime if resistant.

O   **The "red man syndrome" is classically associated with what antibiotic?**

Too rapid an infusion of vancomycin.

O   **What is the drug of choice in a child with the signs and symptoms of whooping cough?**

Erythromycin estolate (10 mg/kg QID PO for 14 days).

○   **In a child with the typical facial features of classic mumps, where else on the body should you look for suggestive signs?**

Look for sternal edema (classic) and examine the testicles.

○   **An 11-year-old child stepped on a nail on his way home from school. The nail pierced through his sneaker and into his foot. His tetanus status is up to date. What is you main concern?**

Infection with Pseudomonas that can lead to osteomyelitis. Pseudomonal infection is soon most commonly in association with hot, moist environments, such as sneakers.

○   **What would be your empiric antibiotic of choice for the boy in the preceding question?**

Ceftazidime (100mg/kg/day as TID) AND nafcillin (150mg/kg/day as QID). Debridement with culture is a cornerstone of therapy.

○   **What is the most common cause of infectious arthritis in patients with sickle cell disease? What joint is most commonly affected?**

Staph. aureus remains the most common cause, as in otherwise healthy children. However, *Salmonella* is more commonly seen in septic arthritis in children with hemoglobinopathies. The hip is most commonly affected.

○   **In a child with the clinical signs and symptoms of encephalitis, what non-invasive test can be used to determine whether herpes simplex is the causative agent?**

An EEG with patterns of periodic lateralized epileptiform discharges (PLEDs). An MRI of the brain is more sensitive.

○   **If the test above is positive, what test can be used to confirm your diagnosis of herpes simplex encephalitis?**

Polymerase chain reaction (PCR) analysis of CSF.

○   **Infection with what agent is commonly seen in children with liver transplants?**

CMV infection is seen in up to 60% of these patients.

○   **What is the antibiotic regimen of choice after an appendectomy?**

Cefoxitin or clindamycin and gentamicin.

○   **In the US what is the recommended time of isolation for a dog or cat to rule out rabies?**

10 days.

○   **What are the 2 causes of visceral larva migrans?**

Toxocara canis and Toxocara cati.

○   **A 15-year-old boy is brought to your office with a complaint of joint pains and general weakness. On physical exam, he has a slight fever and hepatosplenomegaly. The father states that the boy has been really depressed lately for no known reason- "why look how happy he was just 2 weeks ago when he shot his first elk!" The father shows a picture of the son holding onto his kill. What possible diagnosis is the picture a clue to?**

It should make you consider Brucellosis from handling the carcass or from ticks.

○   **Stool culture from the stool of a child reveals Cryptosporidium parvum. How should you treat it?**

Watchful waiting. The disease is usually self-limited and there is no effective antibiotic anyway.

○   **What is the easiest way to distinguish residual formula in the mouth from thrush in an infant?**

Formula is easily scraped away with a tongue depressor, while the same maneuver in a child with thrush might lead to minute bleeding points.

○   **Cerebral calcifications are most commonly associated with what 3 congenital infections?**

Toxoplasmosis, herpes simplex and cytomegalovirus.

○   **Minimal to severe brain dysfunction can be a sequelae of what intrauterine infections?**

Toxoplasmosis, rubella, CMV, and herpes.

○   **Which congenital infections are most common?**

CMV, though only about 5% will show any symptoms.

○   **In a pregnant woman with a parvovirus B19 infection, what test could be used to monitor for possible adverse outcomes?**

Serial fetal ultrasounds and maternal alpha-fetoprotein levels.

○   **What are the most characteristic abnormalities of congenital rubella syndrome?**

Congenital heart lesions (esp. PDA), microphthmalia, corneal opacities, cataracts, glaucoma, and radiolucent bone lesions.

○   **How is neonatal herpes usually contracted?**

Contact with genital secretions at delivery.

○   **What is the treatment of choice for the neonate with an HSV infection?**

Acyclovir, but Vidarabine may be just as effective.

○   **What test should be ordered to insure that a pregnant woman does not have an active hepatitis B infection?**

HBsAg.

○   **What is the characteristic triad of manifestations for late congenital syphilis?**

Hutchinson's triad consists of Hutchinson's teeth, interstitial keratitis, and eighth nerve deafness.

○   **What is the most effective method of reducing fever in a child?**

Acetaminophen (and NSAIDS) can return the set-point to normal. Cool sponge baths can also help.

○   **What organism is responsible for most cases of occult bacteremia in infants and toddlers?**

Streptococcus pneumoniae.

❍ **A child with a positive blood culture to what organism is most likely to develop meningitis?**

Meningiococcus.

❍ **How can the distribution of petechiae help one to evaluate the risk of a serious bacterial infection?**

Petechiae found only above the line of the nipples is rarely found in systemic disease.

❍ **What is necessary for the diagnosis of fever of unknown origin?**

1. History of fever over 1 week,
2. Documentation of fever by health provider,
3. Lack of a diagnosis after one week of investigation.

❍ **What specific substance in the body is the cause of fever?**

PGE_2.

❍ **A pediatric AIDS patient with enlargement of salivary glands, digital clubbing, and generalized lymphadenopathy and an x-ray that reveals a nodular, reticular pattern most likely has what disease?**

Lymphoid interstitial pneumonitis (LIP).

❍ **Which has a worse prognosis for the pediatric AIDS patient, PCP or LIP?**

PCP.

❍ **What is the current treatment of choice for LIP therapy?**

Systemic steroid therapy.

❍ **Why should a child with suspected idiopathic thrombocytopenic purpura (ITP) be tested for HIV?**

Because thrombocytopenia may be the presenting sign for HIV infection.

❍ **How do viral meningitis and bacterial meningitis differ with regards to CSF pressure? CSF leukocytes? CSF glucose?**

The pressure in bacterial infection is increased, whereas it is normal or slightly increased in viral. The leukocytosis is greater than 1000 (up to 60K) in bacterial, and rarely over 1000 in viral meningitis. The glucose concentration is decreased in bacterial meningitis and is generally normal in viral.

❍ **What is the most common cause of bacterial meningitis in a child greater than 2 months old?**

Strep. pneumonia, and *N. meningitidis.*

❍ **What antibiotic agent(s) should you start immediately in a toxic, febrile infant that is less than 3 months old?**

Ceftriaxone or cefotaxime and ampicillin.

❍   **What is the most common cause of death in children with HbSS?**

Infection.

❍   **A premature infant is delivered at 32 weeks of age. How long after delivery should the infant be given his first vaccine?**

Same schedule as a full-term baby.

❍   **Of measles, mumps, and rubella, which is the only vaccine component that is free of egg protein?**

Rubella.

❍   **What are the absolute contraindications to pertussis immunization?**

If the child had either an immediate anaphylactic reaction or an encephalopathy within one week of the previous vaccination.

❍   **An 8-year-old child who has never received any vaccinations is brought to your office. Should this child be given pertussis vaccine?**

No. In children greater than 7 years old, it is not necessary.

❍   **Which children should receive a meningococcal vaccine?**

Children over 2 years of age with either asplenia or complement deficiency.

❍   **Why do so many patients with meningitis become hyponatremic?**

Because a majority of patients with this disease develop some degree of SIADH.

❍   **What is the *sine quo non* of botulism poisoning presentation?**

Bulbar palsy.

❍   **If the mother of a child with erythema infectiosum is infected, what would be her most likely presentation?**

Arthralgia and arthritis.

❍   **Which cephalosporins cover *Listeria monocytogenes*?**

None. That is why ampicillin is usually added to the antibiotic regimen when infection with this organism is a possibility.

❍   **Where does the rash of rocky mountain spotted fever usually start?**

On the wrists and ankles. It then spreads to the trunk and extremities within hours.

❍   **A worried mother calls you concerned that her daughter was exposed to chicken pox at the day care center. If she were exposed, how long would it take for the symptoms to appear?**

Ten to twenty one days.

❍   **What is the most common cause of nosocomial bacteremia?**

Coagulase negative Staphylococcus. This is usually successfully treated with methicillin.

O   **A child is diagnosed with impetigo from group A streptococcus. What sequelae do you have to keep an eye out for?**

Acute post-streptococcal glomerulonephritis. Impetigo does not lead to rheumatic fever.

O   **What is the usual etiologic agent of a hordeolum (stye)?**

Staph. aureus.

O   **For a hordeolum from a Staph infection, what is the therapy of choice?**

Hot soaks, and I & D, if necessary. Routine antibiotic use is not recommended.

O   **What is considered to be the best therapy for patients with uncomplicated cat-scratch disease?**

Symptomatic relief. The use of antibiotic is controversial.

O   **What are the major Jones criteria used to diagnose rheumatic fever?**

Carditis, chorea (Sydenham), erythema marginatum, migratory polyarthritis, and subcutaneous nodules. The diagnosis requires either 2 major or 1 major and 2 minor with evidence of previous strep infection.

O   **What Jones criteria alone is sufficient for the diagnosis of rheumatic fever?**

Sydenham chorea. Deterioration in handwriting and increased clumsiness are commonly seen.

O   **A 10-year-old boy presents to your office with fever, tonsillopharyngitis, and lymphadenopathy. What laboratory tests will confirm your presumed diagnosis?**

CBC and Monospot should be all you need to confirm your suspicion of EBV (infectious mononucleosis).

O   **What would you expect to find on a peripheral blood smear of a patient with an acquired CMV infection?**

Absolute lymphocytosis and atypical lymphocytes.

O   **What is the drug of choice for meningococcal disease?**

Aqueous penicillin G is the ideal, though patients can be started effectively on empiric cefotaxime or ceftriaxone for suspected cases and in patients with penicillin allergy.

O   **How often are fever and a bulging fontanelle in an infant less than 2 months old with meningitis?**

Only about half have a fever, and only a third will have a bulging fontanelle.

O   **How is CNS hemorrhage differentiated from a traumatic tap?**

A traumatic tap will have a decreasing RBC count in each successive tube and will not have crenated RBCs or xanthochromia of the supernatant.

O   **Of bacterial, viral, fungal and tubercular meningitis, which typically presents with the greatest concentration of WBCs?**

Bacterial meningitis.

O   **In what circumstances would it be advisable to re-tap the child with meningitis?**

If there is no clinical response to antibiotic therapy within one to two days, or if cultures indicate that penicillin-resistant *Streptococcus pneumonia* is the causative agent, or with Gram negative meningitis.

O   **Culture of the CSF of your patient with meningitis grows the organism Citrobacter diversus. Aside from appropriate antibiotic therapy, what should be your next step?**

CT or MRI in anticipation of a brain abscess.

O   **Meningitis due to what organism most commonly presents with a sub-dural effusion?**

H. influenzae.

O   **Should people who have had contact with patients with meningococcal meningitis be given prophylactic antibiotics?**

Yes. Rifampin is recommended.

O   **What is, overall, the most common cause of aseptic meningitis?**

Enteroviruses.

O   **Generally speaking, how do exudates of viral conjunctivitis differ from bacterial conjunctivitis?**

Viral is serous, and bacterial is mucopurulent or purulent.

O   **What is the cause of epidemic keratoconjunctivitis?**

Adenovirus.

O   **What is the initial therapy of gonococcal ophthalmia neonatorum?**

Ceftriaxone or cefotaxime and saline irrigation of the eye until resolution of the discharge.

O   **Clinically, how can you distinguish orbital cellulitis from periorbital cellulitis?**

Extra-ocular muscle dysfunction, decreased pupillary reflexes, decreased visual acuity and changes in globe position are seen only in orbital cellulitis.

O   **With a child you suspect has an otitis media from the history, but are unable to visualize the lumen secondary to cerumen obstruction, how should you proceed?**

Remove the cerumen and visualize the membrane.

O   **What is the most common cause of hearing deficits in children?**

Secretory otitis media.

O   **What is the drug of choice for streptococcal pharyngitis?**

Penicillin V.

O   **After initiation of therapy for streptococcal pharyngitis, when should children be allowed back into school?**

After 24 hours have elapse.

❍   **What is the classic cause of herpangina?**

Coxsackievirus A16.

❍   **Does trismus more commonly occur with a peritonsillar abscess or peritonsillar cellulitis?**

Peritonsillar abscess.

❍   **Currently, what is the most common cause of epiglottitis?**

Group A Strep. The widespread use of the HiB vaccine has brought the number of Haemophilus induced epiglottitis cases down dramatically.

❍   **Are steroids effective in acute laryngotracheitis?**

Yes. The use of Dexamethasone (0.3-0.6 mg/kg) can lead to decreased need for intubation and more rapid improvement.

❍   **How often is sinus tenderness found in patients with sinusitis?**

Almost never.

❍   **What sinuses are most commonly involved in sinusitis?**

Ethmoid and maxillary sinuses.

❍   **What are the most common causes of acute sinusitis in children?**

Pneumococcus, H. influenzae non-typeable, and Moraxella catarrhalis (same as otitis media).

❍   **Why does therapy for TB take several months, when other infections usually clear in a matter of days?**

Because the mycobacteria divide very slowly and have a long dormant phase, during which time they are not responsive to medications.

❍   **What is the most common side effect of rifampin?**

Orange discoloration of urine and tears.

❍   **What negative outcome can be avoided by supplementing pyridoxine in patients receiving isoniazid?**

Peripheral neuritis and convulsions.

❍   **Name at least three infectious diseases that give false positive treponemal tests (FTA, MHA-TP, TPI) for syphilis.**

Yaws, pinta, leptospirosis, rat-bite fever (Spirillum minus) and lyme disease.

❍   **Name at least three diseases that give false positive non-treponema (VDRL, RPR) tests for syphilis.**

Infectious mononucleosis, connective tissue diseases, tuberculosis, endocarditis, and intravenous drug abuse.

❍   **What are the organisms most commonly thought to be associated with Guillain-Barré Disease?**

CMV, EBV, Coxsackie virus, Campylobacter jejuni, and Mycoplasma pneumoniae.

❍   **What is the appropriate diagnostic study to perform in order to distinguish lung sequestration from other changes on the pediatric chest x-ray?**

Angiography.

❍   **In what disease is cerebrospinal fluid albuminocytologic dissociation seen and what does it mean?**

Guillain-Barré Disease. An increase in cerebrospinal fluid protein without a corresponding increase in cerebrospinal fluid white cells is referred to as albuminocytologic dissociation.

❍   **Patients with HIV infections who go on to develop AIDS are most commonly infected with what organisms?**

Pneumocystis carinii, cytomegalovirus, candida, aspergillus, nocardia, cryptococcus, and mycobacteria.

❍   **Children with severe combined immunodeficiency disease tend to get what kinds of infectious diseases?**

Bacterial, viral, and fungal infections in general, and Pneumocystis carinii infections in particular.

❍   **Children who have cellular immunodeficiencies tend to get infections due to what organisms?**

Mycobacteria, nocardia, cytomegalovirus, varicella zoster virus, cryptococcus, candida, and Pneumocystis carinii.

❍   **Children with hypogammaglobulinemia tend to get infections with what organisms?**

The usual bacterial pathogens and pseudomonas.

❍   **Children with sickle cell disease most commonly are affected with what organisms?**

Streptococcus pneumoniae, Haemophilus influenzae B, and particularly sever Mycoplasma pneumoniae infections.

❍   **How is the diagnosis of histoplasmosis made in a child?**

By culture or staining from sputum, broncho alveolar lavage or tissue, and by a positive serology.

❍   **How is the diagnosis of coccidiomycosis made in a child?**

By culture or staining of sputum, broncho alveolar lavage or tissue, and by a positive serology.

❍   **How is the diagnosis of pulmonary blastomycosis made?**

By culture from sputum, bronchial washing or tissue.

❍   **How does one diagnose invasive aspergillosis?**

By biopsy.

❍ **How is an aspergilloma diagnosed?**

By chest x-ray.

❍ **How does one go about making the diagnosis of allergic broncho pulmonary aspergillosis?**

Patients will have eosinophilia, Aspergillus fumigatus in the sputum and serum IgE to aspergillus.

❍ **What is the evaluation of foreign body in the lung?**

Chest x-ray and bronchoscopy.

❍ **What is the evaluation for candida of the lung?**

Fresh sputum or transtracheal aspirate should reveal yeast and pseudohyphae. Mycelia and blastospores will be seen in established colonization, so a tissue exam is needed for definitive proof.

❍ **What are some of the most convenient ways to make the diagnosis of Mycoplasma pneumoniae?**

Cold agglutinin levels of ≈1:32 with consistent clinical findings will make presumptive diagnosis. A complement fixation level to Mycoplasma pneumoniae may be seen of ≈ than 1:256, or Mycoplasma pneumoniae specific IgA or IgM will be elevated.

❍ **What are the most common causes of non-infectious stomatitis?**

Behcet's syndrome, Stevens-Johnson syndrome, cancer chemotherapy, and Kawasaki syndrome.

❍ **What culture media are used to grow Neisseria gonorrhea and what is the appropriate treatment for the usual venereal presentations?**

Thayer-Martin or chocolate agar. The appropriate therapy is 125 mg of ceftriaxone intramuscularly one time. All such patients should be studied for chlamydia and syphilis infections as well.

❍ **What culture medium is used to isolate Corynebacterium diphtheriae and what antibiotic should be used for treatment?**

Corynebacterium diphtheriae should be cultured on either Loeffler's medium, tellurite agar, or silica gel pack. Patients should be treated with equine diphtheria anitoxin and either erythromycin or penicillin.

❍ **What is the differential diagnosis for a patient who on first consideration appears to be suffering from tetanus?**

Dental abscess, rabies, hypocalcemic tetany, antipsychotic drugs, or the extrapyramidal effects of compazine.

❍ **What organisms are known to cause renal and perinephric abscesses?**

The most common organisms are Staphylococcus aureus, Escherichia coli, Proteus spp., Pseudomonas spp., and enterococcus.

❍ **Name at least five causes of parotitis in pediatric patients.**

An incomplete list of causes of parotitis include bacteria in general, viruses, especially mumps, echovirus, coxsackie A, lymphocytic choriomeningitis virus, parainfluenza 1 and 3, cytomegalovirus, Epstein-Barr virus, and HIV. Other causes include mycobacteria, histoplasmosis, post-typhoid fever, cat scratch disease, dehydration, collagen-vascular disease, cystic fibrosis, ectodermal dysplasia, familial dysautonomia, sarcoidosis, drugs, poisoning (including lead, copper and mercury), sialolithiasis, and tumors.

○   **What are the common bacterial causes of parotitis in newborns?**

Staphylococcus aureus, Escherichia coli, and Pseudomonas aeruginosa.

○   **What are the most common etiologic agents of parotitis in older children?**

Staphylococcus aureus and streptococci.

○   **Prior to a dental extraction, what prophylactic antibiotic should be given to a child with a tendency to develop endocarditis based on an underlying cardiac lesion?**

Amoxicillin, ampicillin, or clindamycin one hour before the procedure.

○   **If a patient with underlying heart disease that has a tendency towards the development of endocarditis is undergoing a genito-urinary or gastro-intestinal procedure, what prophylactic antibiotic should be administered?**

Intravenous or intramuscular ampicillin and gentamicin thirty minutes prior to the procedure followed by ampicillin or amoxicillin eight hours after the procedure. Alternatively, intravenous vancomycin and gentamicin completed 30 minutes prior to the procedure. For a low risk procedure where the patient remains conscious, amoxicillin may be given one hour before the procedure.

○   **What is the differential diagnosis of a renal abscess in a neonate?**

Renal hamartoma or congenital cyst.

○   **What is the differential diagnosis of a renal abscess in an older infant or child?**

A Wilm's tumor, a lymphoma, an angiomyolipoma, hemorrhagic infarct, hematoma, and acute focal pyelonephritis (acute lobar nephronia).

○   **When a child presents with more than one infected joint simultaneously, what organisms should be considered as the likely culprits?**

Staphylococcus aureus, salmonella or gonorrhea.

○   **When a child has an underlying cardiac condition which predisposes him/her to endocarditis, what events and procedures do not require endocarditis prophylaxis?**

Dental procedures without gingival bleeding; injection of local intraoral anesthetic (except intraligamentary injections); shedding primary teeth; tympanostomy tube insertion; endotracheal intubation; flexible bronchoscopy, with and without biopsy; cardiac catheterization; gastrointestinal endoscopy, with and without biopsy; cesarean section; and, if there is no infection present, urethral catheterization; dilation and curettage; uncomplicated vaginal delivery, therapeutic abortion; sterilization procedures and insertion or removal of an intrauterine device.

○   **Name ate least five infectious agents associated with erythema nodosum.**

Erythema nodosum has been associated with many infectious and some non-infectious processes. Some of its better known associates are Group A streptococcus, meningococcus, syphilis, Mycobacterium tuberculosis, and Mycobacterium leprae, as well as histoplasmosis, coccidiomycosis, blastomycosis and herpes simplex virus. Some of the less common associates of erythema nodosum include Chlamydia trachomatis, Chlamydia psitacci, Corynebacterium diphtheriae, campylobacter, Haemophilus ducreyi, yersinia, Bartonella henselae, trichophyton, filariasis, sarcoidosis, and various drugs.

○   **What would be the most common clinical situation in which to encounter an infection with Flavobacterium meningosepticum?**

This organism is seen most frequently in neonatal meningitis and in infections in the immunocompromised host. It is treated with vancomycin.

○   **The inflammation associated with tuberculous meningitis classically affects what cranial nerves?**

Cranial nerves 3,6,7, and the optic chiasm.

○   **What agent causes a meningitis that gives a crawling sensation?**

Angiostrongylus cantonensis.

○   **What are the immediate and long term infectious disease considerations following bone marrow transplantation?**

Agents which cause infectious complications immediately following the bone marrow transplant include bacteria and fungi in general. In the long term, these patients have infections secondary to Pneumocystis carinii and cytomegalovirus.

○   **Diabetes in children is associated with what infections?**

Staphylococcus, actinomyces, candida and mucormycosis.

○   **Pediatric patients that have received transplantations have an increase in what infections?**

Staphylococcus, pseudomonas, klebsiella, candida, aspergillus, nocardia, Pneumocystis carinii, cytomegalovirus, and varicella zoster virus.

○   **Children with malignancies are known to have an increase in infections due to what agents?**

Pseudomonas, klebsiella, Escherichia coli, cryptococcus, varicella zoster virus, Pneumocystis carinii, mycobactera.

○   **Name five infectious and non-infectious causes of chronic meningitis.**

Mycobacteria, typical and atypical; Borrelia recurrentis and burgdorferi; Treponema pallidum; nocardia, parameningeal foci (including sinusitis, mastoiditis, otitis, osteomyelitis of the skull); enterovirus in agammaglobulinemia; adenovirus in bone marrow transplantation patients; histoplasmosis; coccidiomycosis; blastomycosis; cryptococcosis; aspergillus; and sporotrichosis. Non-Infectious causes include leukemia; central nervous system tumor; Behcet's syndrome; systemic lupus erythematosus; sarcoidosis; foreign body; epidermoid cyst; and non-steroidal anti -inflammatory drugs, especially ibuprofen.

○   **Name three possible causes of an eosinophilic meningitis.**

Angiostrongylus cantonensis, Gnathostoma spinigerum, toxoplasmosis, Taenia solium, Schistosoma spp., Paragonimus westermani, echinococcus, syphilis, tuberculosis, Rickettsia rickettsia, coccidiomycosis, rabies vaccination, intrathecal injection, and foreign body.

○   **A child has a pericardial tap and hemorrhagic fluid is withdrawn. What are the most likely possibilities?**

Trauma, tumor tuberculosis, or histoplasmosis.

O   **Name three possible causes of an enlarged heart, poor myocardial function and dysrhythmia in a pediatric patient.**

Etiologies include myocarditis, congenital heart disease, heart failure, septic shock, endocardial fibroelastosis, anomalous left coronary artery from the pulmonary artery, Pompe's disease, medial necrosis of the coronary arteries, cardiomyopathy, pericarditis, rheumatic fever, systemic lupus erythematosus, rheumatoid arthritis, and ulcerative colitis.

O   **What characteristics categorize a pleural fluid as empyema?**

Greater than 50,000 white cells, glucose ≈ than 30 mg%, and a low pH.

O   **Name three common causes of pleural effusion without empyema in the pediatric age group.**

Staphylococcus aureus, Streptococcus pneumonia, HiB, Streptococcus pyogenes, and Mycoplasma pneumonia.

O   **Name two of the most common infectious causes of an empyema in the pediatric age group.**

Staphlococcus aureus, Streptococcus pneumonia, anaerobes, and tuberculosis.

O   **A person who is deficient in any of the complement components from C5 through C9 is more susceptible to infections by which agents?**

Neisseria species in general, but most especially Neisseria meningiditis.

O   **What are some of the unique aspects of infections associated with agammaglobulinemia?**

Enterovirus infections, parvovirus B19, mycoplasma infections, especially of the joints or the lung, and a prolonged excretion of rotavirus.

O   **What is the appropriate evaluation for immunodeficiency in a patient with chronic pneumonias?**

Immunoglobulin studies, CD4 and CD8 cell counts, and an anergy panel.

O   **What is the most common complication of otitis media?**

Effusion and hearing loss.

O   **What is the most common intracranial complication of otitis media?**

Meningitis. Other intracranial complications include epidural abscess, subdural abscess, brain abscess, encephalitis, lateral sinus thrombosis, communicating hydrocephalus, CSF otorrhea, and petrositis.

O   **What is the most common extracranial complication of otitis media?**

Labyrinthitis, mastoiditis, facial nerve paralysis, subperiosteal abscess, labyrinthine fistulas, perilabyrinthitis, ossicular destruction, cholesteatoma and temporal osteomyelitis.

O   **What are the indications for the prophylaxis of otitis media?**

Prophylaxis should be given after the third episode of otitis media under six months of age, or the fourth episode of otitis media before twelve months of age.

O   **How does the perforation of the tympanic membrane associated with chronic supporative otitis media differ from the perforation associated with acute otitis media?**

Tympanic membrane perforation in chronic suppurative otitis media can be permanent.

❍ **What are the most common causes of acute mastoiditis?**

Group A streptococcus, Streptococcus pneumonia, Staphylococcus aureus, and non-typable Haemophilus influenza.

❍ **What are the most common causes of chronic mastoiditis?**

The most common causes of chronic mastoiditis are Staphylococcus aureus, Pseudomonas aeruginosa dn other gram negative rods, anaerobes and tuberculosis.

❍ **What are the most common intracranial complications of mastoiditis?**

Epidural empyema, brain abscess, meningitis, venous sinus thrombosis, and cerebellar abscess.

❍ **What are the most common extracranial complications of mastoiditis?**

A subperiosteal abscess, a Bezold abscess (an abscess in the submastoid space), facial nerve paralysis, temporal bone osteomyelitis and hearing loss.

❍ **Name two non-infectious, non-malignant and non-inflammatory causes of fever in children.**

Central nervous system dysfunction with brain damage, an isolated form of epilepsy, familial dysautonomia (Riley-Day Syndrome) and drugs.

❍ **What malignancies in children are most likely to present as a fever of unknown origin?**

Leukemia, lymphoma, neuroblastoma, hepatoma, sarcoma, and atrial myxoma.

❍ **What is the relationship between the frequency of Haemophilus influenzae B infections and HLA type?**

HLA B12 is associated with an increase in Haemophilus influenzae B infections while HLA b w 40 is associated with few Haemophilus influenzae B infections.

❍ **Name four immunizations that are associated with post-vaccine aseptic meningitis.**

Measles, polio, rabies, and vaccinia.

❍ **Name the two bacteria that sound and act like fungi.**

1. Nocardia.
2. Actinomyces.

❍ **If Creutzfeldt-Jakob disease (CJD) is a disease whose average age of presentation is 60 years, why has it suddenly become a concern of pediatricians?**

CJD was first described int he 1920's. It can be sporadic (no know cause), environmentally acquired (including pituitary hormones or dura mater grafts) or familial (due to mutations on chromosome 20). The recently diagnosed 21 patients in England were all under 50 years of age with and average age of 27 years. The "new variant" (nv) of CJD has in common with the classic CJD the features of progressive dementia, ataxia, and mild clonus. The unique characteristic of nvCJD are onset with psychiatric and/or sensory symptoms and an absence of characteristic electroencephalograph findings. The nvCJD seems to be associated with consumption of prion-contaminated beef.

❍   **What four classes of contacts of a patient with meningococcal disease require prophylaxis?**

People who live in the same household, attendees of the same child care or nursery school in the previous seven days, those who have been directly exposed to the index case's secretions, such as by kissing or sharing of food, and health care providers whose mucous membranes were unprotected during resuscitation or intubation of the patient.

❍   **Why isn't the meningococcal vaccine in routine use in the United States?**

Serogroups B and C meningococci each cause approximately 50% of the meningococcal disease in the United States. The highest risk age group for meningococcal disease is in children under two years of age. The reason meningococcal vaccine is not routinely used in this country is because serogroup B polysaccharide is not represented in the vaccine and the serogroup C that is present is very poorly immunogenic in children under two years of age.

❍   **What is the most common infectious disease problem in patients with lupus who are not on steroid therapy?**

Urinary tract infections and urosepsis.

❍   **What infectious disease problem is both characteristic of and potentially devastating in patients with lupus, whether on steroids or not on steroids?**

Meningitis.

❍   **How often is herpes simplex virus cultured from the cerebrospinal fluid of a pediatric patient or an adult with HSV encephalitis? How often is it cultured from the cerebrospinal fluid of a neonate with HSV encephalitis?**

Herpes simplex virus may be cultured from the cerebrospinal fluid of a child six months of age or older or an adult with herpes encephalitis only 5% of the time, whereas a neonate with HSV encephalitis will grow the virus from the CSF 50% of the time.

❍   **What rapid diagnostic test is now available to diagnose herpes simplex virus encephalitis in patients of all ages and how reliable is it considered to be?**

HSV polymerase chain reaction (PCR) on cerebrospinal fluid is considered to be highly sensitive and specific in the diagnosis of HSV encephalitis.

❍   **What percent of school age children with classic symptoms (dysuria, frequency, urgency) actually have a urinary tract infection?**

10%. The remainder have urethral irritation from such things as pinworms, masturbation, bubble baths or poor hygiene.

❍   **What is the only reliable result from a culture of urine collected by the bag method?**

No growth.

❍   **Any organisms that grow in the culture of a urine specimen obtained by suprapubic aspiration can be considered to represent true infection. In symptomatic children, how many colonies in a urine culture are required to make the diagnosis when the urine specimen is obtained by catheterization?**

At least 10,000 colonies per ml of a single organism.

❍   **What simple measures can be taken to prevent urinary tract infections in children?**

Taking showers instead of baths, avoiding bubble baths, treating pin worms, treating constipation and in sexually active females, post-coital voiding.

O   **What children are candidates for influenza vaccine?**

Any child six months of age or older who is a resident of a chronic care facility; who has a chronic cardiovascular condition; or who has pulmonary, metabolic, hematologic, or an immunologic disorder (including asthma, diabetes, renal failure, sickle cell disease, immunosuppression and HIV infection). Also, children who are receiving aspirin therapy, or are the siblings of children who are in any of these high risk group, should have the influenza immunization as well.

O   **What are the three questions that every victim of a dog bite should be asked?**

1.   Was the attack provoked or unprovoked?
2.   Was the dog known or unknown?
3.   Has the dog had its rabies shots?

O   **Do bite wounds caused by humans usually become infected with one or with multiple organisms?**

The average human bite wound contains 5.4 organisms per wound.

O   **What are the most common organisms found in human bite wounds?**

Staphylococcus aureus, Streptococcus species, and Eikenella corrodens. Anaerobes are also commonly seen.

O   **Children with sickle cell disease are started on prophylactic penicillin by two to three months of age. This should be continued until what age?**

Routine prophylaxis with penicillin has been shown to have no effect on reduction of the risk of invasive pneumococcal infections for children older than five years of age.

O   **In a pediatric patient who is suspected of having meningitis, cranial computed tomography (CT) of the brain should be performed before lumbar puncture under what circumstances?**

When the patient is in a coma, has papilledema or focal neuroligic findings. When head CT is performed, patients should have blood cultures taken and then appropriate empiric anibiotic therapy started prior to the CT.

O   **Is it necessary to treat the male sexual partner of women with vaginal bacterial vaginosis?**

No. Affected women should be treated with oral or intra-vaginal metranidozole or clindamycin.

O   **If a pediatric patient with an acute illness who is receiving a third generation cephalosporin becomes secondarily infected and bacteremic, what organism would be the usual offender?**

Enterococcus.

O   **In the United States, which domestic animal is <u>most</u> <u>commonly</u> infected with rabies: the cat, or the dog?**

The cat. Among wild animals, rabies are most commonly found among raccoons, skunks, foxes, coyotes, and bats.

O   **Would a child be likely to receive a rabies vaccine following a wild rat bite?**

No. Bites from rodents rarely pose a risk of rabies.

❍   **Since 1980, in the United States, what percentage of the 32 cases of human rabies has an associated history of animal bite?**

25%.

❍   **There are twenty indigenously derived cases of rabies in the United States between 1980 and 1996. How many series of post exposure rabies prophylaxis were given in the United States during that same time period?**

40,000 people received post exposure prophylaxis during that time period. Post exposure prophylaxis for rabies consists of 20 international units per kilogram of Human Rabies Immune Globulin (HRIG) and five doses of vaccine.

❍   **Which method is more reliable for the diagnosis of cytomegalovirus (CMV) infection in the newborn--the CMV lgM antibody, or the CMV culture of the urine or saliva?**

The presence of IGM antibody to CMV in the serum of a newborn is diagnostic of a congenital CMV infection. However, the sensitivity of most of these antibody methods is poor, with fewer than half of congenitally infected neonates being detected. The CMV culture has greater sensitivity.

❍   **How many hours must Ixodes scapularis, the deer tick, feed on a human before being able to transmit Lyme Disease?**

Transmission rarely occurs if the infected tick feeds for less than 48 hours.

❍   **Neonates with HSV infection may present with a localized skin, eye and mouth (SEM) infection, a disseminated infection or an encephalitis. What is the mortality rate of infants with disseminated HIV infection who are treated with acyclovir?**

Fifty percent.

❍   **What percentage of patients with localized skin, eye and mouth infection survive and what is the neurological outcome?**

All neonates with SEM treated with acyclovir survive and greater than 90% develop normally.

❍   **What agent is the major cause of parenterally transmitted non-A, non-B hepatitis?**

Hepatitis C virus (HCV).

❍   **What type of Haemophilus influenza most commonly causes otitis media, conjunctivitis, and sinusitis?**

Non-typable Haemophilus.

❍   **Does non-typable Haemophilus influenza ever cause pneumonia, meningitis, septicemia, endocarditis, epiglottitis, septic arthritis, post-partum bacteremia, or neonatal sepsis?**

While Haemophilus influenza B and other typable Haemophilus influenza infections are more likely causes of these invasive diseases, non-typable Haemophilus influenza may infrequently cause them as well.

❍   **Brazilian purpuric fever, a fulminant disease of young children characterized by fever, abdominal pain, vomiting, and the rapid development of purpura and vascular collapse leading to death, is caused by what etiologic agent?**

The non-typable haemophilus influenza of Biotype III, Biogroup aegyptius, is the responsible agent. The disease was first recognized in 1984 and since has been seen to occur in Brazil and Australia.

❍   **In the United States polio vaccine is no longer necessary to give after a person reaches which birthday?**

The 18th birthday.

❍   **Haemophilus influenzae B vaccine is not necessary after which birthday?**

The fifth birthday.

❍   **Pertussis vaccine is not recommended after which birthday?**

The seventh birthday.

❍   **Name three immunizations which are necessary at any age if they have not previously been given.**

The measles, mumps, and rubella (MMR), the tetanus-diphtheria vaccine, and, though not generally appreciated, the hepatitis B vaccine (HBV).

❍   **Is a pregnant mother in the household a contraindication to the immunization of a child in the house and, if so, to which vaccine?**

A pregnancy in the household is not a contraindication to vaccinating any household member other than the pregnant person herself. Pregnancy is a contraindication to live vaccines in general.

❍   **Would a time lapse of two years between the second and third dose of hepatitis B vaccine be an indication to restart the series?**

NO vaccine series ever has to be restarted, no matter what the time lapse between doses.

❍   **T/F: all vaccines may be given simultaneously.**

True. (The only exception to this rule is that cholera and yellow fever may not be given at the same time.)

❍   **What impact does breast feeding by the mother have on immunizations of the baby?**

All vaccines may be given to a baby who is breast feeding and all vaccines may be given to a mom who is breast feeding a baby.

❍   **May a child with contraindication or precaution against the use of DPT be given a DTaP?**

DTaP is contraindicated in anyone who may not use DPT. The patient may however by given the TD or Td.

❍   **If a child has received a course of chemotherapy, does the child need to be revaccinated?**

No.

❍   **If a child has had a bone marrow transplantation, will her or she need to be revaccinated?**

A child who has had a bone marrow transplant will receive some or all of the immunity of the donor. After recovery, consider giving the most important vaccines such as MMR and Td.

❍ **Following an immunoglobulin or blood product administration, how long should a patient wait before receiving a measles vaccination?**

It depends. If a child has received washed red blood cells, no wait whatsoever is required. If a child has received packed red blood cells, a five month interval is required. Children who have received tetanus immune globulin or immune serum globulin, either for Hepatitis A prophylaxis or international travel and patients who have received Hepatitis B immune globulin, are required to wait three months for the next measles vaccination. Various other immune globulins and blood products require longer waits. The longest waits are following the receipt of respiratory syncytial virus (RSV)--IGIV (a nine month wait) and intravenous immune globulin (IGIV) for Kawasaki Disease (eleven months).

❍ **By all accounts, polymerase chain reaction (PCR) has an impressive diagnostic potential. It is reputed to have extraordinary sensitivity. One copy of an organism's DNA can be amplified to 1 billion copies with thirty heating and cooling cycles. How reliable is this technique?**

In a study of seven laboratories blindly tested with a specimen containing 10^3 Mycobacterium tuberculosis organisms, the rates of positive results ranged from 3% to 77% and the rates of false negative results ranged from 2% to 90%. PCR test results should be interpreted with caution. The accuracy and validity of PCR testing is expected to improve considerably over the coming years.

❍ **T/F: A culture from a patient is reported as growing coagulase negative staphylococci. This should be interpreted to mean staphylococcus epidermidis.**

False. There are 15 different coagulase negative staphylococci that have been reported to cause diseases in or to colonize humans. An additional sixteen non-human coagulase negative staphylococci exist.

❍ **The laboratory report reads "Streptococcus viridans." What is wrong with that report?**

There is no such thing as Streptococcus viridans. The class of organisms being referred ot is rightly called Viridans streptococci. Viridans streptococci are alpha hemolytic streptococci which are composed of at least eight separate species which cause diseases in man. Examples of Viridans streptococci include: S. milleri, S. constellatus, S. anginosus and S. mutans. While most laboratories will not normally speciate a Viridans streptococci for you because they may simply be contaminants, if they are seen in two or more blood cultures or grow in pure culture from a deep site, it is appropriate to ask for speciation. The species of the organism can point to the etiology of the disease. Certain Viridans streptococci are associated with endocarditis, while others are associated with such things as carcinoma and brain abscess.

❍ **A six-year-old child presents with a history of having had a PPD placed three weeks ago which was 4 mm in induration, measured by a reliable colleague. A repeat PPD was placed one week ago and the child's forearm demonstrated 14 mm of induration. This PPD was measured by the same physician. Which PPD should be accepted as reflecting the correct amount of induration.**

The second, or "boosted" response, is accepted as the reliable response. It is routine for many institutions to test their employees with two PPD's, separated by two weeks, in order to take advantage of this phenomenon.

❍ **A six-year-old child presents with history classic for giardia and has a three-year-old brother who was documented to the same. A complete stool work-up is performed and after the first day, the laboratory reports the identification of rotavirus. What is the most likely explanation?**

The six-year-old probably has both rotavirus and giardia, and probably caught them both from his three-year-old sibling. Like venereal diseases, more than one infectious agent is often transmitted at a time. Two pathogens or more are found in the stool of patients symptomatic with acute gastroenteritis at least 15% of the time.

❍ **An eighteen month old presents with an exudative pharyngitis, fever and mildly abnormal liver function tests. You suspect mononucleosis. What study would you send?**

An EBVlgG and IGM (lgG and lgM antibody to viral capsid antigen or VCA). The chances that a mono spot will be positive in the presence of mononucleosis between 0 and 2 years of age is practically zero. The chances that a mono spot is positive between the second birthday and the fourth birthday is approximately 30%. Specific Epstein-Barr virus antibodies are much more useful for making the diagnosis in the first four years of life.

❍ **A ten month old presents with the signs and symptoms of pneumonia, which is confirmed by chest x-ray. What are the chances that this pneumonia is due to Mycoplasma pneumoniae?**

About 2%. Mycoplasma pneumoniae is hardly ever seen in the first year of life. It increases steadily as a cause of pneumonia in children into early adulthood. A convenient way to remember the chances of a child's pneumonia being due to mycoplasma is to assign a 2% chance per year of age into the twenties. By the mid-twenties, as many as 35-45% of all pneumonia is secondary to Mycoplasma pneumoniae.

❍ **Pasteurella multocida infection from an animal bite is best treated with which antibiotic?**

Augumentin.

❍ **The intervention most likely to be successful in the treatment of onychomycosis of the toenail is: a) removal of the toenail or b) antifungal therapy for four to eighteen months.**

Drug therapy with Itraconazole (Sporanox) is the easiest and shortest term of the various antifungal drug regimens. Treatment can be given for one week each month for three to four months. Other medications that are useful include terbinafine, ketoconazole, and griseofulvin. Therapy with griseofulvin can take as long as eighteen months.

❍ **Name two common urinary pathogens that do not give a positive urine nitrate test.**

Enterococcus and Staphylococcus saprophyticus. Acinetobacter also fails to give a positive urine nitrate test.

❍ **What unusual but important CNS side effect can be seen with ibuprofen usage?**

Aseptic meningitis.

❍ **Group B Streptococcus is known to have both an early and a late onset presentation in neonatal sepsis and meningitis. What other organism does the identical thing?**

Listeria monocytogenes.

❍ **What common minor surgical procedure is associated with a decreased incidence of pyelonephritis in males?**

Circumcision.

❍ **What percentage of the time do infants with documented pyelonephritis fail to demonstrate pyuria?**

Approximately 50% of the time.

❍ **What is the incidence of occult bacteremia in infants between six and twenty-four months of age with temperature higher than 40 degrees centigrade and a white blood count >15,000/cu.mm?**

Approximately fifteen percent.

❍ **How likely is it that a child with fever and petechiae has meningococcal sepsis or meningitis?**

Seven to ten percent.

O   **A child with a fever of unknown origin, a lack of tears, an absent corneal reflex, and a smooth tongue (lacking fungiform papillae) has what condition?**

Familial dysautonomia.

O   **What could be concluded about the spinal fluid of a three day old infant with a CSF white count of 15 and a CSF protein of 90?**

That it is normal. At birth the CSF white count can be as high as 29. It may not fall to the expected "adult" normal of 6 or 7 until a month of age. The CSF protein can be up to 175 at birth and may take as long as three months to fall to the expected upper limit of normal of 45.

O   **What is the risk and where is the risk of salmonella coming into a household in an ordinary package of a dozen eggs?**

In some studies, as many as 30% of commercial eggs are contaminated with salmonella. The organism can be found on the surface of the shell, may penetrate the egg itself, or may contaminate the egg yolk, having been transmitted from an ovarian infection.

O   **What are the chances that salmonella will be introduced into a household on contaminated meats?**

Up to 50% of poultry samples, 15% of pork and 5% of beef have been demonstrated to be contaminated with salmonella.

O   **Bartonella henselae is one of the causes of Parinaud's oculoglandular syndrome (a combination of conjunctivitis and ipsilateral preauricular adenitis) and is the most common cause of chronic lymphadenopathy in children. With what animal is this organism associated?**

The cat. It is the agent of cat scratch disease.

O   **While on the farm, Coxiella burnetii is most commonly associated with sheep. In the city a parturient cat can aerosolize enough organisms n a closed space to be infective to people for days. What illness does Coxiella burnetii cause?**

Q Fever. This usually presents as an atypical pneumonia.

O   **One day after sitting in a hot tub, a three-year-old child and her mother develop papular and pustular skin lesions. What is the most likely explanation?**

Pseudomonas aeruginosa dermatitis has been reported to occur in healthy individuals following immersion in hot tubs. There may be a few scattered lesions or extensive involvement. Patients may also have malaise, fever, vomiting, sore throat, conjunctivitis, rhinitis, and swollen breasts.

O   **What are the two most common organisms known to be transmitted by unpasteurized Mexican cheese?**

Brucella and listeria.

O   **What is the most productive source of positive cultures for patients with Brucellosis?**

While blood, abscess and tissue cultures may be useful, bone marrow is the most productive source of positive cultures.

O **Which hemoglobin provides the greatest innate resistance to falciparum malaria?**

Erythrocytes of patients that are heterozygous for sickle cell hemoglobin (sickle cell trait) are resistant to malaria.

O **What is the most common infectious disease complication of both measles and influenza?**

Pneumococcal pneumonia.

O **What rickettsial disease can be mistaken for chickenpox in inner city children?**

Rickettsialpox caused by Rickettsia akari is characterized by an initial skin lesion followed by headache, fever, chills and a vesicular rash. It is transmitted by the mouse mite.

O **Which rickettsial infection is most common in the United States?**

Rocky Mountain Spotted Fever caused by Rickettsia.

O **What is the most important therapeutic action to be taken in the teenager with infected abortion?**

Evacuation of the retained products of conception.

O **In the treatment of a patient with cellulitis, what therapeutic maneuver is arguably as important as antibiotic therapy?**

Elevation of the affected part.

O **What prophylactic antibiotic should be given systemically to burn victims?**

None. Prophylactic agents with antibacterial activity should be given topically. Chief among these is Silvadene.

O **What is the most likely focus of infection in a patient who presents with gram negative enteric bacteremia?**

Urinary tract infection.

O **What is the most likely focus of infection in a patient who presents with periorbital cellulitis unassociated with skin trauma?**

Sinusitis.

O **A previously healthy child has had an accidental overdose of oral iron; she appears to be septic. What is the most likely organism to cause her sepsis?**

Yersinia enterocolitica. The growth of Y. enterocolitica appears to be enhanced after exposure to excess iron. This, combined with intestinal damage to the mucosa by the iron, may play a role in pathogenesis.

O **In the United States, 50-100 cases of Clostridium tetani (tetanus) occur each year. What percentage of these cases occur in newborns?**

None. No cases of neonatal tetanus have been reported in the United States in recent years.

O **A 3 month old infant presents with poor feeding, constipation, and hypotonia. There is a recent history of ingestion of honey. While you suspect infant botulism, you cannot rule out the possibility of sepsis. What class of antibiotics would you <u>not</u> give to this patient?**

Aminoglyosides. Gentamicin and related drugs can add to the blocked motor nerve terminals, and lead to respiratory failure in these patients with botulism.

O   **T/F: It is fairly common for children to become infected with tuberculosis following casual exposures.**

False. Primary infection in children usually occurs following a prolonged close contact with an untreated adult who has cavitary disease.

O   **A 7-year-old child is diagnosed with primary pulmonary tuberculosis and is treated appropriately with four drugs. An organism collected by gastric aspirate proves to be sensitive to three of the four drugs. Following six months of therapy, the chest x-ray appears unchanged from six months ago. What is wrong?**

Nothing. It can take many months for the chest x-ray abnormalities in pulmonary tuberculosis to show improvement. The child's symptoms, however, should have resolved and the sedimentation rate should be normal with effective therapy.

O   **In normal children, what is the most common clinical manifestation of disease due to non-tuberculous mycobacteria?**

The most common form of non-tuberculous mycobacteria is lymphadenitis of the submandibular or anterior cervical nodes. The usual agent is M. avium intracellulare complex and M. scrofulaceum.

O   **A child from the Philippines has a hypo-pigmented patch that is lacking in sensation. What is the most likely cause of his problem?**

Leprosy (Mycobacterium leprae).

O   **A teenager presents with an irritating cough which is becoming gradually worse. The boy's father had a similar problem, which was treated with erythromycin and resolved after seven days. PPD's on both the father and the son have been negative. What are the three most likely etiologic agents for this problem?**

Mycoplasma pneumonia, Chlamydia pneumonia, and Bordetella pertussis.

O   **What part of the body should you examine to confirm that a vesicular rash is related to chickenpox?**

The scalp. Vesicular and crusting lesions in the scalp are typical of chicken pox. It is extremely unlikely that other causes of vesicular lesions on the skin would be associated with scalp lesions.

O   **It is well known that children with chickenpox may eventually have an episode (or episodes) of herpes zoster. Will herpes zoster appear following an immunization with chickenpox vaccine?**

Yes. It occurs at approximately one-third to one-fifth the frequency that it does following the natural illness, but it is a distant complication of the vaccine as well.

O   **What is the earliest age at which a child may be immunized for influenza?**

At 6 months of age.

O   **While older infants and children with respiratory syncytial virus infection (RSV) usually present with cough and wheezing, some infants may present with what other symptom?**

Apnea.

❍ **What is the name of the viral illness that presents predominantly with pharyngitis and conjunctivitis?**

Pharyngoconjunctival fever. It is caused by adenovirus.

❍ **Since only a minority of children who present with fever and petechiae have meningococcemia, what etiologic agent accounts for the bulk of the remaining cases?**

The enteroviruses, including the Coxsackieviruses, and the ECHOviruses.

❍ **A ten month old infant presents with fever, diarrhea, and mild irritability. A spinal tap shows 68 white cells, no red cells, normal protein, normal glucose, and a CSF latex agglutination that is negative for all bacterial pathogens tested. What is the most likely diagnosis?**

Rotavirus. A septic meningitis is not uncommon in children with rotavirus gastroenteritis.

❍ **What parasitic agent should be included in the differential diagnosis when mononucleosis and CMV are considered?**

Toxoplasmosis. Everything EBV and CMV can do, toxoplasmosis can do.

❍ **When itchy lesions are seen on the palms and/or soles, what blood sucking ecoparasite should be high in the differential diagnosis?**

Sarcoptes scabiei, the etiologic agent of scabies.

❍ **Aside from drainage of the cyst, what is the primary concern of the surgeon during surgical treatment of echinococcosis?**

Care should be taken during the operative procedure not to spill any of the infected cystic fluid, as this could lead to dissemination of the infection and the establishment of multiple other cysts.

❍ **Which intestinal parasites are known to cause anemia as their major manifestation?**

Hookworms.

❍ **Which strains of Neisseria meningitis are responsible for epidemics of meningitis?**

Groups A and C usually epidemic meningitis, and groups B, W and Y are usually responsible for endemic disease.

❍ **Which strain of meningococcus is most commonly responsible for meningitis?**

Group B is the most common cause of non-epidemic meningococcal disease.

❍ **Is there a vaccine available for group B meningococcus?**

No.

❍ **What are the common pathogens for meningitis in the neonates?**

Streptoccus group B and E. coli.

❍ **What is the most common sequel of pediatric bacterial meningitis?**

Hearing impairment.

○   **What other deficits may develop following bacterial meningitis?**

Mental retardation, seizure, and spastic weakness.

○   **What are the sequelae of viral meningitis?**

None, usually.

○   **What are the CSF characteristics of tuberculous meningitis?**

Lymphocytic pleocytosis, very high protein (several hundred to a thousand mg/dl), and very low glucose.

○   **What is the management of herpes simplex encephalitis?**

Early treatment with acyclovir, anticonvulsants for seizures and general supportive care.

○   **What is the most common cause of encephalitis in neonates?**

Enterovirus.

○   **What is the recommended treatment for neurosyphilis?**

Intravenous penicillin G. Follow up CSF examinations are mandatory.

○   **What complication may arise from aggressive penicillin treatment of neurosyphilis?**

Jarisch Herxheimer reaction.

○   **At which stage of Lyme disease does neurological involvement occur?**

The second and third stages.

○   **Which is the vector responsible for the transmission of Lyme disease?**

Deer tick (Ixodes dammini).

○   **What important feature in a patient's history should be sought when a diagnosis of Lyme disease is being considered?**

History of erythema chronicum migrans (ECM), which present in nearly 60-80% of patients early in this disease.

○   **What are the main differences between the European and the American patterns of Lyme disease?**

The European variety has more peripheral nervous system involvement, with relatively fewer joint and cardiac complications.

○   **What is the currently recommended treatment for Lyme disease?**

For early, localized disease in children over 7 years of age, doxycycline. Amoxicillin may be used for all ages. These same drugs are used for early-disseminated disease, facial palsy, and arthritis. Recurrent arthritis, carditis and CNS disease is treated with ceftriaxone or penicillin.

○   **What is Weil's disease?**

A less common variety of leptospirosis. It presents with icterus, marked hepatic and renal involvement, along with a bleeding diasthesis.

O   **How is brucellosis spread?**

Through the ingestion of contaminated milk and milk products. It may also be spread by contact with an infected animal (usually cattle), including respiratory.

O   **What are the typical features of Zidovudine associated myopathy?**

AZT is known to cause myopathy when used in high doses over prolonged periods. There is typically severe myalgia, and striking atrophy of the gluteal muscles.

O   **Name some common causes of peripheral neuropathy in AIDS.**

Peripheral neuropathy has been postulated to be directly related to HIV, concomitant infections such as cytomegalovirus (CMV), side effects of drugs such as ddI, ddC, and 3TC, and nutritional deficiencies such as B_{12} deficiency.

O   **What is the most common cause of intracranial mass lesions in HIV disease?**

Intracranial toxoplasmosis. About 20-30% of AIDS patients with positive serology for toxoplasmosis will develop toxoplasma encephalitis. The second most common intracranial mass lesion is lymphoma.

O   **What is the current recommended treatment for intracranial toxoplasmosis in HIV disease?**

This is usually a combination therapy with sulfadiazine, pyrimethamine, and folinic acid.

O   **What is the rationale for using folinic acid in the treatment of intracranial toxoplasmosis with pyrimethamine, and sulfadiazine combination?**

Folinic acid is thought to decrease the incidence of bone marrow suppression.

O   **What percentage of patients with HIV disease develop CNS lymphoma?**

Approximately 2% of AIDS patients will develop primary CNS lymphoma. Up to 0.6% will present with primary CNS lymphoma concurrent with a diagnosis of AIDS.

O   **Which virus is considered responsible for Tropical Spastic Paraparesis (TSP)?**

Human T cell Lymphotrophic Virus type 1.

O   **What are the modes of transmission of HTLV-1?**

Vertical: Mother to child.

Horizontal: Through sexual contact, and blood transfusion.

O   **How is botulism contracted?**

Through the consumption of contaminated foods, by injury from non sterile objects (wound botulism), and (in infants) from intestinal colonization by Clostridium botulinum.

O   **What are botulism's principle clinical features?**

A descending paralysis with complete ophthalmoplegia, bulbar and somatic palsy.

O   **Which is the organism responsible for causing Bornholm's disease?**

Coxsackie viruses are a group of enteroviruses that are responsible for the epidemic myalgia (Bornholm's disease) where pleurodynia is also a common feature. Specifically the disease is thought to occur due to a Coxsackie group B virus.

❍   **Name three paralytic diseases caused by an infectious agent other than polio.**

Paralytic rabies, botulism and tick paralysis.

❍   **To which group of viruses does polio belong?**

The polio virus is enterovirus like Echovirus and Coxsackie virus.

CARDIOVASCULAR

○ **Are aortic aneurysms more common in males or in females?**

Ten times more common in men. Other risk factors are hypertension, atherosclerosis, diabetes, hyperlipidemia, smoking, syphilis, Marfan's disease, and Ehlers-Danlos disease.

○ **What is the most common cause of aortic regurgitation in children?**

Aortic valve prolapse associated with a congenital ventricular septal defect.

○ **How is atrial flutter treated?**

Urgent conversion requires DC cardioversion. A patient may be started on digoxin (slows the ventricular response by prolonging conduction time through the AV node) followed by an agent such as quinidine or procainamide (to suppress the arrhythmia).

○ **What is the most common cause of atrial fibrillation in childhood?**

This is most often the result of a chronically stretched atrial myocardium. Atrial fibrillation occurs most commonly in older children with rheumatic mitral valve disease.

○ **What is the mechanism that most commonly produces SVTs?**

Re-entrant tachycardias using an accessory pathway in infants, though AV node re-entry becomes more common in childhood.

○ **What is the treatment for a stable SVT that is not caused by digitalis toxicity or WPW syndrome?**

Vagal stimulation (submersion of face in iced saline or ice bag to the face); vagotonic maneurens (valsalva, straining, breath-holding); rapid intravenous push of adenosine; quinidine, procainamide or propranolol; or verapamil.

○ **What is the key feature of Mobitz I (Wenckebach) 2° AV block?**

A progressive prolongation of the PR interval until the atrial impulse is no longer conducted. If symptomatic, atropine and transcutaneous/transvenous pacing is required.

○ **What is Mobitz II 2° AV block, and how is it treated?**

A constant PR interval in which one or more beats fail to conduct. Treat with atropine and transcutaneous/transvenous pacing.

○ **A patient presents to the hospital 1 month after placement of a mechanical prosthetic valve with fever, chills, and a leukocytosis. Endocarditis is suspected. Which type of bacterium is most common?**

Staphylococcus aureus or *Staphylococcus epidermidis (coagulase-negative)*.

○ **What is the most common side-effect of Σ-blockers?**

Fatigue occurs early in treatment; depression occurs later.

❍   **Documentation of three BP results in a fully grown adolescent obtained at one week intervals must show an average greater than 140 mm Hg systolic or 90 mm Hg diastolic for the correct diagnosis of hypertension. What single reading can be considered sufficient for the diagnosis of hypertension without necessitating further investigations?**

When a patient's single reading is greater than 110 mm Hg diastolic, a diagnosis can be made. Another conclusive indicator of hypertension is when end organ damage occurs with a lower reading.

❍   **What are the side-effects of thiazide diuretics?**

Hyperglycemia, hyperlipidemia, hyperuricemia, hypokalemia, hypomagnesemia, and hyponatremia.

❍   **A patient presents with a history of episodic elevations in BP. She complains of headache, diarrhea, and skin flushing. What is the diagnosis?**

Pheochromocytoma.

❍   **Which drug can be used for all hypertensive emergencies?**

Sodium nitroprusside (not drug of choice for eclampsia). Sodium nitroprusside assists in relaxing smooth muscle through the production of cGMP. As a result, there is decreased preload and afterload, decreased oxygen demand, and a slightly increased heart rate with no change in myocardial blood flow, cardiac output, or renal blood flow. The duration of action is 1–2 minutes. Sometimes, a ß-blockade is required to treat rebound tachycardia.

❍   **What is the most common complication of nitroprusside?**

Hypotension. Thiocyanate toxicity accompanied by blurred vision, tinnitus, change in mental status, muscle weakness, and seizures is more prevalent in patients with renal failure and after prolonged infusions. Cyanide toxicity is uncommon. However, this type of toxicity may occur with hepatic dysfunction, after prolonged infusions, and in rates greater than 10 mg/kg per minute.

❍   **Define a hypertensive emergency in a fully grown adolescent patient.**

An elevated diastolic blood pressure that is > 115 mm Hg with associated end organ dysfunction or damage.

❍   **How quickly should the blood pressure be lowered in a hypertensive emergency?**

The BP should be lowered gradually over 2-3 hours to a systolic of 140-160 mm Hg and a diastolic of 90-110 mm Hg diastolic. To prevent cerebral hypoperfusion, the BP should not be decreased more than 25% of the mean arterial pressure.

❍   **Define uncomplicated hypertension.**

A diastolic blood pressure that is < 115 mm Hg with no symptoms of end organ damage. Uncomplicated hypertension does not require acute treatment.

❍   **What are the signs and symptoms of hypertensive encephalopathy?**

Nausea, vomiting, headache, lethargy, coma, blindness, nerve palsies, hemiparesis, aphasia, retinal hemorrhage, cotton wool spots, exudates, sausage linking, and papilledema.

❍   **What is the <u>most</u> <u>common</u> cause of myocarditis in US children?**

Viruses (especially adenovirus and Coxsackie virus group B). Other causes include bacteria (diphtheria, meningococcus and tuberculosis), fungi, protozoa (Chagas' disease), spirochetes (Lyme disease), and Kawasaki disease.

❍   **What is the <u>most</u> <u>common</u> cause of mitral stenosis?**

Rheumatic heart disease.

❍   **Is mitral valve prolapse (MVP) more common in males or in females?**

Females have a stronger genetic link to the disease. 2-5% of the population has MVP.

❍   **What is the hallmark sign of mitral valve prolapse?**

A midsystolic click sometimes accompanied by a late systolic murmur. MVP is largely a clinical diagnosis. An ECG is performed to assess the degree of prolapse. Other clinical findings include a laterally displaced diffuse apical pulse, decreased S1, split S2, and a holosystolic murmur radiating to the axilla.

❍   **What physical finding is usually indicative of acute pericarditis?**

Pericardial friction rub. The rub is best heard at the left sternal border or apex with the patient in a forward sitting position. Other findings include fever and tachycardia.

❍   **Acute pyogenic pericarditis is <u>most</u> <u>commonly</u> caused by which organisms?**

Staphylococcus aureus, *Neisseria meningitidis* and *Haemophilus influenza type B*.

❍   **When diagnosing pericardial effusion, how much fluid has to be present in the pericardial sac for visualization by an echocardiography and by an x-ray?**

At least 15 mL for an echocardiography. 250 mL for an x-ray.

❍   **What does an x-ray of a pericardial effusion reveal?**

A water bottle silhouette.

❍   **At what volume does pericardial effusion affect the intrapericardial pressure?**

80-200 mL. However, the rate of accumulation is more important than the amount of accumulation. If accumulated slowly the pericardium can tolerate up to 2000 mL of fluid.

❍   **What is the treatment for pericarditis without effusion?**

A 2 week treatment of aspirin q 4 hours is recommended if no contradictions exist and if effusion is not present. Ibuprofen, indomethacin, or colchicine are other alternatives. The use of corticosteroids is controversial, as recurrent pericarditis is common when doses are tapered.

❍   **What are the <u>most</u> <u>common</u> signs and symptoms of a pulmonary emoblus?**

Tachypnea (92%), CP (88%), dyspnea (84%), anxiety (59%), tachycardia (44%), fever (43%), DVT (32%), hypotension (25%), and syncope (13%).

❍   **What is the <u>most</u> <u>common</u> CXR finding in PE?**

Elevated dome of one hemidiaphragm. This finding is caused by decreased lung volume, which occurs in 50% of patients with PEs. Other common findings include lack of lung markings in the area perfused by the occluded artery, pleural effusions, atelectasis, and pulmonary infiltrates.

O   **Which test is considered the gold standard for a diagnosis of deep vein thrombosis (DVT)? Of pulmonary embolies (PE)?**

The gold standard for DVT is venography. The gold standard for the diagnosis of PE is the pulmonary angiography.

O   **Rheumatic heart disease is the <u>most</u> <u>common</u> cause of stenosis of what 3 heart valves?**

Mitral, aortic (along with congenital bicuspid valve), and tricuspid.

O   **Which is most likely to be pathologic in children: an S_3 or an S_4?**

An S_4.

O   **When measuring a pulsus paradoxus, what is considered a normal difference in systolic blood pressures (with inspiration versus expiration)?**

Up to 8-10 mmHg.

O   **Which congenital heart lesions commonly present with cyanosis in an infant's first day of life?**

All the abnormalities that start with a T. Tetralogy of Fallot, Transposition of the great vessels, Total anomalous pulmonary circulation, Truncus arteriosus, and Tricuspid valve atresia (and Ebstein's malformation of the Tricuspid valve).

O   **What is the usual presentation of children with a ventricular septal defect?**

A systolic murmur in the first days of life with no signs related to their condition. They usually resolve spontaneously.

O   **How do infants with atrial septal defects usually present?**

The majority of these children are totally asymptomatic, and the defect usually is not diagnosed until they are school age.

O   **A short PR interval and a delta wave are characteristic of what cardiac anomaly?**

Wolff-Parkinson-White (WPW) syndrome. This is due to a reentry phenomenon along the Bundle of Kent.

O   **Which patients with mitral valve prolapse (MVP) should receive prophylactic antibiotics to protect against subacute bacterial endocarditis?**

Patients with MVP and a systolic murmur.

O   **How does the size of a VSD correlate with the risk of infective endocarditis?**

It doesn't. The risk is independent of size.

O   **T/F: You can rule out subacute bacterial endocarditis (SBE) after you have obtained two negative blood cultures?**

False. False negatives occur 10-30% of the time in two cultures. For this reason, three blood cultures are recommended.

❍ **How common do children with SBE present with cutaneous manifestations?**

Not very common. These manifestations are seen late in the disease, so they are not commonly seen in the appropriately treated patient.

❍ **A 16-year-old boy comes to your office for a pre-participation sports physical. What three findings during the physical exam can help you identify those patients at risk for sudden cardiac arrest?**

Presence of dysrhythmia, a pathologic murmur, and marfanoid features.

❍ **What test can be used to identify vasovagal neuroregulatory syncope as the cause of syncope in children with a history of "falling out"?**

The tilt-table test.

❍ **What test can be used to differentiate congenital heart disease from primary pulmonary parenchymal disease in a newborn with cyanosis?**

The hyperoxia test. There is little to no difference in arterial oxygen content between breathing room air and 100% oxygen with cyanotic congenital heart disease

❍ **On a chest x-ray of a child, what bony abnormality would lead you to suspect coarctation of the aorta?**

Bilateral rib notching.

❍ **What bony abnormalities are seen in the chest x-rays of children with Down syndrome?**

You may see 11 ribs

❍ **What are the common cardiac complications of juvenile rheumatoid arthritis?**

Pericarditis and (rare) myocarditis.

❍ **What are the common cardiac complications of Marfan syndrome?**

Aortic and mitral insufficiency, mitral valve prolapse (MVP), and dissecting aortic aneurysm.

❍ **What are the common cardiac complications of sickle cell anemia?**

High output cardiac failure, cardiomyopathy and cor pulmonale.

❍ **What congenital cardiac diseases will present with increased pulmonary markings on a chest x-ray?**

Transposition of the great vessels, total anomalous pulmonary venous return (and truncus arteriosus).

❍ **An "egg shaped" heart is a characteristic x-ray finding for what congenital heart malformation?**

Transposition of the great arteries.

❍ **What are the differential diagnoses for a widely split S_2?**

ASD, tetralogy of Fallot (TOF), pulmonary stenosis, right bundle branch block (RBBB), total anomalous pulmonary venous return.

○   **In classifying a heart murmur's intensity, what differentiates a III from a IV?**

The absence (III) or presence (IV) of a thrill.

○   **What are the osculatory findings in an ASD?**

A loud first heart sound, sometimes a pulmonic ejection click, a second heart sound that is widely split and fixed in all phases of respiration, and a systolic ejection murmur (best heard at the left middle and upper sternal border). A short, rumbling mid-diastolic murmur may be heard at the left lower sternal border.

○   **Describe the most common 'innocent' murmur?**

Medium-pitched, "musical" or vibratory systolic ejection murmur best heard at LLSB without radiation.

○   **How common is an 'innocent' murmur?**

Very. Up to 30% of children have one, with peak incidence between 3-7 years of age.

○   **What is the 13th lead in a 13 lead ECG?**

V_3R or V_4R. These are right precordial leads which evaluate the extent of right ventricular hypertrophy.

○   **What is the test of choice to examine for the presence of vegetations in a child with endocarditis?**

Transesophageal echocardiography.

○   **An ECG shows the following findings: RSR' in V_3R and V_1, prolonged P-R interval, tall P waves, a QRS axis of -60 degrees and signs of RVH. What is your diagnosis, doc?**

AV canal defect (a.k.a. AV septal defect, endocardial cushion defect).

○   **What is the most common cardiac malformation?**

VSD. This accounts for about 25% of all heart diseases. Prognosis depends largely on size of the defect- if small it may close spontaneously (usually before 4 years of age).

○   **A 10-year-old child with a history of VSD is about to have an impacted tooth removed. What antibiotic should he be given prophylactically to prevent endocarditis?**

Amoxicillin 50 mg/kg one hour before the procedure and 25 mg/kg six hours after the first dose. If the patient has a penicillin allergy, use clindamycin 20 mg/kg one hour before the procedure and 10 mg/kg six hours after the first dose.

○   **What is the treatment of choice for a patent ductus arteriosus (PDA)?**

Surgical ligation and division, regardless of age.

○   **What compound causes the ductus arteriosus to constrict right after birth?**

Oxygen, which is a vasoconstrictor. (Of course you knew that)

○   **When is it most effective to administer indomethacin to newborns with patent ductus arteriosus?**

During the first 24-48 hours of life, with a second and third dose at 12 and 36 hours, following the initial dose.

❍   **What percentage of patent ductus arteriosi that were initially closed with indomethacin reopen?**

25%. It is more likely to reopen if therapy is started beyond the first week of life.

❍   **What is the treatment of choice for a child with severe aortic stenosis?**

Balloon valvuloplasty if peak systolic gradient between the LV and aorta is > 60 mmHg.

❍   **How does squatting help children with hypoxia secondary to their tetralogy of Fallot (TOF)?**

It increases their systemic vascular resistance.

❍   **You are on call in the NICU when a newborn with severe coarctation of the aorta suddenly starts deteriorating and is acidotic. What do you do initially?**

Infuse prostaglandin E_1 and administer oxygen.

❍   **What test confirms the clinical suspicion of PDA?**

2-D echocardiogram detects up to 90% .

❍   **What is the most reliable way to diagnose neonatal pulmonary hypertension?**

Right heart catheterization.

❍   **What is the normal QRS axis in a newborn?**

+135 to +180 degrees. This reflects their right ventricular dominance.

❍   **A 3-year-old child present with premature atrial contractions (PAC's). Should this be a cause of concern?**

They are usually benign, except in children less than 1-year-old, or those on digitalis.

❍   **Quick, name the anomalies found in tetology of Fallot (TOF).**

Pulmonary stenosis, VSD, dextroposition of aorta with septal override, and RVH.

❍   **What are the most common complications of TOF prior to correction?**

Cerebral thromboses, brain abscess, bacterial endocarditis and CHF.

❍   **What is the shunting procedure currently employed to correct the cyanosis in TOF?**

The modified Blalock-Taussig shunt. This aortopulmonary shunt is a Gore-Tex conduit which anastomoses the subclavian and pulmonary arteries (homolateral branch).

❍   **What therapy can be instituted to decrease the incidence of coronary abnormalities in children with Kawasaki syndrome?**

IV immune globulin.

❍   **What medication has been shown to decrease the fever and discomfort associated with an acute attack of Kawasaki syndrome?**

High dose aspirin therapy.

O   **What laboratory findings differentiate Kawasaki disease from measles?**

Children with Kawasaki syndrome tend to have an increased WBC count, elevated ESR, elevated liver function and pyuria.

O   **What congenital cardiac defects are commonly seen in children with Down syndrome?**

Endocardial cushion defect, ASD, VSD.

O   **What congenital cardiac defects are commonly seen in infants with fetal alcohol syndrome?**

ASD, VSD.

O   **What congenital cardiac defects are commonly seen in patient with autosomal dominant polycystic kidney disease?**

Mitral valve prolapse (MVP).

O   **What is the procedure of choice for treatment of transposition of the great arteries?**

The Jatene (or Switch) operation.

O   **What is the 5 year survival rate of infants and children who undergo a complete heart transplantation?**

70-85% with immunosuppressive agents.

O   **What is the primary cause of congestive heart failure (CHF) in infancy and childhood?**

Congenital heart disease.

O   **A patient with congenital heart disease taking digoxin and Lasix, presents in CHF; what are the potential causes?**

1. Untreated or unrecognized infection
2. Anemia
3. Arrhythmias
4. Inadequate or excessive digitalis dose
5. Hypokalemia
6. Traumatic injury

O   **What diseases lead to a pulsus paradoxus greater than 20 mm Hg?**

Cardiac tamponade, asthma, CHF.

O   **What does a high pulsus paradoxus indicate?**

Circulatory compromise.

O   **What are the classic presenting features of pericarditis in children?**

Positional sharp substernal chest pain, abdominal pain, tachycardia, tachypnea, dyspnea, fever, friction rub.

O   **What are the potential complications of pericarditis?**

Myocarditis, pericardial effusion, pericardial tamponade.

○ **What is the mortality rate from myocarditis?**

35%

○ **What are the ECG findings in myocarditis?**

1. Diffuse nonspecific ST-T wave changes
2. AV blocks
3. Ventricular ectopy
4. Prolonged QT interval

○ **What is the cause of sudden death in myocarditis?**

Dysrhythmias. Treat ventricular arrhythmias with lidocaine, supraventricular tachyarrhythmias with digoxin, and complete atrioventricular block with a temporary pacemaker.

○ **How is acute myocarditis managed?**

Treat the CHF, restrict fluids, diuresis, oxygen, strict bed rest, and inotropic support if needed.

○ **What are the ECG findings in a patient with a significant pericardial effusion?**

1. Low voltage
2. Electrical alternans

○ **What are the findings in an infant with acute CHF?**

1. Irritability
2. Poor feeding
3. Lethargy
4. Failure to thrive
5. Tachycardia
6. Tachypnea
7. Hyperactive precordium
8. Gallop rhythm
9. Rales
10. Hepatomegaly

Peripheral edema and neck vein distention are noted only in older children.

○ **What are the most common bacteria seen in a purulent pericardial effusion?**

1. Staphylococcus aureus
2. Streptococcus pneumoniae
3. Haemophilus influenza

○ **What condition in children is infective endocarditis most often associated with?**

Congenital heart disease (40% of cases).

○ **A patient is diagnosed with infective endocarditis. She has a history of recent dental surgery. What is the most likely organism?**

Viridans streptococcus. Viridans streptococcus is a family of organisms including such microbes of streptococcus mutans, streptococcus salivarius, etc.

O   **A child with congenital heart disease develops infective endocarditis postoperatively, what is the most likely organism?**

Staphylococcal species.

O   **In a child previously healthy child without congenital heart disease, what is the most common cause of infective endocarditis.**

Staphylococcus aureus.

O   **In what percentage of cases of bacterial endocarditis will blood cultures be positive?**

90%.

O   **If antibiotics are required before the organism has been identified, which agents should be used?**

Aminoglycoside (gentamicin 5-7.5 mg/kg/day) + penicillinase-resistant penicillin oxacillin/ nafcillin.

O   **A child presents with chest pain and a new murmur. Which cardiac conditions should be suspected?**

Hypertrophic obstructive cardiomyopathy and aortic stenosis.

O   **What are the five major Jones criteria for diagnosing rheumatic fever?**

Carditis, migratory polyarthritis, chorea, erythema marginatum, and subcutaneous nodules.

O   **Which of the major criteria is the most commonly seen?**

Polyarthritis.

O   **Describe the rash present in rheumatic fever.**

Non-pruritic, fine, lacey in appearance with central blanching and a serpiginous pattern.

O   **What is the most common cardiac defect in children and adolescents with rheumatic heart disease?**

Mitral insufficiency.

O   **What are the cardiac complications of Kawasaki disease?**

Myocarditis and coronary artery aneurysms.

O   **What percent of untreated patients with Kawasaki's disease will develop coronary artery aneurysms?**

15% to 25%. The coronary artery damage can lead to thrombosis or sudden death after acute symptoms have resolved.

O   **What are the common causes of acquired third-degree AV block?**

Myocarditis, endocarditis, rheumatic fever, cardiac muscle disease, cardiac tumors, and postoperative cardiac surgery.

O   **What is the most common dysrhythmia seen in the pediatric age group?**
Supraventricular tachycardia (SVT)

❍ **What is the dosage used in cardioverting a child?**

0.5 to 1 Joules/kg increasing up to 2 Joules/kg.

❍ **What is the most common cause of SVT in infants?**

Congenital heart disease (30%). Other causes include fever, infection, or drug exposure (20%), and unknown etiology (50%).

❍ **Twenty-five percent of SVT is associated with what syndrome?**

Wolf-Parkinson-White.

❍ **What problem can occur by using digoxin to treat SVT in a patient with the WPW syndrome?**

Digoxin can shorten the refractory period in the bypass tract and enhance conduction in the accessory pathway, leading to a rapid ventricular response and ventricular fibrillation.

❍ **What are the most common causes of atrial fibrillation and flutter?**

Congenital heart disease, rheumatic fever, dilated cardiomyopathy, hyperthyroidism.

❍ **What is the treatment of choice in an unstable patient with atrial fibrillation and flutter?**

Immediate cardioversion with 0.5 J/kg.

❍ **What is the treatment for stable atrial fibrillation?**

Digitalization.

❍ **Why should atrial flutter be treated in a patient with congenital heart disease?**

Because this patient's risk of sudden death is four times higher than normal.

❍ **What is the mortality in untreated congenital prolonged QT syndrome?**

80%.

❍ **By what age should a child's ECG resemble an adults?**

> 3 years of age.

❍ **What are the possible etiologies for ventricular tachycardia?**

Electrolyte imbalance, metabolic disturbances, cardiac tumors, drugs, cardiac catheterization or surgery, congenital heart disease, cardiomyopathies prolonged QT syndrome, and idiopathic.

❍ **What is the normal QTc value?**

0.45 in infants, 0.44 in children, 0.43 in adolescents.

❍ **What is the treatment for premature atrial contractions (PACs)?**

No treatment is required in an asymptomatic patient but frequent PACs should be evaluated to rule out myocarditis.

O   **When should premature ventricular contractions (PVCs) be treated?**

Treat those that cause or are likely to cause hemodynamic compromise.

O   **What is the initial treatment for symptomatic second and third degree heart block?**

Atropine 0.01 to 0.03 mg/kg. A minimum dose of 0.1 mg should be used in children to avoid atropine-induced paradoxical bradycardia.

O   **What is the treatment for ventricular fibrillation (VF)?**

Defibrillation with 1 to 2 Joules/kg/dose.

O   **What is the dose of epinephrine in ventricular fibrillation and asystole?**

0.1 mg/kg/dose q 3-5 minutes (1:10,000).

O   **What is a "tet spell?"**

Episodes of paroxysmal hypoxemia which are usually self-limited and last less than 15 to 30 minutes, although they may last longer. The spells are seen more often in the morning but may occur during the day and may be precipitated by activity, a sudden fright, or injury or may occur spontaneously without apparent cause. The tachypnea and cyanosis are due to an increase in right-to-left shunting and concomitant decrease in pulmonary blood flow. The exact mechanism by which this occurs is unknown.

O   **What is the treatment for a "tet spell?"**

Place in the knee-chest position which increases peripheral resistance in the lower extremities, which in turn, promotes increased pulmonary blood flow. Place the patient on oxygen and give morphine sulfate 0.1 mg/kg IV. If these measures fail, use propranolol to a maximum total dose of 0.1 mg/kg.

O   **In the pre-term infant, what is the most common cause of congestive heart failure?**

Persistent patent ductus arteriosus.

O   **What is the most common cause of cardiac chest pain in an infant or child?**

Anomalous pulmonary origin of a coronary artery.

O   **What is the most common atrial septal defect seen and what does it involve anatomically?**

Most often involves the fossa ovalis, is midseptal, and is of the ostium secundum type.

O   **What are the most notable cardiac auscultatory findings in children with atrial septal defects?**

Normal or split first heart sound, accentuation of the tricuspid valve closure sound, a midsystolic pulmonary ejection murmur and a wide, fixed split second heart sound.

O   **What is the typical CXR findings of a patient with atrial septal defect?**

Enlargement of the right atrium and ventricle, dilated pulmonary artery and its branches, and increased pulmonary vascular markings.

O   **What is the confirmatory test of choice for atrial septal defect?**

Echocardiography with color Doppler flow and contrast echocardiography.

O **When should surgical repair be considered for patients with atrial septal defect and when is the optimal timing for such treatment?**

Surgical repair should be carried out in all patients with atrial septal defect who have evidence of a left-to-right shunt where there is a pulmonary-systemic flow ratio equal to or greater than 1.5:1.0 found on cardiac catheterization, ideally carried out at while the patient is between ages 2 – 4. Surgical therapy should not be carried out in patients with small defects and trivial left-to-right shunts (less than 1.5:1.0) or in patients with severe pulmonary hypertension without a significant left-to-right shunt.

SEDATION AND ANALGESIA

○ **Explain the differences between the terms Opium, Opiate, and Opioid.**

Opium: From the Greek word for juice, applies to the juice extracted from the seeds of the poppy plant, the source for over 20 alkaloids.

Opiate: Any substance that is derived from the opium plant and can induce sleep, the naturally occurring medications from the opium plant are morphine and codeine.

Opioid: Any synthetic substance not derived from opium but that can induce narcosis. Synthetic opioids are meperidine (Demerol), and fentanyl (Sublimaze).

○ **What is the most common adverse reaction caused by local anesthetics?**

Contact dermatitis is the most common local adverse reaction and is characterized by erythema and pruritus that could progress to vesiculation and oozing.

○ **What is the half-life of acetaminophen (Tylenol)?**

Its half-life is 2-3 hours and is unaffected by renal disease as acetaminophen is metabolized in the liver.

○ **What is the indication for naloxone (Narcan) use?**

Naloxone (Narcan) is a narcotic antagonist used to treat or prevent respiratory depression or hypotension known or suspected to be caused by opioids/opiates.

○ **How may naloxone be administered?**

Although the intravenous route is preferred, the same dosage is effective almost as rapidly following endotracheal, intramuscular or subcutaneous administration at a dose of 0.1 mg/kg or 2.0 mg/dose if > 20 kg or 5 years, and can be repeated once in 2-3 minutes if there is no response.

○ **In what specific clinical situations should naloxone be used?**

Naloxone should be used to reverse CNS depression in suspected narcotic overdose, neonatal opiate depression and coma of unknown origin.

○ **What are the contraindications to using succinylcholine (Anectine)?**

Succinylcholine is contraindicated in patients with a personal history or a family history of malignant hyperthermia, skeletal muscle myopathies, or known hypersensitivity to the drug. It should also not be used in patients with a history of pseudocholinesterase deficiency. It should be avoided in infants and children with ventricular arrhythmias in which you suspect hyperkalemia.

○ **On what specific sites in the CNS do the benzodiazepines act and where are they located?**

Benzodiazepine receptors are present in many regions of the brain including the thalamus, limbic structures and the cerebral cortex. They form part of a GABA receptor-chloride ion channel complex, and binding of benzodiazepines to this receptor facilitates the inhibitory actions of GABA, which are exerted through increased chloride ion conductance.

○ **Compare the three benzodiazepines commonly used.**

The clinical effects of diazepam are shorter than lorazepam because it dissociates more rapidly from receptor sites than diazepam, however the elimination half-times are longest for diazepam.

Medication	Elimination half time in minutes
diazepam	20-35
lorazepam	10-20
midazolam	1-4

○ **Describe the state induced with the use of ketamine (Ketalar)?**

Ketamine produces a state of dissociative anesthesia in which the patient remains conscious but has marked catatonia, analgesia and amnesia.

○ **What is the most commonly sited contraindication for ketamine use?**

Ketamine should not be used in patients with blunt head injury as causes an increase in intra-cranial pressure.

○ **How is intravenous ketamine administered in the pediatric patient?**

At a dose of 1-2 mg/kg per initial dose, given over 60 seconds, producing 5-10 minutes of anesthesia and used in increments of 1/2 of an initial dose if needed to maintain anesthesia.

○ **What are the common symptoms during recovery from intravenous ketamine?**

It causes disorientation and hallucinations during recovery. These symptoms are seen less in younger patients.

○ **How can the side effects of ketamine be lessened during recovery?**

The concomitant use of a benzodiazepine can lessen the side effects commonly seen during emergence.

○ **What are five non-pharmacologic methods used to reduce pain in pediatric patients?**

Biofeedback, desensitization, distraction, exercise and play are non-pharmacological interventions with demonstrated efficacy.

○ **What is the principle behind biofeedback, and when is it useful?**

Biofeedback teaches the child with pain to distinguish between relaxed and tense body states. It is useful when pain is temporarily associated with stress or tension.

○ **What is the dose and route of administration of fentanyl (Sublimaze) when used in the neonate?**

In the neonate, fentanyl can be given IV or IM at a dose of 1-2 micrograms/kg infused slowly over 1 minute.

○ **What is the fentanyl lollipop and what is its main side effect?**

The lollipop is a pediatric pre-anesthetic medication to be used by children as a self-administered drug. Some series report up to 50% incidence of vomiting making it impractical in children with "full stomachs" such as in an emergency department.

❍   **When using midazolam (Versed) in patients with renal or hepatic dysfunction how should dosing be adjusted?**

If a patient has renal or hepatic dysfunction or is receiving concomitant narcotics, the dose should be decreased by 25-30%.

❍   **Describe the pharmacokinetics of codeine.**

Codeine has adequate oral absorption and is metabolized in the liver to morphine. It has a half-life of 2.5-3.5 hours and is excreted in the urine.

❍   **Why should IV fentanyl be infused slowly?**

Rapid IV infusion of fentanyl can result in skeletal muscle and chest wall rigidity, leading to impaired ventilation, respiratory distress and eventual apnea.

❍   **What is the half-life of morphine?**

In neonates: 4.5-13.3 hours (mean of 7.6 hours). In children: 2-4 hours.

❍   **How potent is fentanyl, when compared to morphine?**

Fentanyl is 50-100 times more potent.

❍   **What are the contraindications to using eutectic mixture of local anesthetics (EMLA) cream?**

Contraindications include known hypersensitivity to lidocaine (Xylocaine), prilocaine or local anesthetics of the amide type. Also, patients with idiopathic or congenital methemoglobinemia should not be given these topical agents.

❍   **What is the mechanism of action of acetaminophen?**

Acetaminophen inhibits the synthesis of prostaglandins in the central nervous system and peripherally blocks pain impulse generation. It also produces antipyresis by inhibiting the hypothalamic heat regulating center.

❍   **What is the toxic dose of acetaminophen?**

150 mg/kg.

❍   **Why should codeine _not_ be given intravenously?**

When given intravenously, codeine causes a large histamine release which leads to palpitations, hypotension, bradycardia, and peripheral vasodilatation.

❍   **Compare the cardiovascular adverse effects of fentanyl when compared to morphine.**

Fentanyl has less hypotensive effects than morphine due to minimal or no histamine release.

❍   **Is it appropriate to use eutectic mixture of local anesthetics on mucous membranes?**

No, because it has increased absorption across mucus membranes which can lead to toxic levels.

❍   **What is the maximum daily dose of ibuprofen (Motrin, Advil)?**

40 mg/kg, up to a 3 grams maximum.

○   **How much sugar, and what kind, is found in each 5 ml suspension of ibuprofen?**

2.5 gm of sucrose. This is important if you plan to use this suspension in a diabetic patient.

○   **What are some of the misconceptions about pain in children?**

One of the misconceptions about pain in children is that pain perception in children is decreased because of biologic immaturity and that children have a higher tolerance to pain. Other misconceptions are that children have little or no memory of pain and that not only are they more sensitive to the side effects of analgesics, but that they are at special risk for addiction to narcotics. These beliefs are false.

○   **Name four ways the pain of subcutaneously injected lidocaine can be reduced?**

1. Use a solution buffered with sodium bicarbonate.
2. Administer slowly.
3. Administer with a small needle, e.g., <30 gauge.
4. Use a warmed solution.

○   **Discuss pain conduction in the neonate.**

In the neonate, as in the adult, unmyelinated C fibers transmit nociceptive information peripherally. Nerve pulse transmission in incompletely myelinated A-d fibers is delayed, not blocked, until myelination has been completed postnatally. The shorter distances necessary for impulse travel offset any delay in conduction velocity.

○   **Which two common paralytic agents are non-depolarizing?**

Pancuronium (Pavulon) and vecuronium (Norcuron).

○   **How do non-depolarizing blocking paralytics exert their effects?**

The non-depolarizing blocking drugs compete with acetylcholine for cholinergic receptor sites on the postjunctional membrane, but lack the transmitter action of acetylcholine. They do not relieve pain and do not effect consciousness.

○   **In many prepubertal children, what appears in the urine after the patient receives succinylcholine?**

Myoglobinuria. About 40% of prepubertal children exhibit this effect; however, it is not related to the apparent severity of the fasciculations.

○   **How long does anesthesia last from a perineural injection of lidocaine?**

When used alone it lasts 60-75 minutes and when used in combination with epinephrine, anesthesia lasts up to two hours.

○   **How long does it take for a local injection of lidocaine to exert its effect?**

Its effect is immediate.

○   **What are endorphins?**

Endogenous morphine.

○   **What is the dose of ketorolac?**

Ketorolac, when given intramuscularly, is done at an initial dose of 0.5 to 1 mg/kg as a loading dose (30-60 mg in an adult), then 0.25 to 0.5 mg/kg every 6 hours (15-30mg in an adult). IV administration is dosed at approximately one-half of the IM dose. Ketorolac is also available orally for adolescents and adults, and is given at a dose of 10 mg every 4-6 hours as needed. It is intended for short term use only. Its use in children has not yet been officially approved.

❍   **What are the routes of administration of chloral hydrate?**

Never intravenous. Chloral hydrate may only be given PO or PR.

❍   **What are the contraindications to using chloral hydrate?**

Chloral hydrate is contraindicated in patients with hepatic or renal impairment.

❍   **What is the maximum dose of locally injected lidocaine?**

7.0 mg/kg/dose with epinephrine every 2 hours or 4.0-5.0 mg/kg/dose without epinephrine every 2 hours.

❍   **What are Mu receptors?**

A specific subtype of opioid receptors that are responsible for supraspinal analgesia, euphoria, and respiratory and physical dependence effects.

❍   **Describe the anesthetic agent propofol (Diprivan).**

Propofol is chemically unrelated to any other anesthetic drugs, it most closely resembles the alcohol family and has sedative properties which are similar to the alcohols. It is anecdotally called *milk of amnesia*. It may cause apnea.

❍   **Compare and contrast pancuronium (Pavulon) and vecuronium (Norcuron).**

Vecuronium (Norcuron) has a shorter duration of action that pancuronium (Pavulon). The vagolytic property of vecuronium is 20 times less than pancuronium.

	Duration of Maximum Effect	Half-life	Elimination	Dose
Pancuronium (Pavulon)	60 minutes	90-150 minutes	Renal	0.1 mg/kg
Vecuronium (Norcuron)	30 minutes	70 minutes	Hepatic	0.1 mg/kg

PULMONARY

○ **What should you suspect if a patient has symptoms similar to those associated with emphysema but he/she is very young and is not a smoker?**

Σ-1-antitrypsin deficiency. Without Σ-1-antitrypsin, excess elastase accumulates resulting in lung damage. Treatment for this condition is the same as emphysema. An Σ-1 proteinase inhibitor may also be useful.

○ **A 14-year-old high school freshman attended three days of classes at his new high school last week before it was shut down because of the potential of asbestos exposure. The boy currently exhibits a non-productive cough and says his chest hurts. Does this boy have asbestosis?**

Although a non-productive cough and pleurisy are symptoms of asbestosis, other signs, such as exertional dyspnea, malaise, clubbed fingers, crackles, cyanosis, pleural effusion and pulmonary hypertension, should be displayed before making a diagnosis of asbestosis. In addition, asbestosis does not develop until 10-15 years after regular exposure to asbestos.

○ **What procedures should be performed to confine aspiration in a patient who is continuously vomiting and at risk for aspiration pneumonia?**

Lie the patient on his right side in Trendelenburg. This will help confine the aspirate to the right upper lobe.

○ **How can aspiration be prevented when intubating?**

By appropriate use of rapid sequence induction, including minimizing unnecessary ventilation and applying cricoid pressure during intubation.

○ **Where does aspiration generally occur as revealed by chest x-ray?**

The lower lobe of the right lung. This is the most direct path for foreign bodies in the lung.

○ **What pH of aspirated fluid suggests a poor prognosis?**

pH < 2.5.

○ **A 16-year-old triathlete develops wheezing when exercising. Describe a relevant treatment program for this individual.**

Beta agonist prior to exercise is still initial management therapy. A sodium cromoglycate (cromolyn sodium) inhaler is the prophylactic medication of choice. Leukotriene inhibitors are currently being tested to this effect as well, and may become the standard of care. Sodium cromoglycate stabilizes mast cells that are involved in the early and late phase bronchoconstrictive reactions of asthma. Sodium cromoglycate is a prophylactic treatment and is not effective once the attack has begun.

○ **What x-ray markings usually result in a patient with a long history of bronchial asthma?**

Increased bronchial wall markings and flattening of the diaphragm. The bronchial wall markings are caused by epithelial inflammation and thickening of the bronchial walls.

○ **What pulmonary function test is the most diagnostic for asthma?**

FEV1/FVC. The amount of air exhaled in 1 second, in comparison to the total amount of air in the lung that can be expressed, is determined by performing this test. A ratio of under 80% is diagnostic of asthma. Peak flow monitors are helpful in monitoring asthma at home.

❍   **Is wheezing an integral part of asthma?**

No. Thirty-three percent of children with asthma will have only cough variant asthma with no wheezing.

❍   **Which is more effective for relieving an acute exacerbation of bronchial asthma in a conscious patient, nebulized albuterol or albuterol MDI administered via an aerosol chamber?**

They are equally efficacious.

❍   **A child is born to two parents who are both asthmatic. What is risk factor of the child having asthma as well?**

Up to 50%.

❍   **What are the <u>most</u> <u>common</u> extrinsic allergens that affect asthmatic children?**

Dust and dust mites.

❍   **What treatment should be initiated for a patient with acute asthma who does not improve with humidified O_2, albuterol nebulizers, steroids, or anticholinergics?**

Subcutaneous epinephrine, 0.3 cc of 1:1,000. (0.01 cc/kg to a max of 0.3 cc)

❍   **What kind of medical family history are asthmatic patients most likely to have?**

Asthma, seasonal allergies, and/or atopic dermatitis.

❍   **Which type of exercise usually triggers an asthmatic episode in patients with exercise-induced asthma?**

High intensity exercise for more than 5-6 minutes.

❍   **What is the role of salmeterol in the asthmatic patient?**

It is used for the long term management of these patients and not in the acute setting. Because of its long half-life, it may be ideal for chronic use in nocturnal break-through exacerbations.

❍   **Sympathomimetic agents are used to treat asthma. What enzyme is activated by these agents?**

Adenyl cyclase.

❍   **What reaction is catalyzed by adenyl cyclase?**

Adenyl cyclase catalyzes ATP to cyclic AMP.

❍   **What effects do increased levels of cAMP have on bronchial smooth muscle and on the release of chemical mediators, such as histamine, proteases, platelet activation factor and chemotactic factors, from airway mast cells?**

Relaxes smooth muscle and decreases the release of mediators. Recall that the effects of cAMP are opposed by cGMP. Thus, another treatment approach can be provided by *decreasing* the levels of cyclic GMP via the use of anticholinergic (antimuscarinic) agents, such as ipratropium bromide.

O   As discussed above, stimulation of Σ-adrenergic receptors increases cAMP availability and results in smooth muscle relaxation. Which flavor of ß-adrenergic receptors primarily control bronchiolar and arterial smooth muscle tone?

ß2-adrenergic receptors.

O   Terbutaline is administered SQ for asthma in what dose?

0.01 mL/kg of 1 mg/mL terbutaline up to 0.25 mL, (i.e., 0.25 mg), which may be repeated once in 20-30 minutes.

O   Is theophylline useful in the emergency management of a severely asthmatic pediatric patient?

No. It has not been shown to affect further bronchodilatation in patients fully treated with Σ-adrenergic agents. However, theophylline can be used successfully for inpatient management of asthma and may be started in the hospital.

O   If corticosteroids are prescribed, how should prednisone be dosed?

1-2 mg/kg/day in two divided doses; no tapering is necessary if duration of therapy is 5 day or less.

O   What effect does acidosis have on treatments with Σ-adrenergic agonists?

Decreased efficacy.

O   If one prefers the most simplified algorithm for determining loading dose of theophylline, what are the appropriate doses for a patient who has not been given any theophylline recently? A patient who has recently been given a dose of theophylline?

1) No recent dose: Load with 7 mg/kg theophylline.
2) Recent dose: Load with 5 mg/kg theophylline.

O   What is the appropriate parenteral dose of methylprednisolone (Solu-Medrol) to administer to a pediatric patient with status asthmaticus?

1-2 mg/kg every 6 hours.

O   If mechanical ventilation is required for such a patient, what is an appropriate setting for the initial tidal volume?

10 mL/kg.

O   What is the most common postoperative respiratory complication?

Atelectasis. Respiratory failure and aspiration pneumonia are other postoperative complications.

O   What percentage of patients who have had abdominal surgery also develop atelectasis?

> 25%.

O   Atelectasis accounts for what percentage of postoperative fevers?

90%.

O   Why do we care about postoperative atelectasis?

If it persists for more than 72 hours, pneumonia may develop. Perioperative mortality rates are then 20%. Incentive spirometry is an important therapy for the prevention of atelectasis.

O   **A chest x-ray shows "honeycombing," atelectasis, and increased bronchial markings. What is the diagnosis?**

Bronchiectasis. Bronchography will show dilations of the bronchial tree, but this method of diagnosis is not recommended for routine use.

O   **Bronchiectasis occurs most frequently in patients with what conditions?**

Patients with cystic fibrosis, immunodeficiencies, lung infections, or foreign body aspirations.

O   **Which is the <u>most</u> <u>common</u> type of pathogen in bronchiolitis?**

RSV. It generally affects infants younger than 2 years old. Bronchiolitis is rarely seen in adults.

O   **A 2-year-old patient presents with a sudden harsh cough that is worse at night, wheezing, and rhonchi/inspiratory stridor. What is the diagnosis?**

Croup (also known as laryngotracheitis). This condition is usually preceded by an URI and most frequently caused by the parainfluenza virus. A barking seal cough is a characteristic of croup.

O   **In treating a patient with a common cold, you prescribe an oral decongestant. Is it necessary to also suggest an antitussive?**

Most coughs arising from a common cold are caused by the irritation of the tracheobronchial receptors in the posterior pharynx by postnasal drip. Postnasal drip can be cleared up with decongestant therapy, thereby eliminating the need for cough suppressant therapy.

O   **What are the <u>most</u> <u>common</u> etiologies of a chronic cough?**

Postnasal drip (40%), asthma (25%), and gastroesophageal reflux (20%). Other etiologies include bronchitis, bronchiectasis, bronchogenic carcinoma, esophageal diverticula, sarcoidosis, viruses, and drugs.

O   **Which condition must be ruled out when childhood nasal polyps are found?**

Cystic fibrosis.

O   **What age group is afflicted with the most colds per year?**

Kindergartners win the top billing with an average of 12 colds per year. Second place goes to preschoolers with 6-10 per year. School children get an average of 7 per year, and adolescents and adults average only 2-4 per year.

O   **What is the duration of a common cold?**

3-10 day self-limited course.

O   **Which age group usually contracts croup?**

6 months to 3 years. Croup is characterized by cold symptoms, a sudden barking cough, inspiratory and expiratory stridor, and a slight fever.

O   **A newborn presents with poor weight gain, steatorrhea, and a GI obstruction arising from thick meconium ileus. What test should be performed?**

The "sweat test," which detects electrolyte concentrations in the sweat. The infant may have cystic fibrosis. Cystic fibrosis is an autosomal recessive defect affecting the exocrine glands. As a result, electrolyte concentrations increase in the sweat glands.

○   **What result from the sweat chloride test is considered positive for cystic fibrosis?**

> 60 mEq/L.

○   **What is the classic triad of cystic fibrosis?**

1. COPD.
2. Pancreatic enzyme deficiency.
3. Abnormally high concentration of sweat electrolytes.

○   **What is the <u>most</u> <u>common</u> presentation of newborns with cystic fibrosis?**

GI obstruction due to meconium ileus.

○   **What is the percentage of effusions that are associated with malignancy?**

25%.

○   **Which age group typically gets epiglottitis?**

The 3-7 year age group, although any group can get epiglottitis.

○   **What is the difference between the "cough of croup" and the "cough of epiglottitis"?**

Croup has a seal like "barking" cough, while epiglottitis is accompanied by a minimal cough. Children with croup have a hoarse voice while those with epiglottitis have a muffled voice.

○   **What is the "thumb print sign"?**

A soft tissue inflammation of the epiglottis on a lateral x-ray of the neck.

○   **Should a 7-year-old who has never received her Hib vaccine be vaccinated now?**

No, most children are immune by the age of 5.

○   **How is fetal lung maturity assessed?**

By measuring the ratio of lecithin to sphingomyelin (L/S). An L/S ratio greater than 2 and the presence of phosphatidyl glycerol verifies that the fetal lungs are mature.

○   **Are aspirated foreign bodies more likely to be found in the right or left bronchus?**

Right.

○   **What is the definition for massive hemoptysis?**

Coughing, not vomiting, of more than 300 mL of blood in 24 hours.

○   **Life threatening hemoptysis should be suspected when there is:**

1. A large volume of blood.
2   The appearance of a fungus ball in a pulmonary cavity via chest x-ray.
3. Hypoxemia.

O   **What are Kerley B lines?**

X-ray findings found in pulmonary edema. Fluid in the lung causes waterlogged interlobular septa that become fibrotic with time. These show up as lines and shadows on an x-ray.

O   **Which type of bacteria is <u>most</u> <u>commonly</u> found in lung abscesses?**

Anaerobic bacteria.

O   **Which single antibiotic is the most effective for treating uncomplicated lung abscess?**

Clindamycin.

O   **T/F: Flora of lung abscesses are usually polymicrobial.**

True.

O   **Which age group is usually afflicted by pertussis?**

Infants younger than 2.

O   **Where does pain from pleurisy radiate?**

The shoulder, as a result of diaphragmatic irritation.

O   **Which is the <u>most</u> <u>common</u> community-acquired pneumonia?**

Pneumococcal pneumonia. Streptococcus pneumonia are actually normal flora. Treatment includes penicillin G or erythromycin.

O   **Pneumatoceles, thin-walled air-filled cysts, on an infant's x-ray are a sign of which type of pneumonia?**

Staphylococcal pneumonia.

O   **What are the <u>most</u> <u>common</u> causes of Staphylococcal pneumonias?**

Drug use and endocarditis. This pneumonia produces high fever, chills, and a purulent productive cough.

O   **What are the extrapulmonary manifestations of mycoplasma?**

Erythema multiforme, pericarditis, and CNS disease.

O   **What is the most frequent etiology of nosocomial pneumonia?**

Pseudomonas aurignosa. There is a high mortality associated with pneumonia caused by *Pseudomonas.* It most frequently occurs in immunocompromised patients or patients on mechanical ventilation.

O   **A 14-year-old comes to your office bragging, between coughs, about a 3 day Young Republicans convention she attended last week in Las Vegas. She is nauseous and coughing; she has chills and a fever of 103.5°F. She also has a minor gait problem and splints his chest when he breaths. Should you be concerned about your own health as she has just given a mighty cough in your direction?**

This patient most likely has Legionnaires' disease. Unless you attended the same convention in Las Vegas, you are unlikely to catch this pneumonia from her. *Legionella pneumophila* contaminates the water in air conditioning towers and moist soil. It is not spread from person to person.

O **Describe the classic chest x-ray findings in a patient with mycoplasma pneumonia.**

Patchy diffuse densities involving the entire lung are most common. Pneumatoceles, cavities, abscesses, and pleural effusions can occur, but are uncommon.

O **Describe the classic chest x-ray findings in Legionella pneumonia.**

Dense consolidation and bulging fissures. Expect elevated liver enzymes and hypophosphatemia.

O **Match the pneumonia with the treatment.**

1. *Klebsiella pneumoniae*   a. Erythromycin, tetracycline, or doxycycline.
2. *Streptococcal pneumoniae.*   *b.* Penicillin G.
3. *Legionella pneumophila.*   c. Cefuroxime and clarithromycin.
4. *Haemophilus influenza pneumonia.* d. Erythromycin and rifampin.
5. Mycoplasma pneumonia.

Answers: (1) c, (2) b, (3) d, (4) c, and (5) a.

O **A 17-year-old college student is home for winter break and comes to your office complaining of a 1 1/2 week history of a non-productive dry hacking cough, malaise, a mild fever, and no chills. What is the diagnosis?**

Mycoplasma pneumoniae, also known as walking pneumonia. Although this is the most common pneumonia that develops in teenagers and young adults, it is an atypical pneumonia and is most frequently found in close contact populations (e.g., schools and military barracks).

O **Describe the different presentations of bacterial and viral pneumonia.**

Bacterial pneumonia is typified by a sudden onset of symptoms, including pleurisy, fever, chills, productive cough, tachypnea, and tachycardia. The most common bacterial pneumonia is Pneumococcal pneumonia.

Viral pneumonia is characterized by gradual onset of symptoms, no pleurisy, chills or high fever, general malaise, and a non-productive cough.

O **What is the most common cause of pneumonia in children?**

Viral pneumonia. Infecting viruses include influenza, parainfluenza, RSV, and adenoviruses.

O **What is the most common lethal, inheritable disease in the white population?**

Cystic fibrosis, an autosomal recessive disease occurring in 1/2,000 births.

O **Which two antimicrobial agents are broadly effective against organisms that cause both typical and atypical pneumonias?**

Azithromycin and clarithromycin.

O **What percentage of upper-respiratory infectious agents are non-bacterial?**

Non-bacterial agents account for over 90% of pharyngitis, laryngitis, tracheal bronchitis, and bronchitis.

O   **If a patient has a patchy infiltrate on a chest x-ray and bullous myringitis, what antibiotic should be prescribed?**

Erythromycin for mycoplasma.

O   **What secondary bacterial pneumonia often occurs following a viral pneumonia?**

Staphylococcus aureus pneumonia.

O   **What 3 findings should be present to consider a sputum sample adequate?**

1.   > 25 PMNs;
2.   < 10 squamous epithelial cells per low powered field;
3.   a predominant bacterial organism.

O   **Should steroids be used in aspiration pneumonia?**

No.

O   **What is the indication for a chest tube in pneumothorax?**

Over 15% pneumothorax or a clinical indication, such as respiratory embarrassment.

O   **What therapy may increase the body's absorption of a pneumothorax or pneumomediastinum?**

A high inspired FiO_2.

O   **What is the profile of a classic patient with a spontaneous pneumothorax?**

Male, athletic, tall, slim, 15-35 years of age. Pneumothorax does not occur most frequently during exercise.

O   **What accessory x-rays may be obtained for the diagnosis of pneumothorax?**

Expiratory film and lateral decubitus film on the affected side.

O   **Which types of pneumonia are commonly associated with pneumothorax?**

Staphylococcus, TB, Klebsiella, and PCP.

O   **Primary pulmonary hypertension is <u>most</u> <u>common</u> in what population?**

Young females. It is rapidly fatal within a few years.

O   **What heart sounds are heard with pulmonary hypertension?**

A shortened second heart sound split and a louder P2.

O   **What is the major etiology of pulmonary hypertension?**

Chronic hypoxia

O   **T/F: Pulse oximetry is a reliable method for estimating oxyhemoglobin saturation in a patient suffering from CO poisoning.**

False. COHb has light absorbance that can lead to a falsely elevated pulse oximeter transduced saturation level. The calculated value from a standard ABG may also be falsely elevated. The oxygen saturation should be determined by using a co-oximeter that measures the amounts of unsaturated O_2Hb, COHb, and metHb.

O   **What is the half-life of COHb for a patient breathing room air? Breathing 100% oxygen? Breathing 100% oxygen at 3 atm of pressure?**

Source	$FIO_2 = 0.21$	$FIO_2 = 1.0$	$FIO_2 = 1.0$ @ 3 atm
Tintinalli, 4th. Ed., pg 918.	4–5.3 hours	50–80 minutes	23 minutes
Harwood-Nuss, 2nd Ed., pg 1280.	4–5 hours	40–80 minutes	20 minutes
Rosen, 3rd Ed., pg 2675	4–6 hours	90 minutes	30 minutes

Using weighted averages and eliminated the outlying values, it is probably safe to remember these values as ≈ 6 hours, 1.5 hours, and 0.5 hours.

O   **A newborn is breathing rapidly and grunting. Intercostal retractions, nasal flaring, and cyanosis are noted. Auscultation shows decreased breath sounds and crackles. What is the diagnosis?**

Newborn respiratory distress syndrome, also known as hyaline membrane disease. X-rays show diffuse atelectasis. Treatment involves artificial surfactant and O_2 administration through CPAP.

O   **Other than avoiding prematurity, what can be done to prevent newborn respiratory distress syndrome?**

If the fetus is > 32 weeks, administer betamethasone 48–72 hours before delivery to augment surfactant production.

O   **Which type of rhinitis is associated with anxious patients?**

Vasomotor rhinitis. This is a non-allergic rhinitis of unknown etiology that involves nasal vascular congestion.

O   **Which sinuses are fully formed in children?**

Only the ethmoid and the maxillary. Frontal sinuses form by age 10.

O   **What is the indication for long-term tracheostomy?**

When intubation is expected to exceed 3 weeks.

O   **Differentiate between transudate and exudate.**

1. Transudate: Serum protein is < 0.5 and LDH is < 0.6. Most common with CHF, renal disease, and liver disease.
2. Exudate: Serum protein > 0.5, LDH > 0.6. Most common with infections, malignancy, and trauma.

O   **Where do primary TB lesions most often occur in the lung?**

Primary lesions most often occur in the lower lobes of the lung. Reactivation occurs in the apices.

O   **What are the side-effects of INH?**

Neuropathy, pyridoxine loss, lupus-like syndrome, and hepatitis.

❍ **What percentage of tuberculosis is drug-resistant?**

About 15%, but this mainly depends on the geographic location.

❍ **What are the classic signs and symptoms of TB?**

Night sweats, fever, weight loss, malaise, cough, and a greenish-yellow sputum most commonly seen in the mornings.

❍ **Where are some common extrapulmonary TB sites?**

The lymph node, bone, GI tract, GU tract, meninges, liver, and the pericardium.

❍ **Is a URI accompanied by a high fever usually caused by a bacterial or a viral source?**

Bacterial. However, most URI's are viral in origin.

❍ **A patient presents with cough, lethargy, dyspnea, conjunctivitis, glomerulonephritis, fever, and purulent sinusitis. What is the diagnosis?**

Wegener's granulomatosis. This is a necrotizing vasculitis and pulmonary granulomatosis that attacks the small arteries and veins. Treatment is with corticosteroids and cyclophosphamide.

❍ **What serological test is diagnostic for Wegener's granulomatosis?**

c-ANCA in association with appropriate clinical evidence. A renal, lung, or sinus biopsy may also be helpful in making the diagnosis.

❍ **Are sedatives beneficial for anxious asthmatic patients?**

Only if you are trying to kill them. However, sedatives are appropriate for use during Rapid Sequence Intubation (RSI).

❍ **What is the major side effect associated with the inhalation of N-acetylcysteine?**

Cough and bronchospasm, most likely due to irritation from the low pH (2.2) of the aerosol solution.

❍ **What is the effect of macrolide antibiotics (erythromycin, clarithromycin) on mucus hypersecretion?**

Some macrolide antibiotics have the ability to down regulate mucus secretion by an unknown mechanism. This is thought to be due to an anti-inflammatory activity.

❍ **What are the signs of a large obstructing foreign body in the larynx or trachea?**

Respiratory distress, stridor, inability to speak, cyanosis, loss of consciousness, death.

❍ **What are the symptoms of a smaller (distally lodged) foreign body?**

Cough, dyspnea, wheezing, chest pain, fever.

❍ **What is the procedure of choice for foreign body removal?**

Rigid bronchoscopy. Fiberoptic bronchoscopy is an alternate procedure in adults, not in children. If bronchoscopy fails, thoracotomy may be required.

❍ **What are the common radiographic findings in foreign body aspiration?**

Normal film, atelectasis, pneumonia, contralateral mediastinal shift (more marked during expiration), and visualization of the foreign body

❍ **T/F: Aspiration of fluids with pH less than 5 produces chemical pneumonitis.**

False. Aspirate pH less than 2.5 produces chemical injury.

❍ **What is the antibiotic choice for gastric acid aspiration?**

None.

❍ **What is the role of corticosteroids in gastric acid aspiration?**

None.

❍ **What is the main priority in treating gastric acid aspiration?**

Maintenance of oxygenation. Intubation, ventilation, and PEEP (positive end expiratory pressure) may be required.

❍ **What are the radiographic manifestations of acid aspiration?**

Varied, may be bilateral diffuse infiltrates, irregular "patchy" infiltrates, or lobar infiltrates.

❍ **What is the usual source of infected aspirated material?**

The oropharynx.

❍ **What pleuropulmonary infections may occur after aspirating infected oropharyngeal material?**

Necrotizing pneumonia, lung abscess, "typical" pneumonia, empyema.

❍ **What is the predominant oropharyngeal flora in outpatients?**

Anaerobes. Community acquired aspiration is usually anaerobic. The most common aerobes involved are streptococcus species.

❍ **What is the antibiotic of choice for outpatient acquired infectious aspiration pneumonia?**

Either clindamycin, high dose penicillin or unasyn.

❍ **What is the bacteriology of patients with inpatient acquired infectious aspiration pneumonia?**

Mixed aerobic and anaerobic organisms. Unlike outpatients, *Staphylococcus aureus*, *Escheria coli*, Pseudomonas aeruginosa, and Proteus species are common.

❍ **T/F: Aspiration of liquid gastric contents with pH greater than 2.5 produces no clinical consequences.**

False. Hypoxemia, bronchospasm and atelectasis may develop, but usually resolve within 24 hours.

❍ **What are the consequences of aspirating small (non-obstructing) food particles?**

Inflammation and hypoxemia, may result in chronic bronchiolitis or granulomatosis.

O   **Name the commonly aspirated hydrocarbons.**

Gasoline, kerosene, furniture polish, lighter fluid.

O   **What are the effects of hydrocarbon aspiration?**

Hypoxemia, intrapulmonary shunting, pulmonary edema, hemoptysis, respiratory failure.

O   **What is the role of emesis induction or gastric lavage in hydrocarbon ingestion?**

These maneuvers are not recommended as the patient may aspirate during regurgitation.

O   **Lipoid pneumonia is associated with chronic aspiration of what?**

Mineral oil, also animal or vegetable oils, oil-based nose drops.

O   **What is the annual U.S. mortality from drowning?**

9000. There are 500 near drowning for each drowning.

O   **What is the definition of drowning?**

Death due to suffocation by submersion in water.

O   **Can drowning occur without aspiration of water?**

Yes. 10% of victims die from intense laryngospasm.

O   **How much fluid can be drained from the lungs after drowning in fresh water?**

Little, as hypotonic fresh water is rapidly absorbed from the lung, unlike salt water which is hypertonic and is retained. There is no difference in outcome.

O   **What is the priority in treatment of near drowning?**

Maintenance of oxygenation.

O   **When is the Heimlich maneuver applied directly after a near drowning?**

When foreign body aspiration is suspected.

O   **What are the indications for intubation and ventilation after near drowning?**

Apnea, pulselessness, altered mental status, severe hypoxemia, respiratory acidosis.

O   **Resistance to airflow in the airway is inversely proportional to what?**

The fourth power of the airway radius.

O   **What is the most common etiology of croup or laryngotracheobronchitis?**

Parainfluenza virus.

O   **What is the most common organism isolated from patients with bacterial tracheitis?**

Staphylococcus aureus.

○ **How do retropharyngeal abscesses arise?**

Lymphatic spread of infections in the nasopharynx, oropharynx, or external auditory canal.

○ **What is the most common type of tracheo-esophageal fistula?**

Blind esophageal pouch with a fistulous connection of the trachea to the distal esophagus.

○ **The croup score is used to assess the degree of respiratory distress accompanying an illness. Which symptoms are evaluated in the score?**

Stridor, cough, air entry, flaring/retractions, and color.

○ **Why does a newborn with bilateral choanal astresia present with severe respiratory distress that is relieved by the insertion of an oral airway?**

Because the newborn is an obligatory nose breather.

○ **According to Poiseuille's law, if the radius of the conducting airway is reduced from 4 mm to 2 mm, by how much will the airflow resistance increase?**

Sixteen-fold.

○ **The funnel-shaped narrowing of the glottis and subglottic airway, commonly known as steeple sign, is observed in what type of extrathoracic airway obstruction?**

Croup or laryngotracheobronchitis.

○ **Name one of the conditions which makes a child a likely candidate for tonsillectomy.**

Recurrent tonsillar abscesses.

○ **A six-year-old male complains of dysphagia and fever. Tonsillar exudates and anterior cervical adenitis are noted. What sign differentiates Group A strep from other causes of pharyngitis?**

A sandpaper-like rash.

○ **A 4-year-old child has high fever, hoarseness, and increased stridor of 3 hours duration. He has a low fever and sore throat earlier in the day. He is ill appearing, with a temperature of 40 degrees C, inspiratory stridor, drooling and intercostals retractions. He prefers to sit up. What is the most likely diagnosis?**

Epiglottitis.

○ **What are the McConnochie criteria for the diagnosis of bronchiolitis?**

1. Acute expiratory wheezing
2. Age 6 months or less
3. Signs of viral illness, such as fever or coryza
4. Without pneumonia or atopy
5. The first such episode

○ **What is the most common pathogen isolated in children with bronchiolitis?**

Respiratory syncytial virus.

❍   **Foreign body aspiration occurs most commonly in which age group?**

1-3 years of age, with slight male predominance.

❍   **Name the most common offender in foreign body aspiration.**

Organic substances such as nuts and corn.

❍   **What will be the predominant symptom of a child who has aspirated a foreign body which is lodged in his/her trachea?**

Stridor.

❍   **The predominant auscultatory finding in a child with a foreign body lodged in the right mainstem bronchus:**

Expiratory wheezing.

❍   **An 11-month old male presents with rhinorrhea, cough and increasing respiratory distress. Treatment with bronchodilators have produced equivocal results. He is now in obvious distress with retractions, grunting, prolonged expiratory time, inspiratory and expiratory wheezes. Chest x-rays shows a tracheal shift to the left and hyperexpansion of the right chest. What is the most likely diagnosis?**

Foreign body aspiration.

❍   **Cor pulmonale resulting from chronic airway obstruction is thought to be due to what?**

Chronic alveolar hypoventilation and the resulting increase in pulmonary vascular resistance.

❍   **The total work of breathing is divided into two parts. Name them.**

1)   To overcome lung and chest wall compliance.
2)   To overcome airway and tissue resistance.

❍   **Total work of breathing in neonates and infants is lowest at what respiratory rate?**

35-40/minute.

❍   **Why are infants more susceptible to inflammatory changes in the airway?**

Because the airway in infants is smaller, and is also much more compliant.

❍   **Grunting is usually more prominent in what type of respiratory pathology?**

Typically in smaller airway disease such as bronchiolitis, or in diseases with loss of functional residual capacity such as pneumonia or pulmonary edema because grunting is an effort to maintain positive airway pressure during expiration.

❍   **What is Sampter's Triad?**

Asthma, nasal polyps, and aspirin allergy.

❍   **What are the criteria associated with severe asthma and likelihood of hospital admission?**

A pretreatment PEFR <25% predicted, pulsus paradoxus > 10 mm Hg on presentation, failure of PEFR to rise > 15% after treatment, or posttreatment PEFR <60% predicted or SaO2 <93%.

❍ **What is the dose of epinephrine in acute asthma?**

mg/kg SC or epinephrine 1:1000, repeated q 20 minutes as needed.

❍ **What is the dose of nebulized albuterol?**

0.1-0.15 mg/kg of a 2 mg/5 ml solution.

❍ **What is the dose of Prelone (prednisolone) in acute asthma?**

1-2 mg/kg/day of a 15 mg/5 ml solution.

❍ **What are the high yield indications for chest radiography in suspected pneumonia?**

Tachypnea, rales, decreased breath sounds, stridor, retractions, or cyanosis.

❍ **What is the best single predictor of pneumonia in children?**

Tachypnea.

GASTROINTESTINAL

❍ **Distinguish, by location, between anal cryptitis, anal fissure, anorectal abscess, and fistula in ano.**

Cryptitis, fissures, and perianal abscess typically occur in the posterior midline. Deep abscesses can point to areas far from the anus. Goodsall's rule declares that fistulas opening anteriorly go straight to the anal canal, while fistulas opening posteriorly may follow a circuitous route.

❍ **What are some common conditions that mimic acute appendicitis?**

Mesenteric lymphadenitis, PID, Mittlesmertz, gastroenteritis, and Crohn's disease.

❍ **What conditions are associated with an atypical presentation of acute appendicitis?**

Situs inversus viscerum, malrotation, hypermobile cecum, long pelvic appendix, and pregnancy (1/2200).

❍ **What are the most frequent symptoms of acute appendicitis?**

Anorexia and pain. The classical presentations of anorexia and periumbilical pain with progression to constant RLQ pain are present in only 60% of the cases.

❍ **What percentage of acute appendicitis cases have an elevated WBC count?**

An elevated leukocyte count and an elevated absolute neutrophil count are present in 86% and 89% of the cases, respectively.

❍ **What intraabdominal pathology should be assumed in a pregnant female with right upper quadrant pain until proven otherwise?**

Acute appendicitis.

❍ **What does an ultrasound show in acute appendicitis?**

A fixed, tender, non-compressible mass, but only in 75-90% of these cases.

❍ **Which method is more sensitive for locating the source of GI bleeding, a radioactive Tc-labeled red cell scan or an angiography?**

A bleeding scan can detect a site bleeding at a rate as low as 0.12 mL/minute, while angiography requires rapid bleeding (i.e., greater than 0.5 mL/min).

❍ **A patient with an "acid stomach" develops melena and vomits bright red blood. Is esophagitis a feasible cause?**

No. Capillary bleeding rarely causes impressive acute blood loss. Arterial bleeding—from a complicated ulcer, foreign body, or Mallory-Weiss tear—or variceal bleeding are much more probable.

❍ **Repeated violent bouts of vomiting can result in both Mallory-Weiss tears and Boerhaave's syndrome. Differentiate between the two.**

1. <u>Mallory-Weiss</u> <u>tears</u> involve the submucosa and mucosa, typically in the right posterolateral wall of the GE junction.

2. <u>Boerhaave</u> <u>syndrome</u> is a full-thickness tear, usually in the unsupported left posterolateral wall of the abdominal esophagus.

❍   **Recurrent pneumonias, especially in the right middle lobe or the superior segments of the bilateral upper lobes, are indicative of what syndrome?**

Aspiration associated with motor diseases and gastroesophageal reflux.

❍   **A 6 month old infant is constipated, flaccid, and only stares straight ahead. He is not running a fever. However, his mother is especially worried because he won't take his bottle—not even for her "honey on the tip of the bottle" trick. Diagnosis?**

Infantile botulism. Infants ingest spores that are in the environment, most commonly in honey. The spores then grow and produce toxins within the host.

❍   **How does infantile botulism differ from food-borne botulism?**

Infantile botulism is caused by the spores of *C. botulinum* while adult food-borne botulism arises from the ingestion of *C. botulinum* neurotoxins.

❍   **What is the antidote for botulism poisoning?**

Trivalent A-B-E antitoxin. This antidote is not required for infantile botulism.

❍   **Gallbladder stones are generally formed of:**

Cholesterol. The diagnostic test of choice is ultrasound. This technique may show stones, sludge bile plugging, or dilated bile ducts.

❍   **A patient with a history of gallstones presents with an acute, postprandial right upper quadrant pain. What's the KUB likely to show?**

Nothing specific. Only around 10% of gallstones are radiopaque. Complications of cholelithiasis, such as emphysematous cholecystitis, perforation, and pneumobilia are uncommon but useful findings.

❍   **A child with sickle-cell disease presents with fever, shaking chills, and jaundice. What is the diagnosis?**

Charcot's triad suggests ascending cholangitis. The precipitating cause is probably pigment stones resulting from chronic hemolysis.

❍   **A 12-year-old male complains of 2 days of rice water stools, muscle cramps and extreme fatigue. He looks pale, dehydrated, and very ill. The patient states that he has just returned from India. What is the diagnosis?**

Cholera. The incidence of cholera in the US is 1/10,000,000. Cholera usually develops in travelers returning from endemic areas, such as India, Africa, southeast Asia, southern Europe, Central and South America, and the Middle East. This disease can be prevented if the water ingested during the trip is purified and raw, and unpeeled fruits/vegetables and seafood are avoided altogether.

❍   **How does the pathology of Crohn's disease differ from that of ulcerative colitis?**

Crohn's is a trans-mucosal, segmental, granulomatous process, while ulcerative colitis is a mucosal, juxtapositioned, ulcerative process.

❍ **A young man with atraumatic chronic back pain, eye trouble, and painful red lumps on his shins develops <u>bloody</u> <u>diarrhea</u>. What is the point of this question?**

To remind you of the extraintestinal manifestations of inflammatory bowel disease, such as ankylosing spondylitis, uveitis, and erythema nodosum, not to mention kidney stones.

❍ **At least one-third of the patients with Crohn's disease develop kidney stones. Why?**

Dietary oxalate is usually bound to calcium and excreted. When terminal ileal disease leads to decreased bile salt absorption, the resulting fattier intestinal contents bind calcium by saponification. Free oxalate is "hyper-absorbed" in the colon, resulting in hyperoxaluria and calcium oxalate nephrolithiasis.

❍ **Complications of Crohn's include perirectal abscesses, anal fissures, rectovaginal fistulas, and rectal prolapse. What percentage of patients with Crohn's disease have perirectal involvement?**

Approximately 90%.

❍ **What are the odds that a patient with severe ileal disease will be cured by surgery?**

Virtually zero. Crohn's invariably recurs in the remaining GI tract. In contrast, total proctocolectomy with ileostomy is curative procedure for ulcerative colitis.

❍ **What hereditary diseases evident in infancy may cause cirrhosis?**

Glycogen storage disease, cystic fibrosis, galactosemia, fructose intolerance, tyrosinemia, and acid cholesterol esterhydrolase deficiency.

❍ **Are there any useful therapies for the rapid renal failure that can accompany cirrhosis?**

Unfortunately not. The hepatorenal syndrome still has a mortality rate that approaches 100%.

❍ **What stool studies are crucial for evaluating acute diarrhea?**

Statistically speaking, acute diarrhea is so common and typically self-limited that most cases require no testing, just oral rehydration. In sick patients or those at risk for complications, (i.e., at the extremes of age, recently hospitalized, or the immunocompromised), enteroinvasive infection should be ruled out with a stool guaiac and test for fecal leukocytes. Gram's or methylene blue stains are comparable. Also consider checking for ova and parasites.

❍ **Which diarrheal illnesses cause fecal leukocytes?**

The usual culprits are *Shigella, Campylobacter*, and enteroinvasive *E. coli*. Others include *Salmonella, Yersinia, Vibrio parahaemolyticus*, and *C. difficile*. Fecal WBCs are absent in toxigenic and enteropathogenic infection, even with such a virulent organism as *Vibrio cholera*. Viral and parasitic infections rarely produce fecal WBCs.

❍ **Name the most probable cause of diarrhea in a 6-month old in day-care.**

Viral diarrhea caused by *Rotavirus* is the most common. Also test for *Giardia* and *Cryptosporidia* because these agents have recently been added to the list of day-care-associated diarrheal illnesses.

❍ **What is the most common cause of bacterial diarrhea?**

E. coli (enteroinvasive, enteropathogenic, enterotoxigenic).

❍ **Which is the most common form of acute diarrhea?**

Viral diarrhea. It is generally self limited, lasting only 1- 3 days.

O   **Diarrhea that develops within 12 hours of a meal is most probably caused by what?**

An ingested pre-formed toxin.

O   **When does traveler's diarrhea typically occur?**

3-7 days after arrival in a foreign land.

O   **What is the treatment for traveler's diarrhea?**

Traveler's diarrhea is caused by *E. Coli*; the preferable treatment is with Bactrim.

O   **What is the definition of chronic diarrhea?**

Passage of greater than 200 g of loose stool per day for over 3 weeks.

O   **The most common symptom of esophageal disease is:**

Pyrosis (heartburn).

O   **What are the indications for the surgical removal of a GI foreign body?**

GI obstruction, GI perforation, the toxic properties of the material, and whether its length, size, and shape will prevent the object from passing safely.

O   **What size objects rarely pass through the stomach and require endoscopic retrieval?**

Objects longer than 5 cm and wider than 2 cm.

O   **Radiographs should be performed on all patients suspected of swallowing coins to determine the presence and location of the foreign body. How will the coin appear on a x-ray in the AP view?**

Coins in the esophagus lie in the frontal plane. Coins in the trachea lie in the sagittal plane.

O   **What is the management of button batteries that have passed the esophagus?**

In the asymptomatic patient, repeat radiographs. The symptomatic patient and patients in whom the battery has not passed the pylorus after 48 hours require an endoscopic retrieval.

O   **Foreign bodies lodge at what esophageal levels in the pediatric patient?**

Typically at levels of the cricopharyngeus muscles. The thoracic inlet, aortic arch, tracheal bifurcation, and lower esophageal sphincter are also possible lodging sites.

O   **X-rays are crucial for finding suspected swallowed foreign bodies. In kids, what physical findings can tip you off?**

Besides the child's distress, a red or scratched oropharynx, dysphagia, a high fever, or peritoneal signs may be evident. In addition, subcutaneous air suggests perforation.

O   **Which type of hepatitis is usually contracted through blood transfusion?**

Hepatitis C. Eighty five percent of post transfusion hepatitis is caused by hepatitis C.

❍   **A poor prognosis is associated with which two LFTs in acute viral hepatitis?**

A total bilirubin > 20 mg/dL and a prolongation of the prothrombin time > 3 seconds. The extent of transaminase elevation is not a useful marker.

❍   **Match the following hepatitis serologies with the correct clinical description.**

1.   HBsAg (-), and antiHBs (+)
2.   IgM HBcAg (+), antiHBs (-)
3.   IgG HBcAg (+), antiHBs (-)
4.   HBeAg (+)

a.   Ongoing viral replication, highly infectious.
b.   Remote infection, not infectious.
c.   Recent or ongoing infection; a high titer means high infectivity, while a low titer suggests chronic, active infection.
d) Prior infection or vaccination, not infectious.

Answers: (1) d, (2) c, (3) b, and (4) a.

HBeAg (+):   "e" = "Eeek! I'm infectious!" for e ANTIGEN, anti-HBe implies decreased infectivity.
IgG HBcAg (+): "G" = Gone.
IgM HBcAg (+): "M" = Might be contagious still.
ANTIHBs (+):   "s" = Stopped. Patient has antibodies to surface antigen.

Warning! You must specify whether the antigen or the antibody is present when learning these letter codes; otherwise you will learn these the wrong way around! Go over it ten times in your text of choice so it will make sense. Then, remembering the letters won't be necessary.

❍   **T/F: The "Σ-agent" can cause hepatitis D in a patient without active hepatitis B.**

False. The Σ-agent is an incomplete, "defective" RNA virus that is responsible for hepatitis D. It is an obligate covirus and requires hepatitis B for replication.

❍   **You stick yourself with a needle from a chronic hepatitis B carrier. You've been vaccinated, but have never had your antibody status checked. What is the appropriate post exposure prophylaxis?**

Measure your anti-HBs titer. If it's adequate (> 10 mIU), treatment is not required. If it is inadequate, you need a single dose of HBIG as soon as possible and a vaccine booster.

❍   **Which is more dangerous, a small hernia or a large one?**

Incarceration is more likely with small hernias.

❍   **List three types of internal hernias.**

1) Diaphragmatic hernia.
2) Lesser sac hernia (i.e., through the foramen of Winslow).
3) Omental or mesenteric hernia.

❍   **Distinguish between a groin hernia, a hydrocele, and a lymph node.**

Hydroceles transilluminate and are non-tender. Lymph nodes are freely moving and firm. Hernias don't transilluminate and may produce bowel sounds.

❍   **A patient tells you that 2 days ago his groin bulged. He then developed severe pain with progressive nausea and vomiting. He also has a tender mass in his groin. What shouldn't you do?**

Don't try to reduce a long-standing, tender, incarcerated hernia! The abdomen is no place for dead bowel.

❍   **What simple test can distinguish between conjugated and unconjugated hyperbilirubinemia?**
A dipstick test for urobilinogen, which reflects conjugated (water soluble) hyperbilirubinemia.

❍   **In addition to conjugated hyperbilirubinemia, what liver function abnormalities suggest biliary tract disease?**

Elevated alkaline phosphatase out of proportion to transaminases.

❍   **Currant jelly stool in a child is indicative of what?**

Intussusception.

❍   **What is the most common cause of bowel obstruction in children under 2?**

Intussusception. Usually the terminal ileum will slide into the right colon. The cause is unknown but suspected to be due to hypertrophied lymph nodes at the junction of the ileum and colon.

❍   **What is the treatment for intussusception?**

An air, or barium, enema is both a diagnostic tool and curative (i.e. by reducing the intussusception). If the air enema is unsuccessful, surgical reduction may be required.

❍   **Crampy abdominal pain with mucus in the stool is indicative of what syndrome?**

The irritable bowel syndrome. Patients are afebrile and often improve after passing flatus.

❍   **What is the most common cause of small bowel obstruction?**

Adhesions are the most common cause of extraluminal obstruction, followed by incarcerated hernia. Conversely, gallstones and bezoars are the most common causes of intraluminal obstruction.

❍   **What is the hallmark sign of a perforated viscus?**

Abdominal pain.

❍   **What percentage of patients with a perforated viscus also have radiographic evidence of a pneumoperitoneum?**

60-70%. Therefore, one-third of patients will not have this sign. Keep the patient in either the upright or left lateral decubitus position for at least 10 minutes prior to performing x-rays.

❍   **An ill-appearing patient says her sore throat became worse after a week. She also complains of spiking fevers and central chest burning. What is the diagnosis**

A retro or parapharyngeal abscess with extension to superior mediastinitis.

❍   **Name two endocrine problems that cause peptic ulcer.**

Zollinger-Ellison syndrome and hyperparathyroidism (hypercalcemia).

❍   **A postprandial midabdominal pain is indicative of what ectopic syndrome?**

Peptic ulcer in a Meckel's diverticulum.

❍   **T/F: Antibiotics are unnecessary after an uncomplicated perirectal abscess is incised and drained.**

True, assuming the patient has no underlying immunoincompetence, such as HIV, diabetes, or malignancy. The primary aftercare includes sitz baths beginning the next day.

❍   **Do pilonidal abscesses communicate with the anal canal?**

No. They are virtually always midline and overlie the lower sacrum. Posterior-opening, horseshoe-type anorectal fistulas can find their way to the lower sacrum, but are rarely in the midline. Remember Goodsall's rule.

❍   **Should pilonidal cysts be excised in the office?**

Probably not. Incision and drainage are okay, followed by a bulky dressing, analgesics, and hot sitz baths, which should be initiated the next day. Antibiotics are not typically necessary. Excision should be completed in the OR once the acute infection clears up.

❍   **A patient with chronic and occasionally bloody diarrhea develops severe diarrhea and abdominal pain with marked distention. What "can't-miss" diagnosis is confirmed by these signs?**

Toxic megacolon. This condition is a life-threatening complication of ulcerative colitis.

❍   **What are the peak ages for the onset of ulcerative colitis?**

15-35 years with a smaller incident rate in the seventh decade.

❍   **What are potential gastro-intestinal causes of apnea and bradycardia in neonates?**

Oral feeding, bowel movement, G.E. Reflux, esophagitis and intestinal perforation.

❍   **What substances can mimic upper GI bleeding?**

Red food coloring in cereals, Jell-O, drinks such as Kool-Aid and fruit juices and natural coloring in beets.

❍   **What substance can mimic malena?**

Iron supplements, dark chocolate, spinach, cranberries, grape juice, bismuth, and blueberries.

❍   **Name the infectious causes of hematochezia?**

Salmonella, Shigella, Yersinia enterocolitica, Campylobacter jejuni, Escherichia coli, Clostridium difficile, Aeromonas hydrophilia and Entamoeba histolytica.

❍   **A 10-year-old child presents with a three day history of episodic abdominal pain and hematochezia. Examination reveals a palpable purpuric rash mostly on the lower limbs. Platelet count is normal. What is the most likely cause?**

Henoch-Schonlein Parpura (Anaphylactoid purpura).

❍   **What are the 3 most common causes of upper gastrointestinal bleeding in neonates**

Swallowed maternal blood, gastritis (sepsis? Hypoxia?), duodenitis.

❍   **What test can differentiate neonatal from swallowed maternal blood?**

Apt test (also known as Kleinhauer Betke Test) - which is based on the conversion of oxhemoglobin to hematin when mixed with alkali. Fetal hemoglobin is resistant to alkali (pink reaction) while maternal hemoglobin is denatured (dirty brown).

❍   **Name the more common prescription drugs associated with gastric ulcers in children.**

Salicylates, Nonsteroidal anti-inflammatory agents, Digitalis, Reserpine, Aminophylline, Anticoagulants, and Antimetabolites.

O   **Is there an increased risk for GI bleeding in patients with Turner Syndrome?**

Yes. Turner syndrome is associate with GI vascular malformations and Inflammatory bowel disease.

O   **What is the recommended volume of normal saline for gastric lavage in pediatric patients with GI bleeding?**

3-5 cc/Kg.

O   **What is the comparative usefulness of endoscopy as opposed to an upper GI series in identifying bleeding sources?**

A diagnosis can be made in 90% of cases by using endoscopy, but less than 50% of cases by upper GI series.

O   **Vasopressin intravenously may be useful in the control of variceal bleeding in children. What are the side effects of this drug?**

Bradycardia, vasoconstriction, myocardial ischemia, elevation of systemic blood pressure, oliguria, tissue necrosis, hyponatremia and water intoxication.

O   **At what age does intussusception most commonly occur?**

60% of all cases occur by 12 months of age, and 80% by 24 months.

O   **Which test is best to diagnose a bleeding Meckel's diverticulum?**

Technetium pertechnetate scan, preferably with Pentagastrin or H2 antagonist stimulation.

O   **What are the two best ways to carry an avulsed tooth prior to reimplantation?**

Tooth Socket or stored in milk.

O   **How common is infantile hypertrophic pyloric stenosis?**

Affects approximately 1:150 males and 1:750 females, and is more common in first born males.

O   **Name the three areas of physiologic narrowing in the esophagus, where an ingested coin is likely to lodge.**

Below the cricopharyngeal muscle, at the level of the aortic arch, and just below the diaphragm.

O   **What is the classical metabolic picture in infants with pyloric stenosis?**

Hypochloremic alkalosis.

O   **What is the incidence of intestinal obstruction in newborn infants?**

Approximately 1:1500.

O   **What is the most common mechanical reason for malrotation?**

Failure of the cecum to move into the right lower quadrant, so that the bands fixing it to the posterior abdominal wall cross over and may obstruct the duodenum.

❍ **When does midgut volvulus usually present?**

50% of cases in 1st week of life and 80% within the first month.

❍ **Do infants with malrotation, always present with bilious vomiting?**

No. About 25% of infants under 2 months, present with nonbilious emesis.

❍ **What is the incidence of meconium ileus in newborn infants with cystic fibrosis?**

Meconium ileus is most commonly seen in infants with cystic fibrosis, but less than 10% of infants with cystic fibrosis have meconium ileus.

❍ **What are the typical radiographic findings in meconium ileus?**

Lack of air in the distal colon; distended loops of small bowel associated with bubbles of stool and air-described as a ground-glass appearance or Neuhauser's sign.

❍ **How common is diabetes mellitus in patients with cystic fibrosis?**

It is 40 to 200 times higher than in the general pediatric population. This may be very difficult to control, especially in DKA.

❍ **How common is rectal prolapse in children with cystic fibrosis?**

It occurs in almost 20% of patients and is the presenting sign of CF in half or these.

❍ **What could happen to patients with cystic fibrosis during periods of increased physical activity and heat stress?**

Hyponatremia dehydration due to the high losses of sodium in sweat.

❍ **Name the 3 leading causes of acute pancreatitis in children.**

Viral infections; drugs and trauma.

❍ **What is the most common clinical finding in children with acute pancreatitis?**

Epigastric tenderness with decreased bowel sounds.

❍ **What is the age of patients when ulcerative colitis in childhood is usually diagnosed?**

Between 5 and 16 years of age.

❍ **What are the most common presenting signs and symptoms of ulcerative colitis?**

Stool mixed with mucus and blood; lower abdominal cramping which is most intense during defecation.

❍ **What is the most common organic causes of chronic/recurrent abdominal pain in children?**

Genitourinary-Approximately 10% of children age 5-10 years have chronic/recurrent pain. Of these less than 10% have an organic cause.

❍ **How common is retrocecal appendix?**
19-20% - according to most recent reviews

❍   **Name the most common non-infectious causes of chronic diarrhea in children.**

Food allergy, food intolerance, chronic nonspecific diarrhea (CNSD), lactase deficiency, irritable colon, encopresis, metabolic/malabsorption disease, ulcerative colitis, regional enteritis, and Hirschsprung's disease.

❍   **When you suspect that a child has CNSD, what are the "four Fs" to which you should pay special attention?**

Fiber, Fluid, Fat and Fruit juices.

❍   **Pedialyte is frequently used for oral hydration in infants. What is the composition of this solution?**

Na   -   45 meq/L
K   -   20 meq/L
Cl   -   35 meq/L
HCO_3 -   30 meq/L
Glucose   -   25 g/L

❍   **Is this oral solution appropriate for rehydration?**

Pedialyte is appropriate and may lead to less osmotic diarrhea. However, the American Academy of Pediatrics recommends a solution containing at least 75 to 90m Eq Na per liter for rehydration. REHYDRALITE and the WHO solution are two such solutions.

❍   **What is the most common reason for "spitting up" in young infant?**

Overfeeding! Parents frequently report that the child is vomiting

❍   **A two week old male infant presents with persistent emesis and dehydration. Blood electrolytes reveal significant hyperkalemia. What potentially lesion must be ruled out?**

Congenital adrenal hyperplasia (CAH)

❍   **What anti-emetic is recommended in the infant who presents with emesis?**

Trick question! Antiemetics are strongly discouraged because of the incidence of side effects.

❍   **Two children from the same family present with severe nausea and vomiting about 4-6 hours after eating. What are the most likely causes?**

S.aureus toxins, Bacillus cereus, heavy metals.

❍   **Two children from another family develop paraesthesias a few hours after eating. What causes should you consider?**

Fish (scombroid and ciguatera poisoning); Shellfish (neurotoxic & domoic acid poisoning); Monosodium glutamate. (Chinese Restaurant Syndrome)

❍   **What is a common G.I. complication of nephrotic syndrome?**

Spontaneous bacterial peritonitis

○ **Is perforation following appendicitis more common in children than in adults?**

Yes, because localization of abdominal pain is more difficult. Also, the omentum is not as well developed and cannot wall off the inflamed appendix.

○ **What are some lesions that can present as a mass protruding the rectum?**

Rectal polyp, rectal prolapse, and procidentia

○ **Give the DDX of an inguino-scrotal mass.**

Inguinal hernia, hydrocele, hydrocele of a cord, and retractile testes

○ **What are the common causes of unconjugated hyperbilirubinemia in the neonatal age group?**

Physiological jaundice, blood group incompatibility, and breast-milk jaundice.

○ **At what level of serum bilirubin will a newborn appear icteric?**

5-7 mg/dl.

○ **In older children?**

2-3 mg/dl.

○ **What are the most common causes of unconjugated hyperbilirubinemia in childhood?**

Sickle cell anemia and other hemolytic disorders, ie, hereditary spherocytosis, hereditary elliptocytosis.

○ **What clinical investigations would you consider for the initial work-up of a case of unconjugated hyperbilirubinemia?**

Serum bilirubin and direct fraction, Coombs' test, Hematocrit, and RBC morphology/Retic count.

○ **What is the span of the liver at birth?**

4.5 - 5 cm.

○ **The Kasai procedure (hepatoportoenterostomy), an operative procedure used in cases of biliary atresia which are deemed correctable, is most successful when done before how weeks of life?**

Eight.

○ **What are two of the most significant sequelae of the Kasai procedure?**

Cholangitis, and gram-negative sepsis.

○ **What pathognomonic eye-sign is noted in almost all patients of Wilson's disease with neurological symptoms?**

Kayser-Fleisher rings.

○ **What is the best screening test for Wilson's disease?**

Serum Ceruloplasmin level (decreased).

○ **What agent is commonly used in the treatment of Wilson's disease?**

D-Penicillamine (chelates copper).

O   **Beyond what duration is the use of Total Parenteral Nutrition (TPN) in newborns, especially prematures, associated with cholestasis?**

Two weeks.

O   **The consumption of what agent has been implicated in the incidence of Reye's syndrome in children with an influenza-like illness?**

Aspirin.

O   **What age group is Reye's syndrome seen most commonly?**

4 - 12 years.

O   **What is the major lethal factor in children with Reye's syndrome?**

Increased intracranial pressure, secondary to cerebral edema.

O   **Name some drugs associated with hepatic injury in children?**

Acetaminophen, Sulfonamide, Erythromycin, Ceftriaxone, INH, Valproic acid, Phenytoin.

O   **What are some causes of fulminant hepatic failure?**

Viral hepatitis
Hepatotoxic drugs and chemicals
Circulatory shock
Metabolic liver diseases like Wilson's or galactosemia

O   **What are the common causes of biliary colic?**

Gall stones caused by hemolytic diseases like spherocytosis, infections like Salmonellosis, and parasitic infestations like ascariasis.

O   **What is the definition of portal hypertension?**

Elevation of portal pressure above 10 - 12 mm of HG.

O   **What common NICU procedure might result in portal hypertension?**

Umbilical catheterization.

O   **What is the most common presentation of childhood portal hypertension?**

Bleeding from esophageal varices.

O   **What is the major risk associated with portocaval shunts, which divert blood flow away from esophageal varices?**

Hepatic encephalopathy.

O   **What is the major indication for liver transplantation in the pediatric age group?**

Biliary atresia.

○ **What metabolic condition manifests with jaundice, hypoglycemia, convulsions, cataracts, and mental retardation?**

Galactosemia.

○ **Do the levels of liver-dependent coagulation factors decrease after birth?**

Yes, they fall 48 - 72 hours after birth, and return to birth levels only by 7 to 10 days of life.

○ **A healthy three-week old female child is brought to the emergency room with complaints of spitting up blood. She was a full-term birth, who has been thriving well on breast milk, and has gained 15oz since birth. CBC and liver enzymes are normal, but the prothrombin time, and partial thromboplastin time are prolonged. What would you do next?**

Administer 1 to 5 mg of Vit K1 intravenously.

○ **Can a newborn manifest Vitamin K deficiency induced bleeding within the first 24 hours of life?**

Yes, if the mother has been on Phenobarbital or Phenytoin. Classic Hemorrhagic Disease of the Newborn is seen between 2 and 7 days of life.

○ **What is the most commonly occurring malignant liver neoplasm in the pediatric age group?**

Hepatoblastoma.

○ **What hepatic condition could manifest with hepatomegaly, failure to thrive, congestive cardiac failure, thrombocytopenia, and a bruit over the right upper abdominal quadrant?**

An angiomatous malformation like hemangioma-endothelioma.

○ **Of the hepatitis viruses A through E, which are transmitted by the feco-oral route?**

Hepatitis A and E.

○ **What recommendations would you make regarding the immunization of a full-term newborn, the HbsAg status of whose mother is not known?**

Administration of HBIg and Hepatitis B vaccine simultaneously, at two different sites.

○ **How long can you defer giving HBIg to a newborn infant?**

12 hours after birth.

○ **How would you classify a person with the following hepatitis serology: HbsAg negative, Anti-HBe positive, Anti-HBc positive, Anti-HBs negative, HBAg negative.**

Infected in the past.

○ **How would you distinguish a person who is immune to hepatitis B as a result of a past infection from one who is immune following a vaccination?**

Both anti-HBs and anti-HBc are seen in serum following an infection, while only anti-HBs is seen following immunization.

❍   **Has the American Academy of Pediatrics recommended universal administration of Hepatitis A vaccine?**

No, it is used only in high-risk children, and in those considering travel to Hepatitis A-endemic areas.

❍   **What is the chief sequel of untreated perinatal acquired Hepatitis B?**

Chronic infection, which might occur in close to 70- 90 % of the cases.

❍   **What is the best indicator of the severity of liver damage, in a case of acetaminophen overdosage?**

Prothrombin time, done at 12-hourly intervals.

❍   **What is breast-feeding jaundice?**

Elevated levels of serum bilirubin, approaching 15-20 mg/dl, seen in the second or third week of life in breast-fed infants who are otherwise healthy.

❍   **What effect is encountered in an infant with conjugated hyperbilirubinemia who is subjected to phototherapy?**

"Bronze baby syndrome" caused by an unusual bronzing of the skin by bilirubin breakdown pigments. This is reversible.

❍   **An infant with biliary atresia is noted on follow-up to be short-stature, and has round, bony prominence at the costochondral junctions. What is the pathology you suspect?**

Vitamin D deficiency, leading to rickets.

❍   **6-12 hours after ingesting a wild mushroom, a child developed vomiting, diarrhea, and abdominal pain which has lasted for the past 3 days. How the child is noted to be jaundiced. What do you suspect?**

Acute liver toxicity from "amanita" mushroom poisoning.

❍   **You see a 10-year-old boy in the ER, with ear ache, and diagnose him as having otitis media. The boy is clearly jaundiced, and his mother informs you that he has the Dubin-Johnson syndrome. What management would you like to offer for his jaundice?**

Nothing, the condition is benign. However, drugs capable of aggravating jaundice should be avoided.

❍   **An 11-year-old girl with cystic fibrosis presents with a one-day history of fever. On examination she is noted to have equal breath sounds on both sides. She has right upper abdominal quadrant pain. Labs reveal leukocytosis, with an increase in serum bilirubin. What do you suspect?**

Acute calculous cholecystitis, seen in up to 4% of patients with cystic fibrosis.

❍   **A patient with portal hypertension presents to the your office with a nose bleed. The patient insists that he lost only about 5cc of blood, yet looks quite pale. CBC reveals a Hb of 8.5 gm/dl with a platelet count of 25, 000cu.mm. How would you explain these hematological findings in this patient?**

Hypersplenism, in which one or more blood cell lines are decreased on blood counts.

❍   **What are xanthomata?**

Depositions of lipid in the dermis and subcutaneous tissue, seen often in chronic cholestasis, when the serum cholesterol levels exceed 500 mg/dl.

O   **A neonate with neonatal hemochromatosis is awaiting liver transplantation. He is presently being managed with desferrioxamine. His anxious mother calls you up, and informs you that her son's diapers are stained brown. What is your diagnosis?**

Desferrioxamine chelates iron, which is then excreted in the urine. When such urine stands for some time, it turns brown in color.

O   **What are some poor prognostic factors for survival in a patient with hepatic encephalopathy?**

Jaundice for more than 7 days before the onset of encephalopathy; a prothrombin time more than 50 sec; a serum bilirubin level more than 17.5 mg/dl.

O   **In what percentage of the population is the gall bladder congenitally absent?**

0.1%.

O   **Esophageal varices are a form of portal-systemic blood shunting. Name some other sites at which such shunts might develop.**

Around the umbilicus (caput medusae), between the middle and inferior hemorrhoidal veins.

O   **What is Charcot's triad?**

The triad of right upper quadrant abdominal pain, fever, and jaundice. This should lead you lead to the suspicion of cholangitis.

O   **Which infectious agents are commonly associated with necrotizing enterocolitis?**

Gram negative enteric bacilli, *E. coli*, Klebsiella pneumonia, and Enterococcus.

CRITICAL CARE

○ **Acute renal failure, Coomb's negative hemolytic anemia, and thrombocytopenia comprise the triad for which syndrome?**

Hemolytic-Uremic Syndrome (HUS).

○ **Aplastic crisis in sickle cell disease is associated with what condition?**

Parvo virus. Primary erythropoietic failure can result in life-threatening anemia in a patient with a significantly decreased RBC life span.

○ **Primary or spontaneous bacterial peritonitis is more frequently seen with patients who have which underlying conditions?**

Nephrotic syndrome, chronic liver disease, and systemic lupus erythematosus.

○ **If you suspect that a patient has herpes simplex encephalitis, what procedures can be done to confirm diagnosis?**

Herpes simplex virus polymerase chain reaction (HSV PCR).

○ **Which MRI findings are suggestive of herpes simplex encephalitis?**

Edema or hemorrhage in the temporal lobes.

○ **What are the features required to diagnose Guillain-Barré Syndrome?**

Progressive motor weakness and areflexia.

○ **What is the hallmark in cerebrospinal fluid which indicate that the patient might have Guillain-Barré Syndrome?**

Albumino-cytologic dissociation, which is found as early as the third day into the illness, but may occur as late as the second or third week.

○ **What is the most common cause of fulminant hepatic failure in the U.S.?**

Acute viral hepatitis.

○ **The liver dysfunction in fulminant hepatic failure is evidenced by what condition?**

Uncorrectable coagulopathy, jaundice and encephalopathy. All three occur together in an illness of less than eight weeks duration.

○ **What is the most potent therapy for the temporary treatment of hyperkalemia?**

Insulin, plus hypertonic dextrose.

○ **The most feared complication associated with extracorporeal membrane oxygenation (ECMO)?**

Intracranial hemorrhage.

O   **Decompensated shock is characterized by what conditions?**

Hypotension and low cardiac output.

O   **How long is the blood pressure maintained in hypovolemia caused by hemorrhage?**

The blood volume falls by 25% to 30%.

O   **In an unconscious, non-breathing patient with suspected cervical injury, which maneuver should be used to open the airway?**

Jaw thrust with cervical spine immobilization.

O   **Why shouldn't blind finger sweeps of the mouth be performed for manual removal of a foreign body?**

Because the foreign body may be pushed back into the airway, resulting in further obstruction.

O   **During resuscitation, which drugs can be administered through the endotracheal tube?**

Naloxone, atropine, epinephrine, and lidocaine.

O   **What do the indications for calcium therapy include?**

Documented or suspected hypocalcemia, hyperkalemia, hypermagnesemia, and calcium channel-blocker overdose.

O   **When should atropine be used to treat bradycardia?**

Only after adequate ventilation and oxygenation have been established, since hypoxemia is the most common cause of bradycardia in children.

O   **T/F: Defibrillation is indicated for the treatment of asystole.**

False. Defibrillation is the definitive treatment for ventricular fibrillation or pulseless ventricular tachycardia. The treatment for asystole is epinephrine.

O   **What are the three inotropic agents commonly used in the post-arrest setting?**

Dopamine, dobutamine and epinephrine.

O   **Name some complications associated with intraosseous cannulation and infusion.**

Tibia fracture, compartment syndrome, skin necrosis and osteomyelitis. This has been reported in less than 1% of patients.

O   **What are the most common causes for deterioration of ventilatory status in a stable, intubated patient?**

Endotracheal tube dislodgment, occlusion, pneumothorax and equipment failure.

O   **Hypoxemia with a normal alveolar-arterial oxygen difference is the result of what?**

Hypoventilation.

○   **What are the causes for an increase in the alveolar-arterial oxygen difference?**

Ventilation-perfusion (V/O) mismatch or an alveolar-arterial diffusion abnormality.

○   **Blood gas analysis findings characteristic of a salicylate overdose include what?**

Respiratory alkalosis and an increased anion gap metabolic acidosis.

○   **T/F: Physostigmine is the treatment of choice for a tricyclic antidepressant overdose.**

False. Physostigmine can reverse many of the neurologic manifestations of a tricyclic overdose, but its use is not recommended because of its propensity to cause seizures. It does not reverse the cardiac effects. Good supportive care is the mainstay of treatment.

○   **Name some indications for using digoxin immune F antibody.**

The occurrence of a life-threatening dysrhythmias, ingestion of more than 4mg of digoxin by a child, or digoxin serum levels that are associated with a risk for developing a life-threatening dysrhythmia.

○   **Aside from measures intended to stop seizures, what is the major therapeutic priority in the management of status epilepticus?**

Maintenance of oxygenation, adequate ventilation, and the prevention of hypoxia.

○   **What is the major complication in the treatment for diabetic ketoacidosis?**

Cerebral edema.

○   **When cerebral edema is clinically evident, management should include what?**

Administration of mannitol, reduced rate of fluid infusion and hyperventilation (maintaining PCO_2 <u>above</u> 35 mmHg). An ICP monitor may need to be placed to guide therapy.

○   **What symptoms characterize tumor lysis syndrome?**

Hyperuricemia, hyperkalemia, and hyperphosphatemia.

○   **The major goal of therapy for tumor lysis syndrome is to prevent?**

Acute renal failure. The principles for treatment include alkalinization of the urine, vigorous hydration and diuresis, and prevention of the formation of toxic metabolites.

○   **What is the treatment of choice for a brain tumor edema?**

Dexamethasone.

○   **What is the major toxicity associated with a hydrocarbon ingestion related to?**

Pulmonary aspiration.

○   **What is the blood gas analysis characteristic of a patient with malignant hyperthermia?**

Metabolic and respiratory acidosis.

○   **What should treatment for malignant hyperthermia include?**

A change in the anesthetic agent to remove possible triggers, administration of Dantrolene and the surgical procedure should be terminated.

O   **Cardiac index is calculated by using which parameters?**

Cardiac output x body surface area.

O   **What are two symptoms which characterize heat stroke?**

An altered mental status, and a rectal temperature of > 40 C.

O   **A four-year-old sickle cell patient presents with pallor, weakness, tachycardia and abdominal fullness. What should you suspect?**

Acute splenic sequestration.

O   **How should you treat the patient characterized in the previous question?**

Colloid and whole blood transfusion for correction of hypovolemia, anemia and prevention of circulatory failure.

O   **How many subsequent episodes of acute splenic sequestration be avoided?**

Splenectomy or chronic transfusions.

O   **When are corticosteroids indicated for the treatment of tuberculosis?**

When mediastinal adenopathy causes airway obstruction or pleural fluid causes mediastinal shift.

O   **What clinical lung findings are characteristic of acute hypersensitivity pneumonitis?**

Inspiratory crackles.

O   **Which cardiac anomalies are associated with congenital Rubella?**

Pulmonic stenosis and PDA.

O   **Name some conditions in which both intracranial calcifications and skin lesions are present.**

Toxoplasmosis, Cytomegalovirus and Sturge-Weber Syndrome.

O   **What is the narrowest part of the respiratory tract in children?**

The inferior ring portion of the cricoid cartilage.

O   **Name and define three divisions of the airway.**

Extrathoracic: Nose to the trachea before it enters the thoracic inlet.
Intrathoracic Extrapulmonary: Trachea at the thoracic inlet to the right and left mainstem bronchi before they enter the lungs.
Intrapulmonary: Bronchi within the lungs.

O   **In what phase of respiration is stridor observed?**

Inspiration.

O   **What causes stridor?**

With extrathoracic airway obstruction, the pressure inside the extrathoracic part of the airway is negative relative to the level of atmospheric pressure. This results in further narrowing of the larynx during inspiration and therefore, stridor.

○ **Grunting is observed during what phase of respiration?**

Expiratory- exhalation against a closed glottis.

○ **A neonate has Apgar scores of 8 and 8. He is actively crying, but cyanosis and retractions appear when he is quiet. What is the most likely diagnosis?**

Choanal atresia.

○ **Which anomalies of the great vessels result in airway obstruction?**

1. Right aortic arch with or without a left ligamentum arteriosum
2. Double aortic arch
3. Anomalous innominate or left carotid artery
4. Aberrant right subclavian
5. Anomalous left pulmonary artery

○ **What is the <u>most common</u> cause of cardiac arrest in children?**

Hypoxia.

○ **What are the <u>most common</u> arrhythmias in pediatric patients?**

Sinus bradycardia, Asystole.

○ **What is the drug of choice in the treatment of supraventricular tachycardia?**

Adenosine, at a dose of 0.1 mg/kg. Propranolol, digoxin, and verapamil are also indicated. Verapamil, however, is not indicated in patients less than one year of age because it can cause hypotension.

○ **Why must adenosine be given as a rapid intravenous bolus?**

Its half-life is around 6 seconds.

○ **What is the most common causes of pulseless electrical activity (PEA)?**

Pneumothorax, Pericardial tamponade, Hypoxemia, Acidosis, Hypovolemia.

○ **To achieve more than 90% FIO_2 in a non-intubated patient, which oxygen device should be used?**

Non-rebreather mask.

○ **What do the most common primary diagnoses in pediatric arrests involve?**

The respiratory system.

○ **Name some acceptable modes of intravascular access.**

Intraosseus, peripheral veins, central veins, surgical cut-down.

○ **What are the acceptable routes for central venous access?**

External jugular, internal jugular, subclavian, umbilical (newborns less than 2 weeks of age), and femoral veins.

○   **Is the femoral vein lateral or medial to the femoral artery?**

Medial.

○   **Name some skin manifestations of shock/hypoxemia.**

Circumoral pallor/cyanosis, mottled skin, distal cyanosis, prolonged capillary refill, diminished distal pulses.

○   **What are the signs and symptoms of central nervous system hypoxia?**

Irritability, Diminished response to pain, Seizures, and Lethargy.

○   **A three-year-old presents with signs/symptoms of epiglottitis. Should intravenous access be a priority?**

No. Intravenous access is an absolute contraindication in suspected epiglottitis. The procedure is to put the patient in a comfortable position with supplemental oxygen and minimize the level of anxiety in the patient. All invasive procedures are to be done in the operating room.

○   **In a child who is hypoglycemic and hypotensive, is it appropriate to use a solution containing dextrose for fluid resuscitation?**

No. The use of a glucose containing solution for fluid resuscitation will result in an osmotic diuresis secondary to hyperglycemia.

○   **What is the appropriate treatment for a hypoglycemic child?**

D50W, 1.0 ml/kg through a central line, or D25W, 2.0 ml/kg through a central or peripheral line, use D10 in infants.

○   **What fluids are suitable for the initial treatment of hypotension?**

Normal saline or Lactate Ringers. The dose is 10-20 ml/kg IV.

○   **What are the relative contraindications to the use of a nasopharyngeal airway?**

Suspected airway trauma, adenoidal hypertrophy, and bleeding diatheses.

○   **After intubating a 1 month old baby for respiratory failure, you confirm appropriate tube placement by auscultation. However, CXR reveals the tube is the right mainstem bronchus. Why were you able to hear breath sounds bilaterally?**

In small infants, it is not uncommon to hear transmitted breath sounds. In the patients, the physician is advised not only to auscultate, but also to visualize adequate chest rise bilaterally.

○   **Supplemental oxygen delivery devices include what?**

Nasal cannula, oxygen hood/tent, and masks.

○   **Name some types of oxygen masks?**

Simple mask, partial rebreathing mask, and nonrebreathing mask.

○   **What is the amount of FiO_2 each device can deliver?**

1. Nasal cannula: 30-40%
2. Oxygen hoot/tent: up to 80-90%
3. Simple mask: up to 40%
4. Partial rebreathing mask: up to 60%
5. Nonrebreathing mask: 100%

○   **What is the rate of chest compressions in an infant?**

100-120 times per minute.

○   **Name some hand-bag devices.**

Self-inflating bag, and the anesthesia bag.

○   **What are the major differences between the self-inflating and anesthesia hand-bags?**

Self-inflating: Refills independently of gas flow, is relatively easy to use, the bag must be squeezed for gas to flow into the patient, and can deliver a maximum of 60-90% FIO_2.
Anesthesia bag: Requires adequate air flow to refill, requires a certain degree of expertise and experience to use, there is constant air flow into the patient without the need to squeeze the bag, and can deliver 100% FIO_2.

For the inexperienced physician, the use of the self-inflating bag is the best choice, because it is easy to use. However, the physician must remember to squeeze the bag for gas to flow into the patient.

○   **What comprises the assessment of the circulatory system in the pediatric patient?**

Blood pressure, heart rate, peripheral and central pulses, capillary refill, and skin color.

○   **What is the time-frame for a normal capillary refill?**

Two to three seconds. When assessing capillary refill, make sure the skin is warm Cold ambient temperature will cause prolonged capillary refill, and can be misleading in the assessment of the circulatory system.

○   **Renal output is a good indicator of adequate cardiac output. What can the physician do to assess recent urinary output in a patient?**

Assessment of simple things, like the color of the urine (dark color indicating concentrated urine) and the number of wet diapers can provide the physician with a general idea of recent urinary output.

○   **What are the complications associated with subclavian vein cannulation?**

Hemothorax, pneumothorax, and trauma to the subclavian artery.

○   **What is the initial dose of epinephrine in cardiac resuscitation?**

0.01mg/kg of a 1:10,000 solution. PALS recommend increasing the dose to 0.1 mg/kg of 1:1,000 solution if there is no response to the initial dose. If the intratracheal route is used, the initial dose should be 0.1 mg/kg of a 1:1,000 solution.

○   **What is the dose of atropine given during cardiac resuscitation?**

0.02 mg/kg initial dose. However, the minimum dose is 0.1 mg. Intratracheal dose is the same.

○   **When is sodium bicarbonate indicated in cardiac resuscitation?**

The use of sodium bicarbonate in cardiac arrest is controversial. Current thinking is to use it if there is a documented metabolic with pH < 7.00.

○   **A term newborn is delivered in your office. You check the heart rate and it is approximately 80-120 beats/min. After drying, suctioning, and stimulation, the heart rate remains low. What should the next step be?**

100% oxygen should be given by hood or face mask. Most babies with bradycardia will respond to stimulation or administration of oxygen. Infants that remain bradycardic will need endotracheal intubation, hand-bagging with 100% oxygen, and chest compressions.

○   **What are some major complications of endotracheal intubation?**

Esophageal intubation/perforation, trauma to the teeth, emesis and aspiration, and bradycardia. It is recommended that the physician has atropine ready for administration when intubating an infant or child, because they can develop reflective (vasovagal) bradycardia.

○   **What are the major side effects of lidocaine?**

Lidocaine is used in the treatment of ventricular tachycardia and fibrillation. The recommended dose is 1 mg/kg, followed by a constant infusion of 20-50 micrograms/kg/min. The major side effect is hypotension, therefore, it should be used with caution in patients with myocardial depression. Lidocaine is also used as a sedative prior to intubation in patients with suspected increased intracranial pressure.

○   **What are the indications for calcium?**

Suspected hypocalcemia, hyperkalemia, hypermagnesemia, and calcium channel blocker overdose. Calcium is no longer indicated in the treatment of asystole or electromechanical dissociation.

○   **Is there a difference between calcium chloride and calcium gluconate, in an emergency situation?**

Yes. The liver must first metabolize calcium gluconate before elemental calcium is available. Therefore, calcium chloride is the preferred drug during an emergency. The dose should be 0.2 cc/kg or 10 mg/kg. If a peripheral route is used, the drug should be given slowly. Extravasation of calcium can lead to tissue damage and necrosis.

○   **What is the catecholamine of choice when treating small infants with heart failure?**

Dopamine. In small infants, cardiac output is more dependent on heart rate than stroke volume. Dopamine is an excellent chromotrope, and will have a profound effect on blood pressure and cardiac output by increasing the heart rate. However, dopamine can cause tachyarrhythmias, so its use should be carefully monitored. Unlike in adults, dopamine causes little renal vasoconstriction or vasodilatation in pediatric patients.

○   **When inserting an intraosseous needle into the tibia, in which direction should the needle be placed?**

Caudal, away from the epiphysial plate. This will avoid damage to the growth plate of the tibia.

○   **When is isoproterenol indicated?**

Isoproterenol is ideal for the treatment of bradyarrhythmias and heart block. It can also be used in small infants with heart failure, because of its chronotropic properties. Adverse reactions include tachyarrhythmias and hypotension.

○ **What is the rate for performing chest compressions in a child?**

100 times per minute.

○ **What are the steps in the initial resuscitation of a newborn?**

Dry thoroughly, stimulate, suction, then check airway, breathing, circulation, and temperature control. Newborns are very sensitive to heat loss, so they should be dried immediately after birth, and placed under a radiant warmer to prevent heat loss through the skin. Excessive hypothermia can lead to acidosis and hypoxemia.

○ **What is the acceptable heart rate for a newborn?**

100 beats/min or higher.

○ **List the equipment necessary for intubation.**

Oxygen source, bag and mask, endotracheal tube, suction device, stylet, laryngoscope and blade, pulse oximeter, adhesive tape, appropriate sedative and muscle relaxant, resuscitation medications.

○ **What is the best place to assess heart rate in a newborn?**

The umbilical cord.

○ **You are asked to assist in a precipitous delivery. The newborn is lethargic and unresponsive to tactile stimulation. The mother admits to recent heroin use. How should you proceed?**

The infant is most likely suffering from narcotic induced respiratory depression. Treatment is naloxone hydrochloride given either intravenously, intratracheally, intraosseously, subcutaneously, or intramuscularly, at a dose of 0.1 mg/kg. The first two methods are the routes of choice.

○ **What are the most common causes of bradycardia in a newborn?**

Hypoxemia, hypoglycemia, hypothermia, exposure to narcotics, and sepsis.

○ **A seven day old baby is cyanotic. Physical exam reveals a holosystolic murmur. He remains cyanotic after treatment with 100% oxygen. What is the possible diagnosis and subsequent treatment of choice?**

The patient has a ductus dependent cyanotic congenital heart defect. The treatment of choice is prostaglandin E1.

○ **While hand-bagging a patient, his oxygen saturation drops acutely. What are some of the possible causes?**

Dislodgment of the endotracheal tube, obstruction of the endotracheal tube, pneumothorax, or equipment failure (i.e., bag disconnected from oxygen, etc.)

○ **While hand-bagging a 14-year-old patient, you notice the stomach is getting distended. What steps should you take to remedy the situation?**

Apply gentle cricoid pressure to occlude the esophagus. Insertion of nasogastric or orogastric tube can also be used to decompress the stomach. It is imperative that pressure not be applied to the stomach for decompression, as this can lead to emesis and aspiration.

❍ **Where is the best location to palpate the pulse in an infant?**

The brachial or femoral artery.

❍ **What complications are associated with chest compressions in the newborn?**

Broken ribs, laceration of the liver, pneumothorax, cardiac contusion, pericardial tamponade.

❍ **What is the rate for chest compressions and the administration of ventilation during resuscitation of a neonate?**

100-120 chest compressions per minute and 30 breaths per minute.

❍ **What is the normal systolic pressure in a neonate?**

Greater than 60 mm Hg.

❍ **Which fluids are indicated in the resuscitation of a newborn?**

Normal saline, 5% albumin; ringer's lactate; and whole blood (which can be obtained from the placenta).

❍ **What are the signs of hypovolemia in a newborn?**

Poor response to resuscitation, persistent pallor after appropriate oxygenation, weak pulses, hypotension.

❍ **Which actions are appropriate to provide tactile stimulation on a newborn in order to encourage the patient to cry?**

Flick or slap the sole of foot, or rub the back (preferably with a towel while drying the baby).

❍ **Why is a straight blade recommended for intubating infants and toddlers?**

It provides better visualization of the glottis. The tip of the blade can also be used to physically displace the floppy epiglottis.

❍ **When is cardioversion indicated?**

During SVT, ventricular fibrillation, ventricular tachycardia (VT). For SVT and VT, use synchronized cardioversion.

❍ **What is the age limit for the use of the intraosseous technique?**

6 in some studies but it is now used as a last resort from children to adults.

❍ **A 5-year-old takes several KCL tablets. An EKG shows peaked T-waves, and the presence of U-waves. What is the indicated therapy?**

Calcium chloride, 10mg/kg IV; sodium bicarbonate, 0.5-1.0 mEq/kg IV; glucose and insulin intravenous drip; sodium polystyrene sulfonate (Kayexalate), 1 gm/kg/dose Q2-6 hours PR or PO.

❍ **What three signs suggest that a newborn is responding to resuscitation?**

Increasing heart rate, spontaneous respirations, improving color.

❍   **A 5-year-old boy is found on the medical floor in a coma. What is the differential diagnosis?**

Hypoxemia, hypoglycemia, hypotension, drug overdose, postictal state after a seizure, and/or toxin ingestion.

❍   **What are the initial steps in neonatal resuscitation?**

Positioning, suctioning, tactile stimulation, ventilation.

❍   **What is the compression/ventilation ratio during cardiopulmonary resuscitation when treating pediatric patients who are older than newborns?**

5:1

❍   **Failure to respond to cardioversion is due to what?**

Hypothermia, hypoglycemia, acidosis, hypoxia.

❍   **How can it be determined that an endotracheal tube is in the right place?**

Symmetrical chest rise during inspiration; bilateral breath sounds on auscultation; presence of vapor in the tube; check for placement with a laryngoscope; improved oxygenation detection of CO_2 during expiration, with a CO_2 detector attached to the tube; CXR.

❍   **If a newborn fails to respond to epinephrine, what should be the next step?**

Repeat epinephrine, volume expansion, and sodium bicarbonate. Unlike older pediatric patients where bicarbonate is indicated only in documented metabolic acidosis, the use of bicarbonate is indicated when the patient is not responding to epinephrine, even if there is no documented acidosis.

❍   **What complications may occur as a result of central venous catheterization?**

Infection, air embolism, hemorrhage, injury to the adjacent nerve or artery, and pneumothorax in subclavian and internal jugular catheterization.

❍   **Which drugs are indicated for airway management in patients with suspected increased intracranial pressure?**

For sedation, lidocaine and/or thiopental are good choices, because they both lower intracranial pressure. The use of a nondepolarizing agent should be used for muscle relaxation.

❍   **Which sedatives are recommended for routine intubation?**

Valium 0.1 mg/kg, Midazolam 0.1 mg/kg, Lorazepam 0.1 mg/kg, Morphine 0.1 mg/kg, Fentanyl 1 mcg/kg.

❍   **A 4-year-old is brought to the emergency room with suspected foreign body aspiration. The patient is alert, cyanotic, and grasping for air. What should be the immediate treatment?**

Provide oxygen. As long as the patient is awake medical personnel should not intervene. Patient should be encouraged to continue coughing and breathing.

❍   **After a few minutes, the patient described in the previous question becomes unconscious. What should be the next step?**

Administer 5 back blows, followed by 5 abdominal thrusts until object is dislodged. When treating infants, administer 5 back blows, followed by 5 chest thrusts.

O   **Despite repeated efforts, the object has still not been dislodged. What should be the next procedure?**

An emergency needle cricothyrotomy or tracheostomy.

O   **Which medications cannot be given intraosseously?**

Phenytoin and Chloramphenicol.

O   **Which site is used to evacuate a pneumothorax by using needle thoracentesis?**

The second intercostals space at the midclavicular line, or the fourth intercostals space at the anterior or midaxillary line.

O   **What is the best place to palpate the pulse in children?**

The carotid artery.

O   **Which drug overdoses are associated with cardiac arrhythmias?**

Cocaine, heroin, tricyclic antidepressants, digitalis, calcium channel-blockers, and beta-blockers.

O   **What are indications for endotracheal intubation?**

Oxygenation and ventilation, airway protection, removal of airway secretions, hyperventilation (when increased intracranial pressure is suspected), and cardiovascular instability.

O   **Which laboratory studies can be obtained through an intraosseous needle?**

Electrolytes and blood cultures.

O   **What is the APGAR score?**

A scoring system which measure five physiological variables (heart rate, respirations, muscle tone, reflex irritability, and color), enabling a rapid evaluation of a newborn's physiological status. Named after Virginia Apgar, a British nurse.

O   **You are called to assist in the delivery of a baby because meconium was noted in the amniotic fluid. What steps should you take to prevent meconium aspiration?**

After delivering the head, you should thoroughly suction the mouth, pharynx, and nose. After the baby is delivered, place him/her under a radiant warmer, finish suctioning the upper airway, and intubate and suction the trachea. To suction the trachea connect the endotracheal tube directly to the suction machine. The use of a suction catheter is not recommended because meconium particles may occlude the catheter.

O   **Are there any differences in the "ABC" approach to cardiopulmonary arrest in children (as compared to adults)?**

Only one. The airway and breathing are relatively more stressed in children than is circulation. Except in the child with congenital cardiovascular anomalies, there are few purely cardiac causes of cardiopulmonary arrest. The basic "ABC" algorithm remains sound.

O   **What anatomic site is preferred for IO infusion?**

The preferred IO site is on the anteromedial surface of the tibia, one or two centimeters below the palpable tubercle. This area is relatively flat and easy to locate.

○   **Why is hypothermia a particular concern in the field treatment of small children?**

Children have poorly developed heat regulation mechanisms (e.g. poor shivering), and a relatively larger surface area to volume ratio than adults. Accordingly, infants and small children are more likely to become hypothermic if exposed to the cold for prolonged periods, as may occur during extrication from a motor vehicle crash.

○   **What is the normal IV maintenance amount for a 25 kg child?**

1600 cc/day or 65 cc/hr. The formula is: 4 ml/kg/hr or 100 ml/kg/day for the first 10 kg, 2ml/kg/r or 50 ml/kg/day for the second 10 kg, and 1 ml/kg/hr or 20 ml/kg/day for all further kg.

○   **What is the fluid deficit in a child with mild (<5%), moderate (5-10%) and serve (>10%) dehydration?**

40-50 ml/kg, 60-90 ml/kg, and 100 ml/kg/respectively.

○   **What are high yield criteria for clinical determination of dehydration >5%?**

Capillary refill > 2 seconds, dry mucous membranes, absent tears, and general in appearance.

○   **How does the urine specify gravity help you determine the level of dehydration in a child?**

<1.020 is found in mild dehydration, Σ1.030 in moderate, and >1.035 in severe.

○   **What causes pseudohyponatremia?**

High glucose, triglycerides, or protein.

○   **What are the daily sodium requirements of premature and full term newborns?**

3-4 mEq/kg/d for premature and 1-2 mEq/kg/d for full term.

○   **In which conditions are electrolytes considered high yield?**

Age <6 months, vomiting, tachycardia, dry mucous membrane, and capillary refill >2 seconds. The presence any of these criteria is 100% sensitive for significant abnormalities.

○   **What is the formula for obtaining the true calcium level with hypoalbuminemia?**

Subtract 0.8 mg/dL from total serum calcium for each 1 g/dL decrease in serum albumin below normal.

○   **What are the clinical findings in patient with hypocalcemia?**

Chvostek sign (tapping on facial nerve causes twitch), Trousseau sign (carpal spasm after inflating BP cuff for 3 minutes), hyperactive reflexes, low BP, or CHF.

○   **What is the relationship between acidosis and hyperkalemia?**

A decrease in the pH of 0.1 will increase K+ 0.3-1.3 mEq/L due to the H+/K+ exchange pump.

METABOLIC, ENDOCRINE AND NUTRITION

○ **What are the causes of factitious hyponatremia?**

Hyperglycemia, hyperlipidemia, or hyperproteinemia.

○ **How does hyperglycemia lead to hyponatremia?**

Because glucose stays in the extracellular fluid, hyperglycemia draws water out of the cell into the extracellular fluid. Each 100 mg/dL increase in plasma glucose decreases the serum sodium by 1.6 to 1.8 mEq/L.

○ **What is the most common cause of hypovolemic hyponatremia in children?**

Viral gastroenteritis. Vomiting and/or diarrhea occurs with this condition.

○ **What is the most common cause of euvolemic hyponatremia in children?**

Syndrome of inappropriate secretion of antidiuretic hormone (SIADH). Causes include CNS disorders, medications, tumors, and pulmonary disorders.

○ **What are the signs and symptoms of hyponatremia?**

Weakness, nausea, anorexia, vomiting, confusion, lethargy, seizures, and coma.

○ **What are the most common causes of hypotonic fluid loss leading to hypernatremia?**

Diarrhea, vomiting, hyperpyrexia, and excessive sweating.

○ **What are the signs and symptoms of hypernatremia?**

Confusion, muscle irritability, seizures, respiratory paralysis, and coma.

○ **What are the ECG findings of a patient with hypokalemia?**

Flattened T-waves, depressed ST segments, prominent P- and U-waves, and prolonged QT and PR intervals.

○ **What are the ECG findings for a patient with hyperkalemia?**

Peaked T-waves, prolonged QT and PR intervals, diminished P-waves, depressed T-waves, QRS widening, levels exceeding 10 mEq/L, and a classic sine wave.

○ **What is the first ECG finding for a patient with hyperkalemia?**

The development of tall peaked T-waves at levels of 5.6–6.0 mEq/L, which is best seen in the precordial leads.

○ **What is the quickest way to stabilize the myocardium in a patient with hyperkalemia?**

Administration of calcium gluconate (10%) 10-20 mL, IV with an onset of action of 1-3 minutes.

❍   **What are some causes of hyperkalemia?**

Acidosis, tissue necrosis, hemolysis, blood transfusions, GI bleed, renal failure, Addison's disease, primary hypoaldosteronism, excess po K+ intake, RTA IV, and medication (such as succinylcholine, Σ-blockers, captopril, spironolactone, triamterene, amiloride, and high dose penicillin).

❍   **What are the causes of hypocalcemia?**

Shock, sepsis, multiple blood transfusions, hypoparathyroidism, vitamin D deficiency, pancreatitis, hypomagnesemia, alkalosis, fat embolism syndrome, phosphate overload, chronic renal failure, loop diuretics, hypoalbuminemia, tumor lysis syndrome, and medication, such as Dilantin, phenobarbital, heparin, theophylline, cimetidine, and gentamicin.

❍   **What is the most common cause of hyperkalemia?**

Lab error. Chronic renal failure is the most common cause of "true hyperkalemia."

❍   **What are the most common causes of hypercalcemia?**

In descending order, malignancy, primary hyperparathyroidism, and thiazide diuretics.

❍   **What are the signs and symptoms of hypercalcemia?**

The most common gastrointestinal symptoms are anorexia and constipation. A classic mnemonic can be used to remember them:

Stones: renal calculi.
Bones: osteolysis.
Abdominal groans: peptic ulcer disease and pancreatitis.
Psychic overtones: psychiatric disorders.

❍   **What is the initial treatment for hypercalcemia?**

Patients with hypercalcemia are dehydrated because high calcium levels interfere with ADH and the ability of the kidney to concentrate urine. Therefore, the initial treatment is restoration of the extracellular fluid with 2 times maintenance level of normal saline within 24 hours. After the patient is rehydrated, administer Furosemide in doses of 1 to 3 mg/kg.

❍   **What is the most common cause of hyperphosphatemia?**

Acute and chronic renal failure.

❍   **What are the two primary causes of primary adrenal insufficiency?**

Tuberculosis and autoimmune destruction account for 90% of the cases.

❍   **What are the signs and symptoms of primary adrenal insufficiency?**

Fatigue, weakness, weight loss, anorexia, hyperpigmentation, nausea, vomiting, abdominal pain, diarrhea, and orthostatic hypotension.

❍   **What characteristic lab findings are associated with primary adrenal insufficiency?**

Hyperkalemia, hyponatremia, hypoglycemia, azotemia (if volume depletion is present), and a mild metabolic acidosis.

○   **How should acute adrenal insufficiency be treated?**

Administration of hydrocortisone (2 mg/kg) and crystalloid fluids containing dextrose.

○   **What are the main causes of death during an adrenal crisis?**

Circulatory collapse and hyperkalemia-induced arrhythmias.

○   **What are the causes of acute adrenal crisis?**

It occurs secondary to a major stress, such as surgery, severe injury, or any other illness in a patient with primary or secondary adrenal insufficiency.

○   **What is thyrotoxicosis, and what are the causes?**

A hypermetabolic state that occurs secondary to excess circulating thyroid hormone caused by thyroid hormone overdose, thyroid hyperfunction, or thyroid inflammation.

○   **What are the hallmark clinical features of myxedema coma?**

Hypothermia (75%) and coma.

○   **What is the most common cause of hypoglycemia seen in the ED?**

An insulin reaction in a diabetic patient.

○   **What is the role of phosphate replacement during the treatment of DKA?**

Phosphate can drop rapidly during the correction of DKA so phosphate supplementation should be started early, especially if serum phosphate is <1.0 mg/L.

○   **What is the most important "initial" step for the treatment of DKA?**

Fluid administration with 10 cc/kg normal saline. Over-aggressive fluid administration can lead to cerebral herniation from brain edema.

○   **In the first two years of life, what is the most common cause of drug-induced hypoglycemia?**

Salicylates. Between 2 and 8, alcohol is the most likely cause, and between 11 and 30, insulin and sulfonylureas are the culprits.

○   **Which principle hormone protects the human body from hypoglycemia?**

Glucagon.

○   **What is the most common type of hypoglycemia in a child?**

Ketotic hypoglycemia. Attacks usually occur when the child is stressed by caloric deprivation. This condition usually develops in boys between 18 months and 5 years of age. Attacks may be episodic and are more frequent in the morning or during periods of illness.

○   **What are the neurologic signs and symptoms of hypoglycemia?**

Hypoglycemia may produce mental and neurologic dysfunction. Neurologic manifestations can include paresthesias, cranial nerve palsies, transient hemiplegia, diplopia, decerebrate posturing, and clonus.

○ **What lab findings are expected with diabetic ketoacidosis?**

Elevated ß-hydroxybutyrate, acetoacetate, acetone, and glucose. Ketonuria and glucosuria are present. Serum bicarbonate levels, pCO_2, and pH are decreased. Potassium may be initially elevated but falls when the acidosis is corrected.

○ **Outline the basic treatment for DKA.**

Administer fluids. Start with normal saline (10 cc/kg), followed by potassium (100-200 mEq in the first 12-24 hours). Prescribe insulin, 0.1 units/kg bolus, then 0.1 units/kg/hr infusion. (Ed. Note: Many physicians no longer give bolus.) Add glucose to the IV fluid when the glucose levels fall below 250 mg/dL and give the patient potassium phosphate as supplement.

○ **Distinguish between type A and type B lactic acidosis.**

Type A lactic acidosis is often seen in the ED. The onset of this condition usually occurs because of shock. Type A lactic acidosis is associated with inadequate tissue perfusion and resultant anoxia, and with subsequent lactate and hydrogen ion accumulation. Type B lactic acidosis includes all forms of acidosis in which there are no evidence of tissue anoxia.

○ **What are the complications of bicarbonate therapy in DKA?**

Paradoxical CSF acidosis, cardiac arrhythmias, decreased oxygen delivery to tissue, and fluid and sodium overload.

○ **What is the most common cause of secondary adrenal insufficiency and adrenal crisis?**

Iatrogenic adrenal suppression from prolonged steroid use. Rapid withdrawal of steroids may lead to collapse and death.

○ **An increase of pCO_2 of 10 mm Hg leads to an expected decrease in pH of about:**

0.08.

○ **A decrease of pCO_2 of 10 mm Hg leads to an expected increase in pH of about:**

0.13.

○ **What expected increase in pH is associated with a rise in HCO_3 of 5.0 mEq/L?**

0.08.

○ **What expected decrease in pH is associated with a decrease in HCO_3 of 5.0 mEq/L?**

0.10.

○ **How is the anion gap calculated from electrolyte values?**

Anion gap = $Na–Cl–CO_2$. The normal gap is $12^{+/-}4$ mEq/L.

○ **What is the most common endocrine disorder of childhood and adolescence?**

Diabetes mellitus(DM).

○   **How is the etiology of type I DM different from type II DM?**

Type I DM is associated with Human Leucocyte Antigens (HLA), autoimmunity, and or islet cell antibodies. Type II DM usually involves a genetic mutation resulting in inactive pancreatic and liver enzymes as well as insulin receptor defects.

○   **What are the causes of an oxygen saturation curve's shift to the right?**

A shift to the right delivers more O_2 to the tissue.
The mnemonic "CADET! Right face!" helps in remembering causes of an O_2 shift to the right.

Right =   Release to tissues.

Hyper   Carbia.
              Acidemia.
2,3   DPG.
              Exercise.
Increased   Temperature.

○   **When body waste materials, urine and stool, are enterally recycled, they can cause a _normal anion gap_ metabolic acidosis. Remember:**

U   = ureteroenterostomy,
S   = small bowel fistula,
E   = extra chloride (NH_4Cl or amino acid chlorides 2° TPN),
D   = diarrhea.

C   = carbonic anhydrase inhibitors,
R   = renal tubular acidosis,
A   = adrenal insufficiency,
P   = pancreatic fistula

○   **What are the two primary causes of metabolic alkalosis?**

Loss of hydrogen and chloride from the stomach and overzealous diuresis with loss of hydrogen, potassium, and chloride.

○   **What etiologies are responsible for secondary DM?**

Exocrine pancreatic diseases like cystic fibrosis, pancreatic cancer and Cushing's disease.

○   **What are the peak age groups in children who develop IDDM?**

Between the ages of 5 and 7 and at puberty.

○   **What are the diagnostic criteria for IDDM, NIDDM, and GDM respectively?**

IDDM: Glucose and ketones in the urine with a BGL > 200 mg/dL
NIDDM: FPG > 140 mg/dL and a two hr value > 200 mg/dL during OGTT on more than one occasion
GDM: Two or more of the following during OGTT; FPG > 105 mg/dL, 1 hr > 190 mg/DL, 2 hr > 165
            mg/dL, 3 hr > 145 mg/dL
○   **What is the relationship between HLA-D3 and HLA-D4 with type I DM?**

The presence of these particular HLAs increases the relative risk for developing diabetes by 7-10 fold.

○   **What is the renal threshold for serum glucose before glucosuria develops?**

Approximately 180 mg/dL.

O   **What is the equation for determining serum osmolarity?**

Osmserum = [serum Na+(mEq/L) + K+(mEq/L)] x 2 + (glucose(mg/dL) / (18) + (BUN(mg/dL) / (3).

O   **What condition should be suspected in a child who presents with lethargy, weight loss, and new onset enuresis in a previously toilet trained child?**

New onset DM.

O   **How does a child with DKA present?**

The child will present with vomiting, polyuria, dehydration, Kussmaul breathing and abdominal pain.

O   **What conditions should be considered in the differential diagnosis of metabolic acidosis in children?**

DKA, uremia, gastroenteritis with dehydration, lactic acidosis, salicylate poisoning, and encephalitis (remember MUD PILES).

O   **What condition should be suspected in a child with a serum glucose of 642 mg/dL, mild ketonuria, depressed sensorium and positive Babinski sign?**

Non-ketotic hyperosmolar coma (NKHC).

O   **How do you treat NKHC?**

Dehydration should be corrected using .45%NS with 50% of the deficit being corrected in the first 12 hrs and the remainder corrected in the following 24 hrs. When the BGL approaches 300 mg/dL the fluid should be changed to 5% dextrose in .2%NS with 20 mEq of K+ added to each liter. Insulin therapy should be initiated in the second hr with a loading dose of .05 U/kg of regular insulin followed by .05 U/kg/hr.

O   **How is the insulin requirement different between DKA and NKHC?**

In DKA the rate of insulin infusion is .1 U/kg/hr while in NKHC it is .05 U/kg/hr. The lower dose of insulin in NKHC is due to the dramatic decrease in glucose levels due to rehydration alone.

O   **What do U waves on the EKG suggest in the treatment of DKA?**

Hypokalemia.

O   **What are the dangers of administering HCO_3^- to a child with DKA?**

Alkalosis shifts the oxygen distribution curve to the left ultimately diminishing the release of oxygen to peripheral tissue. Also, use of HCO_3^- can result in a paradoxical cerebral acidosis.

O   **What is paradoxical cerebral acidosis?**

When exogenous HCO_3^- combines with H+, H_2O and CO_2 are formed. The blood brain barrier is more permeable to CO_2 that to HCO_3^- thus CO_2 accumulates in the CNS. Therefore a CNS acidosis will be created while the systemic acidosis is being treated.

O   **What is the Primary life threatening complication in the aggressive treatment of DKA?**

Cerebral edema.

❍   **What signs and symptoms should a physician look for when considering cerebral edema in a patient being treated for DKA?**

Change in mental status, "delirious outbursts", bradycardia, vomiting, decreased reflexes, and changes in pupillary response.

❍   **How should insulin be administered to children?**

The injection is given subcutaneously in a rotating pattern utilizing the thighs, buttocks, and abdomen. Parents should administer insulin for children younger than 10-12 years of age.

❍   **How should parents of a diabetic child monitor BGLs once discharged from the hospital?**

Blood glucose testing should be done at least two times a week. On all other days urine glucose should be monitored prior to each of the major meals as well as prior to the evening snack.

❍   **What is the ideal BGL range in a diabetic child?**

Ideally the BGL should be maintained between 80 - 140 mg/dL. BGLs between 60 - 240 mg/dL are acceptable in children.

❍   **What is the significance of the HbA1C?**

It represents the fraction of hemoglobin that has been nonenzymatically glycosylated. It provides an accurate estimation of the relative BGL over the preceding two to three months.

❍   **What is an acceptable HbA1C in a diabetic child?**

6 - 9% represents good control, 9 - 12% is fair control, above 12% is poor control.

❍   **What does the "honeymoon period" refer to in a newly diagnosed diabetic?**

After a newly diagnosed diabetic is stabilized more than three quarters will experience a significant reduction in insulin requirement as the pancreas makes a final effort to produce insulin.

❍   **What is meant by the term "brittle diabetic"?**

A brittle diabetic refers to a patient who has poor blood glucose control with wide fluctuations in BGLs that require frequent alterations in insulin requirements.

❍   **What percent of pediatric patients have DKA at their first hospital presentation?**

DKA is present at 30% of initial presentations of newly diagnosed juvenile onset diabetics.

❍   **What is the most serious immediate life threatening risk to a child with DKA?**

Dehydration. While patients may have hyperglycemia and metabolic acidosis, dehydration is the most serious life threatening condition.

❍   **When a child in DKA presents to the emergency department, The K+ will be increased, decreased, or normal?**

Total body K+ is depleted though serum levels may be normal. Transcellular shifts during acidosis move K+ extracellular in exchange for H+ ions. The osmotic diuresis due to the hyperglycemia results in overall K+ loss. In addition, the dehydration stimulates aldosterone secretion which further contributes to K+ excretion.

O   **How do established diabetics present differently than new onset diabetics?**

Established diabetics will have the prodrome of polydipsia, polyphagia, and polyuria for less than 24 hrs. New onset diabetics may be symptomatic for days to weeks prior to presentation.

O   **What are the presenting symptoms of DKA in children?**

Abdominal pain, nausea, vomiting, listlessness, lethargy and anorexia.

O   **Deep sighing respirations in a known diabetic are referred to as what?**

Kussmal breathing.

O   **How do you calculate the water deficit in a patient with DKA?**

The fluid deficit is estimated to be approximately 10% of the patient's weight in kilograms.

O   **How should the fluid loss be replaced over the next 24 hrs?**

TIME (hr)   REPLACEMENT FLUID   AMOUNT REPLACEDfirst 8 hrs   .9% normal
saline   1/3 of the 24hr maintenance + 1/2 of the deficitnext 16 hrs   .45% normal saline
                       2/3 of the 24 hr maintenance + 1/2 of the deficit

O   **How do you determine if a child in DKA requires HCO_3^-?**

If the $PCO_2 > (1.5 \times HCO_3^-) + 8$, the respiratory effort is incapable of compensating for the metabolic acidosis therefore HCO_3^- is needed.

O   **When should glucose be added to the IVF in the treatment of DKA?**

When the BGL reaches 300mg/dL the IVF should be changed to D5.45%NS.

O   **How often should you monitor the serum K+ in a child with DKA?**

The K+ should be checked every 4 hours until acidosis is corrected.

O   **Why do DKA patients experience changes in vision following the initiation of therapy?**

Rehydration in conjunction with the correction of hyperglycemia causes fluid shifts in the eyes with reversible lens distortion.

O   **How is hypoglycemia defined?**

A BGL less than 50 mg/dL with or without symptoms.

O   **What is the differential diagnosis for hypoglycemia?**

Malnutrition, acute diarrhea, glycogen storage disease, insulinoma, endogenous administration of insulin or oral hypoglycemics, Wilm's tumor, and sepsis.

O   **What are the hormonal effects of insulin?**

Insulin promotes glucose uptake in muscle and fat while promoting glycogenesis in the liver. Insulin inhibits lipolysis and glycogenolysis.

O   **What are the three biochemical mechanisms used by the liver to prevent hypoglycemia?**

Glycogenolysis, gluconeogenesis and ketogenesis.

❍   **What are the substances that oppose insulin's effects?**

Glucagon, cortisol, epinephrine, and growth hormone.

❍   **What are the signs and symptoms of hypoglycemia?**

They are nonspecific but may include seizures, tremulousness, confusion, palpitations, sweating, and irritability.

❍   **In patients where the diagnosis of hypoglycemia vs. hyperglycemia is uncertain, what should be the initial course of therapy?**

A glucose solution should be administered until a definitive diagnosis can be made. Temporary hypoglycemia can be fatal while temporary hyperglycemia is much less likely to significantly alter the prognosis of the patient.

❍   **What is the differential diagnosis in a child who presents with hypoglycemia without urine ketones?**

Hyperinsulinemia (exogenous or endogenous) or an enzymatic defect in the fatty acid oxidation pathway.

❍   **How is a child with hypoglycemia treated?**

Administer 2.5 ml/kg of 10% dextrose. If convulsions are present increase to 4ml/kg of 10% dextrose. Maintain the BGL using 8 mg/kg/min of a 10% dextrose solution.

❍   **What is the incidence of congenital hypothyroidism world wide?**

1 in 4,000 infants.

❍   **What is the most common cause for hypothyroidism in the neonate?**

Thyroid dysgenesis.

❍   **What is the most common thyroid anomaly in childhood?**

The thyroglossal duct cyst which is remnant of the thyroglossal duct.

❍   **Are infants born with complete thyroid agenesis symptomatic at birth?**

No. Transplacental T4 provides adequate thyroid hormone however the TSH level will still be elevated enough for detection of the abnormality.

❍   **Untreated hypothyroidism in a child leads to what condition?**

Cretinism.

❍   **What are the clinical manifestations of cretinism?**

Severe mental retardation, decreased physical growth leading to dwarfism, macroglossia and a protuberant abdomen.

❍   **A mass at the base of the tongue in a newborn with adequate T4 levels is suggestive of what disorder?**

A sublingual thyroid or a thyroglossal duct cyst.

○   **What is the possible cause for a transient congenital hypothyroidism?**

Maternal antibodies that inhibit TSH binding.

○   **How many times stronger is T3 than T4?**

Approximately three to four times stronger.

○   **What is the predominant protein that binds T4?**

Thyroxin binding globulin (TBG) binds 70% of thyroxine while the remainder is bound by transthyretin and albumin.

○   **What percent of circulating thyroxine is "free"?**

Less than 1%.

○   **What happens to the children with hyperthyroidism when exogenous TRH is administered?**

In a patient with a normal thyroid a concomitant rise in TSH would occur. In patients with hyperthyroidism however, the TRH receptors are blocked thus preventing a rise in TSH levels.

○   **What are the causes for elevated TBG levels?**

Pregnancy, newborn state, estrogens, and heroin.

○   **What enzyme is most commonly associated with a defect in thyroxine synthesis?**

The thyroid peroxidase responsible for the production of H_2O_2.

○   **What are the signs of neonatal hypothyroidism?**

Poor appetite, sluggishness, macroglossia, somnolence, large abdomen, hypothermia, molted skin, constipation, edema, and bradycardia.

○   **What is the treatment for neonatal hypothyroidism?**

Sodium-L-Thyroxine (at 10 - 15 micrograms/kg in neonates).

○   **What is the most common cause of a acquired hypothyroidism?**

Lymphocytic thyroiditis.

○   **What are the clinical manifestations of acquired hypothyroidism?**

Myxedema of the skin, cold intolerance, constipation, low pitched voice, menorrhagia, mental and physical slowing, dry skin, coarse brittle hair, and decreased energy level with increased need for sleep.

○   **What percent of children with lymphocytic thyroiditis have antimicrosomal antibodies?**

Approximately 90%.

○   **Is there a gender predominance in lymphocytic thyroiditis?**

Yes. Girls are affected 4 -7 times more frequently than boys.

○ **What is the most common clinical manifestation of lymphocytic thyroiditis?**

The appearance of a goiter.

○ **Patients with lymphocytic thyroiditis are usually hypothyroid, euthyroid, or hyperthyroid?**

The majority of patients will be euthyroid. However, many will eventually become hypothyroid while only a few will clinically manifest the symptoms of hyperthyroidism.

○ **What is Schmidt's syndrome?**

It is a type II polyglandular autoimmune disease. It involves Addison's disease and IDDM with or without lymphocytic thyroiditis.

○ **What is DeQuervain's disease?**

It is a subacute nonsupporative thyroiditis. Clinical manifestations involve a tender thyroid, fever and chills usually remitting within several months.

○ **What is the etiology of DeQuervain's thyroiditis?**

It is most likely due to a viral infection such as mumps or Coxsackie virus.

○ **What is the differential diagnosis of a congenital goiter?**

Antithyroid drugs or iodine containing medications used during pregnancy, hyperthyroid infants, iodine deficient infants and rarely congenital teratoma.

○ **Which medications are commonly found to result in sporadic goiters?**

Lithium, amiodarone and iodide containing asthma inhalers.

○ **What is a thyrotropin receptor-stimulating antibody?**

It is an antibody commonly found in Grave's disease which binds to the TSH receptor leading to thyroid stimulation and goiter production.

○ **Which HLA is associated with Grave's disease?**

HLA-DR3. The association of this HLA type represents a seven fold relative risk for Grave's disease.

○ **Is Grave's disease more common in boys or girls?**

Girls are affected five times as much as boys.

○ **What are the classical signs and symptoms of Grave's disease?**

Emotional lability, autonomic hyperactivity, exophthalmos, tremor, weight loss or increased appetite with no weight gain, diarrhea, and a goiter in nearly all affected individuals.

○ **How is Grave's disease confirmed by laboratory testing?**

One would find increased bound and free T3 and T4 with decreased TSH. Frequently, there is presence of thyroid peroxidase and TSH receptor stimulating antibodies are present.

O   **What treatment options exist for children with Grave's disease? What treatment is recommended?**

Children can be managed medically with propylthiouracil(PTU) or methimazole, surgically with a subtotal thyroidectomy or with radioiodine therapy. Medical management is the treatment of choice.

O   **What are the differences between PTU and methimazole?**

Methimazole is ten times more potent on a weight basis allowing it to be a once a day medication. PTU is predominately protein bound making it a better choice in pregnant and nursing mothers as its ability to cross the placental membrane is limited.

O   **What are the respective doses of PTU and methimazole?**

PTU is given at 5 - 10 mg/kg/d dived T.I.D. while methimazole is .5 - 1.0 mg/kg/d given either QD. or B.I.D.

O   **How much time must pass before noticing a clinical response when using medical treatment for Grave's disease?**

2 - 3 weeks.

O   **What medication is available to treat the autonomic hyperactivity associated with Grave's disease?**

Propranolol, a beta blocker dosed at .5 - 2.0 mg/kg/d divided T.I.D.

O   **What are the three largest concerns with surgical management of Grave's disease?**

Hyper or hypothyroidism depending on the amount of tissue removed, hypoparathyroidism, and vocal cord paralysis.

O   **What is the most common cause for congenital hyperthyroidism?**

Transplacental passage of thyroid receptor antibodies from a mother with Grave's disease.

O   **Name the unusual condition where an ovarian tumor produces thyroid hormone?**

Struma ovarii.

O   **What common finding is seen in nearly all infants and children with thyroid carcinoma?**

Prior irradiation to the thyroid or adjacent structures.

O   **What is the most common type of thyroid carcinoma in children?**

Papillary thyroid carcinoma. This type of cancer makes up greater than 80% of thyroid cancer in children.

O   **If fine needle aspiration of a thyroid nodule reveals parafollicular cells, what type of carcinoma should be suspected?**

Medullary carcinoma of the thyroid.

O   **What combination of medical illnesses account for multiple endocrine neoplasia (MEN) type IIA?**

Medullary carcinoma of the thyroid, adrenal medullary hyperplasia or pheochromocytoma, and parathyroid hyperplasia.

○ **What is the mode of inheritance of MEN Type IIA?**

Autosomal dominant.

○ **How is MEN Type IIA different from MEN Type IIB?**

Men Type IIB is associated with multiple neuromas. It too is autosomal dominant.

○ **What commonly occurs in the newborn whose mother suffered from hyperparathyroidism during pregnancy?**

Hypocalcemia resulting from suppression of the fetal parathyroids due to the elevated serum calcium in the maternal circulation.

○ **What are the hallmarks of polyglandular autoimmune disease type I?**

Autoimmune hypoparathyroidism, Addison's disease, and chronic mucocutaneous candidiasis.

○ **What percent of children with hyperthyroidism experience a thyroid storm?**

Approximately 1%.

○ **What are the symptoms of child suffering from a thyroid storm?**

Tachycardia, systolic hypertension, tremulousness, delirium and hyperthermia.

○ **How do you manage acute thyrotoxicosis?**

Propranolol at 10 mg/kg IV over 10 - 15 minutes for hypertension and increased metabolic rate. Lugol's iodide, 5 drops PO every eight hrs or Na+ iodide 125 - 250 mg/d IV over 24 hrs will stop thyroxine production.

○ **What measures can be taken to further reduce peripheral conversion of T4 to T3?**

Oral dexamethasone at .2 mg/kg or oral hydrocortisone 5 mg/kg.

○ **What is the differential diagnosis of acute primary adrenal insufficiency?**

Congenital adrenal hypoplasia, autoimmunity, TB, infection, trauma, and adrenal hemorrhage.

○ **What are the clinical manifestations of adrenocortical insufficiency?**

Low blood pressure, muscular weakness, weight loss, anorexia and salt craving.

○ **What emergency should be suspected in patients who present with cyanosis, cold skin, thready pulse, hypotension and tachypnea?**

Addison's crisis.

○ **What conditions have been implicated in precipitating adrenal crisis?**

Infection, trauma, fatigue, and various medications.

○ **Which symptom is most commonly seen in children with Addison's disease?**

Hypoglycemia.

O   **How is adrenal insufficiency diagnosed?**

Plasma levels of cortisol are measured before and after administration of ACTH.

O   **What is the Waterhouse-Friderichsen Syndrome?**

Primary adrenal insufficiency due to adrenal hemorrhage. It is often secondary to meningococcemia induced shock.

O   **What are the causes of secondary adrenal insufficiency?**

Diminished ACTH levels secondary to long term glucocorticoid treatment.

O   **Does the clinical presentation of adrenal insufficiency differ between primary and secondary causes?**

Yes. Primary insufficiency involves both glucocorticoids and mineralocorticoids while secondary insufficiency will only involve glucocorticoids. Primary causes involve the adrenals directly while secondary causes involve the hypothalamic-pituitary axis..

O   **Is hyperpigmentation a common finding with acute adrenal insufficiency?**

No. It is usually seen with chronic primary adrenal insufficiency.

O   **How do you manage a child in acute adrenal insufficiency?**

The two mainstays of therapy include fluid replacement and exogenous glucocorticoids.

O   **What is the maintenance dose of cortisol for infants and children suffering from adrenal insufficiency?**

The daily dose of cortisol for an infant is 5 - 10 mg/d in two to three divided doses. The dose for children and adolescents is doubled.

O   **What is the dose of glucocorticoid to be administered to a child with acute adrenal insufficiency?**

Hydrocortisone 2 mg/kg/dose q6hr. Larger doses may be needed during high stress situations.

O   **What is the most common cause of primary adrenal insufficiency?**

Autoimmune destruction of the adrenal glands.

O   **What percent of children with primary adrenal insufficiency also have another autoimmune endocrinopathy?**

45%. Most involving the thyroid gland.

O   **What is adrenoleukodystrophy?**

It is an autosomal disorder involving defective peroxisomes leading to fatty infiltration of the adrenal glands with concomitant dysfunction. It is commonly associated with CNS abnormalities.

O   **What two autosomal dominant diseases have a high prevalence of pheochromocytomas?**

Neurofibromatosis and Von Hippel-Lindau disease.

○ **What percent of pheochromocytomas in children are malignant?**

2 - 4%.

○ **What percent of pheochromocytomas in children are bilateral?**

Up to 30%.

○ **What laboratory tests will help to make the diagnosis of pheochromocytoma?**

Look for increased total 24 hr urinary catecholamines and their metabolites(i.e., epinephrine, norepinephrine, metanephrine and VMA).

○ **What are the classic signs and symptoms of pheochromocytomas?**

Paroxysmal hypertension, autonomic hyperactivity, headache, visual changes and weightloss.

○ **Which class of antihypertensive drugs are recommended for the temporary treatment of pheochromocytoma associated hypertension?**

Alpha adrenergic blocking agents like phenoxybenzamine and prazosin.

○ **How do you manage a hypertensive crisis in a child with a pheochromocytoma?**

1 mg of IV phentolamine or .5-.8mg/kg/min of sodium nitroprusside.

○ **What is a neuroblastoma?**

It is a malignant catecholamine producing tumor or early childhood. It is most commonly found in the adrenal medulla.

○ **Where is ADH synthesized? Where is it stored?**

ADH is made in the supraoptic and paraventricular nuclei of the hypothalamus. Following production it is stored in the posterior pituitary?

○ **What conditions stimulate the secretion of ADH?**

Increased serum osmolarity, hypernatremia, and decreased right atrial pressure due to hypovolemia or shock.

○ **At what decreased Na+ concentration do children generally become symptomatic?**

When the serum Na+ is less than 120 mEq/L.

○ **What are the six peptide hormones secreted from the anterior and posterior pituitary gland respectively?**

Anterior pituitary hormones include; growth hormone, prolactin, thyroid stimulating hormone, and corticotropin. Posterior pituitary hormones include oxytocin and vasopressin.

○ **What is panhypopituitarism?**

A condition where growth hormone, TSH, ACTH, FSH and LH are all abnormally low due to a non functioning or absent pituitary gland.

O   **What hormones need to be replaced in a patient with panhypopituitarism?**

Hydrocortisone, growth hormone, thyroid hormone, and estrogen or testosterone at puberty.

O   **What syndrome is likely to be present in a 7-year-old child who presents with nausea, vomiting, and a single seizure with laboratory results consistent with hyponatremia and increased urine osmolarity?**

The syndrome of inappropriate antidiuretic hormone (SIADH).

O   **What is SIADH?**

It is a the syndrome of inappropriate ADH(antidiuretic hormone) secretion. It occurs when the plasma vasopressin levels are abnormally elevated for the corresponding plasma osmolarity.

O   **What is the most common cause of SIADH in children?**

Infection. 50% of children with bacterial meningitis have concomitant SIADH.

O   **Name three drugs whose side effects include SIADH.**

Vincristine, vinblastine and cyclophosphamide.

O   **What are the symptoms of SIADH?**

When the serum Na+ is between 110 and 120 mEq/L one may see nausea, vomiting, irritability, confusion and mental status changes. Once the Na+ goes below 110 mEq/L, seizures and coma may occur.

O   **How is the diagnosis of SIADH made in children?**

The physician should look for hyponatremia and decreased serum osmolarity in the presence of increased urine Na+ and urine osmolarity.

O   **How is SIADH treated?**

Most important is treating the underlying condition. Fluid restriction and demeclocycline have been proven to increase serum Na+. In emergent situations, furosemide, in conjunction with 300 ml/M2 of 1.5% NaCl may be used.

O   **What is the emergent treatment for a hyponatremic child suffering from SIADH?**

3 ml/kg of 3% saline Q10-20 minutes until the symptoms resolve. A single dose of 1 mg/kg of furosemide may be used. 5 - 10 mg/kg of phenytoin IV can be used to inhibit ADH secretion as well as help to prophylax against possible seizures. Treating the underlying condition however is still the most important consideration.

O   **What is the danger of correcting the Na+ too vigorously?**

Central pontine myelinolysis.

O   **What is central diabetes insipidus?**

A lack of ADH secretion which results in an inability to concentrate the urine despite functioning kidneys.

○ **What specific disease process should be considered in a child who presents with dehydration, hypernatremia, decreased urine osmolarity and a high level of circulating ADH?**

Nephrogenic diabetes insipidus

○ **How is the diagnosis of diabetes insipidus made in a child?**

By finding hypernatremia, increased serum osmolarity and decreased urine osmolarity .

○ **Are central causes of diabetes insipidus generally acquired or congenital?**

Acquired.

○ **What is the most common mode of inheritance of nephrogenic diabetes insipidus?**

X linked recessive.

○ **If a child presents with hypernatremia and dehydration, how is the free water deficiency calculated?**

Free water = [Na+ measured - 145 mEq/L] x 4 ml/kg x (wt in kg before dehydration).

○ **What is the danger of vigorously hydrating a patient who has hypernatremia due to diabetes insipidus?**

Cerebral edema, seizures and death.

○ **What additional adjuncts can be used in addition to volume replacement in a patient with diabetes insipidus?**

Intranasal administration of DDAVP at 0.4 g/kg.

○ **What should the physician do if the patient fails to respond to the initial dose of DDAVP?**

The patient should be given a second dose from a different bottle. DDAVP may fail due to inappropriate administration or due to outdated preparations that have lost their potency.

○ **What should the physician consider if the patient with diabetes insipidus continues to diurese despite repeated doses of DDAVP?**

The patient most probably has nephrogenic diabetes insipidus which is due to unresponsive kidney receptors for ADH regardless of whether the ADH is endogenous or exogenous.

○ **If nephrogenic diabetes insipidus is assumed, what further pharmacological treatment may be helpful?**

Thiazide diuretics have a paradoxical effect in patients with diabetes insipidus and may work in decreasing fluid losses.

○ **How frequently should the physician monitor the serum Na+ and urine osmolarity when correcting a hypernatremic state in a child with diabetes insipidus?**

At least every two hours.

○ **What is acromegaly?**

A condition resulting from overproduction of growth hormone in children with closed epiphyses.

❍ **How does acromegaly differ from gigantism?**

Acromegaly occurs in children with closed epiphyses while gigantism is found in children whose epiphyses are still open.

❍ **What are the clinical manifestations of acromegaly?**

Coarse facial features, enlarged tongue, enlargement of the distal extremities and hypogonadism.

❍ **What medical modality can be used to suppress exogenous growth hormone production?**

Octreotide, an analogue of somatostatin.

❍ **What pituitary tumor is most common among adolescents?**

Prolactinomas.

❍ **What is the primary hormone responsible for the initiation of puberty in children?**

Gonadotropin-releasing hormone(GnRH).

❍ **What is Cushing's disease?**

Pituitary adenomas leading to increased ACTH secretion with resultant bilateral adrenal hyperplasia and elevated cortisol levels.

❍ **Is Cushing's disease different from Cushing's syndrome?**

Cushing's disease results from pituitary adenomas while Cushing's syndrome is elevated cortisol levels from various causes including; paraneoplastic syndromes, primary adrenal tumors, and exogenous use of cortisol.

❍ **How is Cushing's syndrome diagnosed?**

Using the dexamethasone suppression test. Patients with ACTH dependent Cushing's demonstrate suppression with the larger doses of dexamethasone while those with ectopic tumors cannot be suppressed at any level.

❍ **What is the most common cause of excess cortisol production in infants?**

A functioning adrenocortical tumor.

❍ **What are the clinical manifestations of primary aldosteronism?**

Hyperplasia of the zona glomerulosa leading to hypertension, sodium and water retention, hypokalemia and decreased serum renin levels.

❍ **What is hypergonadotropic hypogonadism in males?**

Primary hypogonadism resulting from a defect in androgen production often leading to pseudohermaphrodism.

❍ **What are the clinical manifestations of primary hypogonadism?**

Failure of development of the secondary sexual characteristics with abnormally small penis and testes.

❍ **What is hypogonadotropic hypogonadism?**

A delayed onset of puberty due to decreased levels of FSH and LH with functioning ovaries or testes.

O   **How is the diagnosis of primary hypogonadism made?**

The levels of FSH and LH are abnormally elevated for the corresponding age. Testosterone levels remain low and show little response to the administration of hCG.

O   **What is the deficient hormone in secondary hypogonadism?**

FSH or LH. The defect is in the pituitary rather than in the testes or ovaries.

O   **What is Kallmann's syndrome?**

Hypogonadotropic hypogonadism with anosmia.

O   **Is the pituitary gland responsible for parathyroid regulation?**

No. Unlike the thyroid gland, the parathyroids are not regulated by the pituitary gland but rather by circulating calcium levels.

O   **What is the most common cause of childhood hyperparathyroidism?**

A single parathyroid adenoma.

O   **What are the clinical manifestations of hyperparathyroidism regardless of cause?**

Anorexia, nausea, vomiting, constipation, polydipsia, polyuria, fever, weight loss, kidney stones and muscular weakness.

O   **Explain the difference between primary and secondary hyperparathyroidism?**

In primary hyperparathyroidism the defect is in the parathyroid gland i.e., an adenoma or hyperplasia while in secondary hyperparathyroidism the elevated PTH is a physiologic response to a low calcium level usually as a result of renal disease.

O   **What are the diagnostic laboratory findings seen in hyperparathyroidism?**

Elevated serum calcium and PTH with concomitant decreased phosphorous levels.

O   **What is Von Recklinghausen's disease?**

Hyperparathyroidism leading to cystic changes in bone due to osteoclastic resorption with fibrous replacement forming non-neoplastic "brown tumors".

O   **What is the most common cause for secondary hyperparathyroidism in children?**

Chronic renal disease. The formation of the active form of vitamin D takes place in the kidney. With diseased kidneys the active form of vitamin D is not made resulting in decreased intestinal absorption of calcium.

O   **What is pseudohypoparathyroidism?**

It is an autosomal recessive disorder characterized by kidney unresponsiveness to PTH, shortened fourth and fifth metacarpals and metatarsals, and short stature all occurring without evidence or parathyroid dysfunction.

○   **What is the glucose concentration in most standard oral rehydration solutions?**

According to the World Health Organization (WHO) 2% is optimal.

○   **What disorder has autosomal dominant inheritance and is associated with episodic weakness or paralysis along with transient alterations in serum potassium?**

Periodic paralysis, which is most commonly associated with episodes of hypokalemia but may occur with hyperkalemia as well. Patients are normal between attacks, however the condition becomes progressively worse in adulthood.

○   **How much water should a newborn baby receive in addition to infant formula or breast feeding?**

In normal situations newborns need no additional free water. In fact excess free water is the major cause for water intoxication in infancy and the development of subsequent hyponatremic seizures.

○   **What are the 3 most common side effects of Depo-Provera?**

Menstrual irregularities, amenorrhea, and weight gain.

○   **A child with adrenal insufficiency also has hyperpigmentation of the skin. Is his adrenal insufficiency most likely to be primary or secondary?**

Primary. This would be due to the increased output of POMC (pro-opiomelanocorticotropin).

○   **What is the cosyntropin stimulation test used for?**

To detect whether there is cortisol present in the adrenal gland.

○   **What is the best test of the hypothalamic-pituitary-adrenal axis?**

Metyrapone test. This inhibits 11-hydroxylase (which converts 11-deoxycortisol to cortisol).

○   **Are girls or boys more likely to be diagnosed early with congenital adrenal hyperplasia (CAH)?**

Girls, due to the presence of ambiguous genitalia.

○   **Which steroid preparation has the highest mineralocorticoid potency?**

Fludrocortisone.

○   **A child with a past history of frequent viral infections is currently displaying the signs and symptoms associated with hypoparathyroidism. What is your presumptive diagnosis?**

DiGeorge syndrome. This is a congenital T-cell deficiency secondary to aberrant embryonic development of the third and fourth branchial arches.

○   **What is the treatment of choice for symptomatic hypercalcemia (>15 mg/dL)?**

Isotonic saline, Lasix (1 mg/kg IV Q6 hrs), and ECG monitoring.

○   **The water deprivation test can be used to diagnose what syndrome?**

Diabetes insipidus

O   **A 3-year-old girl has a cafe-au-lait spot with a "coast of Maine" appearance, polyostotic fibrous dysplasia and precocious puberty. What is your diagnosis?**

McCune-Albright syndrome. This is a disease characterized by autonomous hyperfunction of multiple glands in association with the above mentioned abnormalities.

O   **What is Werner syndrome?**

MEN type I- this is usually comprised of pancreatic islet cell carcinoma, anterior pituitary adenoma (most commonly a prolactinoma), and a parathyroid adenoma.

O   **What is the insulin requirements of post-pubertal individuals?**

0.5-1.0 units/kg/day, obviously with individual adjustment depending on level of activity and caloric intake.

O   **What is the Somogyi phenomenon?**

Rebound hyperglycemia after an incidence of hypoglycemia. It is believed to be due to an increased response of counter-regulatory hormones as a response to insulin-induced hypoglycemia. Tighter glucose control raises the risk of this occurring.

O   **What is the dawn phenomenon?**

Hyperglycemia in the dawn hours (5-9 am) without a preceding hypoglycemic episode. This is thought to be due partly from the early morning rise in growth hormone and cortisol, which you'll recall antagonize the effects of insulin.

O   **How long after the diagnosis of diabetes are microscopic changes detectable in the glomerular basement membrane?**

2 years.

O   **How long after the onset of proteinuria do most diabetics require dialysis?**

About 5 years. The mortality is about 12 years after the onset of proteinuria.

O   **What drugs can be given to protect against deterioration in renal function in patients with diabetic nephropathy?**

ACE inhibitors.

O   **The HbA1C level can be used as an indicator of overall glucose level over what time period?**

The life of a red blood cell - 120 days.

O   **What is the cause of hypoglycemic unawareness?**

The capacity to release catecholamines in response to hypoglycemia can become diminished in patients with diabetes. As the signs and symptoms of hypoglycemia are mostly catecholamine induced, this results in lack of awareness of the low levels of blood sugars by the patient.

O   **What are the indications for bicarbonate therapy for children with DKA?**

Symptomatic hyperkalemia, cardiac instability, and inadequate ventilatory compensation.

O   **In a child with resolving DKA, when do you cease insulin infusion?**

When the blood sugar is <300 mg/dL, pH is > 7.3, and bicarbonate level is > 15 mEq/L.

○ **Is a constitutional delay in reaching puberty or menarche familial?**

Yes.

○ **How can radiographs assist in differentiating between genetic disease and familial short stature?**

They can be used to compare chronological age versus bone age, which will be comparable in familial short stature. There are standards of normal skeletal maturation by radiograph. The rate of bony maturation can be determined by a single bone age determination (i.e. left hand and wrist).

○ **A child is brought in obtunded and with acute hypoglycemia, what should be the first treatment modality?**

IV glucose infusion (2-3 mg/kg of $D_{10}W$ or 1ml/kg of $D_{25}W$).

○ **A newborn with ambiguous genitalia and midline abnormalities (i.e. cleft palate), most likely has a dysfunction of which gland(s)?**

Hypothalamus and pituitary.

○ **What is the most common cause of acquired hypothyroidism in the U.S.?**

Chronic Lymphocytic Thyroiditis (Hashimoto's)

○ **How do most patients with Hashimoto's thyroiditis present?**

Asymptomatic goiter.

○ **What is the prognosis of euthyroid Hashimoto's thyroiditis?**

About half of these patients will have complete resolution, the other half will eventually need thyroxine replacement therapy.

○ **What is the most common cause of hyperthyroidism?**

Grave's disease.

○ **What are the three types of therapy available for children with Grave's disease?**

I^{131} therapy, anti-thyroid medication (Methimazole, carbimazole or Propylthiouracil) or sub-total thyroidectomy.

○ **How concerned should you be over an incidental finding of a solitary thyroid nodule in a 12-year-old?**

Fairly. Though these "incidentaloma" are usually benign in adults, they tend to be cancerous in a much larger percentage of children.

○ **What should be the first test you order for this child with a single thyroid nodule?**

Fine needle aspiration. Only if this is suspicious or inconclusive do you order a thyroid uptake scan.

❍   **In a child with suspected hyperthyroidism, what would you expect to see from the following tests: Total T4, T3 Resin Uptake, and Free Thyroxine Index?**

All would be increased.

❍   **What is the "DKA Triad"?**

Uncontrollable hyperglycemia, ketosis and acidemia.

❍   **What are the diagnostic criteria for DKA?**

Blood glucose >250 mg/dL, an arterial pH <7.3, and a bicarbonate level <15 mEq/L.

❍   **A newborn infant is brought to your office with a history of poor feeding, vomiting and convulsions. What five causes need to be considered?**

Hypoglycemia, hypocalcemia, infection, pyloric stenosis, and metabolic disorder.

❍   **The child in the above question was unresponsive to intravenous glucose and calcium, and septic workup is underway. If you are considering a metabolic disorder, what would be the next appropriate step?**

Obtain plasma ammonia, pH and CO_2 levels. If acidotic, consider organic acidemias. If all are normal, consider galactosemia or aminoacidopathies. A high ammonia and normal pH and CO_2 should make you consider urea cycle defects.

❍   **What is the most common form of inheritance of metabolic disorders?**

Autosomal recessive

❍   **What clinical manifestations are suggestive of inborn errors of metabolism?**

Unexplained mental retardation, convulsions, developmental delay, unusual odors, episodes of vomiting, hepatomegaly and renal stones.

❍   **What are the clinical findings in a child with classic PKU?**

Blond hair and blue eyes are common. A mousy/musty odor on body and in urine. An eczematoid rash, microcephaly, and hyperactive DTR's are also commonly seen.

❍   **What is the criteria for diagnosis of classic PKU?**

Plasma phenylalanine level above 20; a normal plasma tyrosine level; normal tetrahydrobiopterin (BH4); increased urinary levels of phenylpyruvic and o-hydroxyphenylacetic acids (metabolites of phenylalanine).

❍   **T/F: Patients with hyperphenylalaninemia can be treated with only a diet low in phenylalanine?**

False. Some patients with hyperphenylalaninemia have deficiency in the cofactor BH4 (tetrahydrobiopterin) also need BH4 supplementation as well as neurotransmitter precursors to avoid neurological damage.

❍   **What is the cause of death of most children with tyrosinemia?**

Hepatic failure. In children with hepatitis and/or evidence of hepatic failure, tyrosinemia needs to be considered, along with galactosemia, hereditary fructose intolerance and giant cell hepatitis.

❍   **What ethnic group has the highest incidence of tyrosinemia?**

French-Canadian ancestry is found in most reported patients with this disease.

O   **What are the two major forms of generalized albinism (oculocutaneous)?**

Tyrosinase positive (type II), which is most common, and tyrosinase negative (Type I), which is most severe. They are classified according to whether or not a hair bulb can produce melanin when incubated in a medium with tyrosine.

O   **What are the two main clinical manifestations seen in alcaptonuria?**

Arthritis and ochronosis.

O   **What is ochronosis?**

A darkening of tissue. Seen as dark spots on the sclera, cornea and ear cartilage.

O   **High levels of what compound in the urine confirms the diagnosis of alcaptonuria?**

Homogentisic acid.

O   **What two disease entities commonly present with tall, thin body habitus, arachnodactyly, scoliosis, ectopia lentis, and pectus carinatum or excavatum?**

Marfan's syndrome and Homocystinuria Type I.

O   **What clinical and laboratory findings are commonly seen with early-onset severe galactosemia?**

Jaundice, hypoglycemia, liver enzyme elevation (AST and ALT) and *E. coli* sepsis.

O   **What is the most common disorder of tryptophan metabolism?**

Hartnup disorder, a usually benign and often asymptomatic disease.

O   **A mother of a four month old infant has noticed that the diaper is blue when the child has a bowel movement. What causes this?**

This condition is most likely from indicanuria, a condition where tryptophan is poorly absorbed, most commonly from bowel stasis, and oxidized by bacteria and enzymatic action to indican.

O   **What is the most remarkable routine laboratory finding in patients with Maple Syrup Urine Disease (MSUD)?**

Severe metabolic acidosis.

O   **The absence or presence of what three features are used to distinguish the cause of organic acidemias?**

Ketosis, skin manifestations, and characteristic odor.

O   **What is the treatment for a child in a state of acute hyperammonemia?**

Clear the ammonia with benzoate, phenylacetate, arginine, and, if ineffective, then dialysis. Also, keep child from going into catabolic state by supplying all nutrients, electrolytes, fluid and calories.

O   **Routine labs on a premature, SGA(small for gestational age) baby reveals ammonia level of 45uM. What should you do?**

Nothing. A majority of these children have a mild, transient increase. They have no neurological sequelae.

O   **An MRI of the cerebral hemispheres of a 2-year-old boy with macrocephaly shows diffuse degeneration of the white matter. What disease entities should top your list of differentials?**

Canavan Disease (defect in aspartic acid metabolism most common in Ashkenazi Jews) and Alexander disease.

O   **A child is born with a epicanthal folds, a high forehead with shallow supraorbital ridges, low/broad nasal ridge, micrognathia, weakness, seizures and corneal clouding. What two syndromes should you suspect?**

Down's syndrome and Zellweger syndrome

O   **What is the life expectancy of a newborn with Zellweger syndrome?**

A few months.

O   **What causes Zellweger cerebrohepatorenal syndrome?**

Absence of, or reduction in, peroxisomes with peroxisome enzyme abnormalities.

O   **What clinical manifestations are most commonly seen in neonates with disorders of peroxisomes?**

Seizures and hypotonia.

O   **An MRI of 5-year-old hyperactive child's brain shows symmetric demyelinative lesions in the periventricular white matter of the parietal and occipital lobes. This is classic for what disease entity?**

X-linked adrenoleukodystrophy (ALD).

O   **What other test would you want to order in this patient?**

ACTH stimulation test (abnormal in 85%). Diagnosis is confirmed by high levels of very long chain fatty acids in cultured fibroblasts, RBC's and plasma.

O   **What drug can be given to relieve the painful muscle spasms associated with ALD?**

Baclofen (*Lioresal*), 5mg BID up to 25mg QID.

O   **What therapeutic measures are suggested for children with ALD?**

"Lorenzo's Oil" (4:1 glycerol trioleate and glyceryl trierucate) and bone marrow transplantation (in certain circumstances).

O   **When should you consider bone marrow transplantation in children with ALD?**

When there are early neurological changes and the MRI shows brain abnormalities consistent with ALD.

O   **Of Niemann-Pick Disease, Gaucher disease, and Tay-Sachs, which does not have CNS involvement?**

Gaucher. These disease differ in, among other things, where the sphingolipid is stored. In Gaucher disease, it is only in the periphery, in Tay-Sachs only in CNS, and in Niemann-Pick disease it is stored in both.

○ **A newborn has hepatosplenomegaly, a cherry-red spot in the macula, an umbilical hernia, a rash, macroglossia, and coarse facial features. What would you look for on the x-rays of this child?**

Dysostosis multiplex. This is a spectrum of specific x-ray findings seen with certain metabolic abnormalities. Findings include a large calvarium with large sella turcica and vertebral changes with anterior beaking. This child has the infantile form of GM_1 gangliosidosis.

○ **In a physical exam of an infant you notice a cherry-red spot on the macula, but no hepatomegaly. What disease is this most probably due to?**

Tay-Sachs. Although many sphingolipidoses manifest themselves with the cherry red spot on the macula, Tay Sachs is the only one that is limited to the CNS.

○ **Tay-Sachs disease occurs most commonly among people of what descent?**

Ashkenazi Jews.

○ **What are the first signs of Tay-Sachs disease?**

Hyperacusis, decreased eye-contact, hypotonia, and a cherry-red spot of the macula.

○ **What enzyme is deficient in Tay-Sachs disease?**

Hexosaminidase A.

○ **Both A and B isoenzymes of *Hexosaminidase* are deficient in what disease?**

Sandhoff Disease.

○ **What is the defect in Niemann-Pick Disease (Type A)?**

Sphingomyelinase.

○ **What are the initial manifestations of Niemann-Pick Disease (Type A)?**

Failure to thrive and difficulty feeding. These usually appear between three and four months.

○ **What is the expected life span of a child diagnosed with Niemann-Pick Disease (Type B)?**

The child is expected to have a normal life span. This form of sphingomyelinase deficiency is benign as there is no CNS involvement.

○ **What is the defect in Gaucher disease?**

Beta-glucosidase is deficient. This leads to accumulation of glucocerebroside in the reticuloendothelial system.

○ **What is the first sign of Gaucher disease?**

Splenomegaly. Lab findings include anemia, leukocytosis, and thrombocytosis.

○ **Gaucher disease occurs most commonly among people of what descent?**

Ashkenazi Jews (1 in 500, making it 7-8 times more common in this population than Tay-Sachs).

○ **What is the current treatment for Gaucher disease?**

Enzyme replacement therapy. *Ceredase* or *Cerezyme* at 8-30 units/Kg/2 wks IV.

○ **How do infantile and juvenile forms of Gaucher disease differ from classic Gaucher disease?**

They both involve the CNS.

○ **What is the mode of inheritance of Fabry disease?**

X-linked recessive

○ **What is the enzyme deficiency in Fabry disease?**

Alpha-galactosidase

○ **T/F: Mental retardation is not seen in Fabry disease.**

True.

○ **What organ systems are affected by Fabry disease?**

Musculoskeletal (pain in extremities), cardiac (mitral insufficiency), renal (kidney failure), and integumentary (angiokeratomas).

○ **A 6-year-old girl has begun having myoclonic seizures, and is complaining of visual disturbances. Physical exam is unremarkable except for retinitis pigmentosa. You suspect what disease of lipid metabolism?**

Batten disease. Diagnosis is established by noting increased amount of dolichol in the urine.

○ **An 18 month old child is brought in for examination of nodules and painful swelling over many joints. There are not, however, any findings of rheumatoid arthritis. What do you do next?**

Order an assay of WBC's for ceramidase activity to rule out Farber disease.

○ **Children should be considered hypercholesterolemic if their plasma cholesterol is above what percentile?**

75th. Above this they are at risk for heart disease as adults.

○ **What children should be screened for hypercholesterolemia?**

Those with family history of a total cholesterol level >240 mg/dL, and those with other risk factors that make them more susceptible for coronary heart disease.

○ **What is the equation for calculating the LDL cholesterol levels?**

LDL cholesterol = total cholesterol - [HDL cholesterol + (total triglycerides/5)]. Levels greater than 130 are considered elevated (for this equation to be accurate, the triglyceride level must be below 400 mg/dL).

○ **What is the Step 1 (Prudent) diet?**

For dietary management of hyperlipidemia and hypercholesterolemia. In this diet, 30% of total calories should be fat (in all forms, divided equally), with a maximum of 100 mg of cholesterol/ 1000 calories. Not for children under 2.

O   **What is the step II diet?**

As above, only more stringent. Less than 7% of calories as saturated fat, and less than 66 mg cholesterol/1000 calories (max 200mg/24 hrs). The ideal goal in management by dietary means is level below 110 mg/dL.

O   **Why is it not advisable to institute fat-limiting diets in children under 2 years old?**

Their rate of growth demands more calories, including fats. Additionally, their CNS systems are developing and they need the fats for their myelin, among other things.

O   **What is the mainstay of therapy for children with familial hypercholesterolemia (FH)?**

Appropriate diet along with cholestyramine or colestipol resin.

O   *Xanthoma striate palmaris* **is seen in what condition?**

These xanthoma seen on the palm of the hand occur in familial dysbetalipoproteinemia.

O   **Why are patients with Tangier disease at increased risk for coronary heart disease?**

The defects in this disease are abnormal and reduced HDL particles. Thus, these patients do not benefit from the protective effects of HDL.

O   **What is the most common familial disorder of lipoprotein metabolism?**

Familial Combined Hyperlipidemia (FCHL) is now more commonly detected than Familial Hypercholesterolemia. Both are dominantly inherited.

O   **A newborn infant presents with failure to thrive, jaundice, cataracts, ascites, and hepatosplenomegaly. What are these infants at risk for?**

The diagnosis in this child is most likely galactosemia. These infants are at high risk for *E. coli* sepsis, which is often the initial presentation.

O   **What triad is commonly found in patients with galactosemia secondary to a deficiency of galactokinase?**

Cataracts, galactosemia and galacturia.

O   **Of Clinitest, Clinistix or Testape, which urine test will pick up the reducing substance to establish the preliminary diagnosis of galactosemia?**

Clinitest

O   **T/F: Hereditary fructose intolerance can be diagnosed easily by doing a fructose tolerance test.**

False. Such a test may lead to hypoglycemia, shock and death. This is bad. Detection of urinary reducing substances by tests such as Clinitest, followed by chromatography will reveal the elevated fructose.

O   **A 12-year-old child complains of easy fatigue and severe muscle cramps well above that of his peers, after strenuous exercise. What enzyme deficiencies might produce these symptoms?**

Deficiencies of either muscle *phosphoglycerate mutase* or muscle type *lactate dehydrogenase* (LDH).

O   **What is MERRF?**

Myoclonus epilepsy with ragged-red fibers. This is one of the types of infantile myopathies thought to result from deficiencies of enzymes possibly in the mitochondrial respiratory chain. It is diagnosed under the rubric of congenital idiopathic lactic acidosis.

O   **An infusion of what chemical can correct a life-threatening attack of hyperlactic acidemia?**

THAM (tris-hydroxymethol aminomethane) IV.

O   **What clinical symptoms characterize Leigh subacute necrotizing encephalopathy (SNE)?**

Optic atrophy, seizures, vomiting, lactic acidosis, psychomotor retardation, and hypotonia.

O   **What should you suspect in an infant with early morning convulsions with hyperketonemia and hypoglycemia?**

Glycogen synthetase deficiency (GSD type 0)

O   **Generally speaking, what should you suspect in a newborn with ketonuria and acidosis?**

An inborn error of metabolism.

O   **A child with urine that smells like cabbage should be investigated for what inborn error of metabolism?**

Tyrosinemia type I

O   **Patients with disorders of which biochemical pathways are more likely to present with hepatomegaly in the acute stages?**

Disorders of fatty acid or carbohydrate metabolism.

O   **What cholesterol level is considered high for children and adolescents?**

>200

O   **In children, what is the most common form of hyperlipidemia?**

Type IIa (familial hypercholesterolemia with increased cholesterol and LDL)

O   **What type of hyperlipidemia is most likely to present in childhood?**

Type I (hyperlipoproteinemia).

O   **What is the defect in Type IIa hyperlipidemia?**

Lack of functioning LDL receptors.

O   **How does Type I hyperlipidemia usually present?**

Hepatosplenomegaly with recurrent abdominal pain.

O   **What is the most common lipid storage disease?**

Gaucher disease.

❍ **In expectant mothers with PKU who are not maintaining a phenylalanine free diet, what is the risk of fetal injury?**

100%.

❍ **What is the most common cause of a positive PKU blood screen test in a premature infant?**

Hyperphenylalaninemia from transient tyrosinemia of the newborn.

❍ **In premature infants with a positive PKU test, how does administration of vitamin C help?**

It increases metabolism of tyrosine and phenylalanine.

❍ **The child with dark urine in the diaper, ochronosis, and degenerative arthritis likely has what metabolic disorder?**

Alkaptonuria.

❍ **How do you clinically distinguish between Marfan's syndrome and homocystinuria?**

By examining the joints, which are normal to contracted in homocystinuria, and hyperextended in Marfan's syndrome.

❍ **Which has the worse prognosis for the kidneys: cystinuria or cystinosis?**

Cystinosis, as it usually progresses to renal failure

❍ **What causes the "blue diaper" syndrome?**

Tryptophan malabsorption.

❍ **Most females with classic galactosemia treated with galactose-free diets still suffer what complication?**

Ovarian insufficiency.

❍ **What metabolic derangement is commonly seen in hereditary fructose intolerance?**

Hypophosphatemia.

❍ **What EKG findings are classically seen in Pompe disease?**

Very large QRS complexes in all leads and a shortened PR interval, due to the intrinsic cardiomyopathy {note: this disorder is sometimes referred to as Glycogen Storage Disease (GSD) type II}.

❍ **A patient who develops severe cramps after exercise and increasing fatigue is noted to have normal lactate levels and low post-exertional lactate levels. What 2 metabolic diseases should you suspect?**

McArdle disease and Tarui disease.

❍ **What tests are used to diagnose the different organic acidemias?**

Gas chromatography and mass spectrometry.

❍ **Before the commonly described self-destructive behavior seen in Lesch-Nyhan syndrome is seen, what features have already manifested themselves in the first year of life?**

Hypotonia, frequent vomiting, dystonia, and chorea.

❍ **The mother of a child with "the flu" wants to give him Pepto-Bismol to relieve his upset stomach. Should you let her?**

No, because of the theoretical risk of "Reye's syndrome" from the bismuth subsalicylates.

❍ **What is that funky name for the ocular abnormalities seen in Wilson's disease?**

Kayser-Fleischer rings.

❍ **What is the drug of choice for patients with Wilson's disease?**

D-penicillamine.

❍ **In patients with Wilson's disease and hypersensitivity reactions to d-penicillamine, what can you give as an alternate treatment?**

Trientine.

❍ **Why do females with porphyry encounter greater problems than their male counterparts?**

Estrogen is an inducer of ALA-synthase, the rate-limiting step in heme biosynthesis.

❍ **Which metabolic disease in the fetus can lead to maternal acute fatty liver of pregnancy?**

Long chain 3-hydroxy acyl coA dehydrogenase deficiency.

❍ **What metabolic defect can present as hypoketotic hypoglycemia?**

Medium chain acyl coA dehydrogenase deficiency (NCAD).

❍ **Zellweger syndrome is a disorder of what organelle?**

The peroxisome.

❍ **What is "Lorenzo's oil" used to treat?**

Adrenoleukodystrophy (a.k.a. Lou Gehrig's disease).

❍ **What acid base disorder is commonly seen in patients with mutations of mitochondrial DNA?**

Persistent lactic acidosis.

❍ **What is Mela's syndrome?**

Mitochondrial encephalopathy with lactic acidosis and strokes.

❍ **What is the most common procedure to diagnose inborn errors of metabolism prenatally?**

Amniocentesis for amniocyte culture or chorionic villi sampling.

❍ **Can Wilson's disease cause rickets?**

Yes, by causing a phosphaturic state.

O   **What is the definition of malnutrition?**

A nutritional deficit associated with increase risk of adverse clinical events, and decreased risk of such events when corrected.

O   **What is the primary goal of nutritional support in critically ill patients?**

To provide usable substrates to meet energy needs, conserve lean body mass, and restore physiologic homeostasis.

O   **What proportion of critically ill and injured patients are catabolic or hypermetabolic?**

Nearly all.

O   **Are immunocompetence and vital organ function dependent upon nutritional support?**

Absolutely. Both are secondary goals of nutritional support.

O   **What is the predominant energy source used during starvation by a healthy subject?**

Lipids.

O   **How long does the body's reserve of carbohydrates last during starvation?**

Glycogen stores are consumed within 24 hours, less in young children.

O   **Does the metabolic rate increase or decrease during starvation in a healthy subject?**

Decrease.

O   **Are adaptation mechanisms seen with starvation similar to those seen in critically ill patients?**

No. There is impaired protein conservation and a persistent hypermetabolic response in the critically ill patient.

O   **With the onset of critical illness, what factors are thought to raise resting energy expenditure and protein turnover?**

Catecholamines and cortisol.

O   **How does the insulin resistance associated with critical illness affect substrate use?**

Insulin resistance decreases the peripheral use of glucose and increases proteolysis.

O   **Is there any rationale for overfeeding or underfeeding critically ill patients?**

No. Both have been shown to be detrimental. The goal is to meet the metabolic needs of the patient.

O   **What is the utility of anthropometric (e.g., weight change), biochemical (e.g., serum albumin level), or immunologic (e.g., absolute lymphocyte count) indices as a measures of nutritional status in the critical care setting?**

Low. Too many other factors such as fluid retention, changes in protein synthesis priorities, and underlying infections make these indices less reliable than in otherwise healthy patients.

○   **What are the serum half-lives of albumin and prealbumin?**

18 days and 2 to 3 days, respectively.

○   **What two methods are frequently used to assess nutritional status in critically ill patients?**

Indirect calorimetry and nitrogen balance.

○   **As a patient's FIO$_2$ requirements increases, is indirect calorimetry more or less accurate in measuring energy expenditure?**

Less.

○   **What other factors are sources of errors with indirect calorimetry?**

Air leak from endotracheal tubes and the need for extrapolation of measurements to 24 hours.

○   **What is the recommended starting point for protein needs in hypermetabolic critically ill patients?**

Approximately 1-3 g/kg/day.

○   **What is the goal of protein delivery?**

To achieve a positive nitrogen balance.

○   **What is the optimal calorie-to-nitrogen ratio for critically ill patients?**

100:1 to 200:1

○   **What is the recommended starting point for non-protein calories needs for hypermetabolic critically ill patients?**

25 kcal/kg ideal body weight/day.

○   **What is the most common manifestation of excessive carbohydrate administration?**

Hyperglycemia.

○   **Can lipid emulsions be useful in patients needing volume restriction or demonstrating carbohydrate intolerance?**

Yes. Lipids are calorie dense compared to dextrose solutions.

○   **What minimum percent of total calories should be supplied as lipid to prevent fatty acid deficiency?**

Five percent of total calories at minimum.

○   **How long does it take non-stressed patients receiving lipid-free total parenteral nutrition (TPN) to demonstrate evidence of essential fatty acid deficiency?**

Within four weeks. Hypermetabolic patients within ten days.

○   **Can lipids administered parenterally hurt cellular immunity?**

There is data to suggest lipids cause reticuloendothelial dysfunction and immune suppression.

❍   **What clinical symptoms are seen with hypophosphatemia brought on by refeeding a malnourished patient?**

Weakness and congestive heart failure.

❍   **Which form of protein, peptides or amino acids, is more uniformly and efficiently absorbed from the gut?**

Peptides.

❍   **What is the main energy source of enterocyte?**

Glutamine.

❍   **Besides an energy source, what role does glutamine play in the gut?**

It is thought to be important in maintaining intestinal structure and function.

❍   **How much glutamine has been included in standard amino acid solutions used with total parenteral nutrition (TPN)?**

None, due to its instability in parenteral solutions.

❍   **Is glutamine an essential amino acid?**

No. However, during times of metabolic stress, intracellular glutamine stores are markedly depleted indicating supplementation may be beneficial.

❍   **Arginine, a semi-essential amino acid, is considered to be vital to what body system?**

The immune system.

❍   **Can branched-chain amino acids improve the outcome in critically ill patients?**

No. Some suggest it may be helpful in patients with hepatic encephalopathy.

❍   **Have immunoenriched diets, containing substrates such as omega-3 fish oils, arginine, and RNA nucleotides, been found to improve outcome?**

Yes, a number of recent studies suggest improvement using enteral immunoenriched formulas.

❍   **Which is the preferred route for the delivery of nutrition, enteral or parenteral?**

The enteral route, although there is still some debate.

❍   **When should nutritional support be started?**

As soon as a hypermetabolic state (e.g., trauma or sepsis), underlying malnutrition, or an expected delay in resuming an oral diet of > 5-10 days is recognized.

❍   **Has early initiation of enteral feedings been shown to decrease septic complications in trauma patients compared to early parenteral nutrition?**

Yes. It appears those most severely injured gain the greatest benefit.

❍   **What complications are associated with enteral nutrition?**

Complications involving routes of access to the GI tract (e.g., feeding tube displacement or obstruction), the GI tract itself (e.g., nausea, vomiting, diarrhea), or metabolic (e.g., hyperglycemia, hypophosphatemia).

❍ **Has preoperative nutritional support for malnourished patients been shown to reduce postoperative morbidity?**

Yes, for those with severe malnutrition.

❍ **In which patients is parenteral nutritional support indicated?**

When enteral access is unobtainable, enteral feeding contraindicated, or when level of enteral nutrition fails to meet requirements.

❍ **In which patients is intravenous nutritional support unlikely to be of benefit?**

Those expected to start oral intake in 5 to 7 days (3-5 days in infants) or with mild injuries.

❍ **Can lipids be given through a peripheral vein?**

Yes. They are isosmotic, unlike the concentrated dextrose solutions that should be infused centrally.

❍ **Is omega-3 fatty acids (fish oil) or omega-6 fatty acids thought to be anti-inflammatory?**

Omega-3 fatty acids.

❍ **What are some of the complications of parenteral nutrition?**

Those associated with catheter insertion (e.g., pneumothorax), with the indwelling line (e.g., line sepsis, thrombosis), with lipid emulsions (e.g., pancreatitis, reticuloendothelial dysfunction), and GI tract complications (e.g., cholestasis, acalculous cholecystitis).

❍ **Should patients with renal insufficiency have their protein intake restricted?**

Protein restriction is usually only necessary in those patients unable to undergo dialysis.

❍ **T/F: It is not recommended to place patients simultaneously on enteral and parenteral feedings.**

False. On the contrary, a small amount of nutrition delivered enterally may be all that is required to gain the positive effects of this route while the parenteral route supplies the balance of caloric and protein needs.

❍ **What is the most common cause of hyponatremia in infants?**

"Water Intoxication" caused by improper mixing of infant formula.

❍ **What is the major complication of hyponatremia in infants?**

Hyponatremic seizures.

❍ **What are the major complications of hypernatremic dehydration?**

Cerebral edema and hemorrhage.

❍ **Significant elevations of serum potassium levels result in what cardiac rhythm disturbance?**

Ventricular fibrillation.

O   **What are the major clinical manifestations of severe hypokalemia?**

Paralysis and respiratory failure.

O   **What is the major electrolyte abnormality associated with Bartter Syndrome?**

Hypokalemia.

O   **What is the major clinical manifestation of Bartter syndrome?**

Severe failure to thrive.

O   **What are associated findings in Bartter syndrome?**

Metabolic acidosis, normal blood pressure, and elevated plasma levels of renin.

O   **Which type of renal tubular acidosis is associated with Fanconi syndrome?**

Type II - proximal RTA.

O   **What is Fanconi syndrome?**

A syndrome associated with genetically transmitted inborn errors of metabolism (galactosemia, Wilson's disease, tyrosinemia, etc.) or it can be acquired secondary to environmental toxins (lead, mercury, etc.).

Fanconi Syndrome causes rickets associated with multiple defects of the proximal renal tubule (Type II RTA). Most commonly associated with glucosuria, phosphaturia, aminoaciduria, and carnitinuria.

O   **What type of RTA usually presents as an isolated condition?**

Type I - distal RTA.

O   **What are the characteristic acid-base/electrolyte abnormalities associated with type I and type II RTA?**

Hypokalemic, hyperchloremic metabolic acidosis.

O   **What are the characteristic acid-base/electrolyte abnormalities associated with type IV RTA?**

Hyperkalemic, hyperchloremic metabolic acidosis.

O   **What is the underlying cause of type IV RTA?**

Decreased sodium reabsorption secondary to lack of aldosterone effect.

O   **What diseases are associated with type IV RTA?**

Diseases of the adrenal gland; most commonly Addison's disease and Congenital Adrenal Hyperplasia.

O   **A bolus of which type of fluid should be used in the initial resuscitation of a dehydrated infant or child?**

An isotonic solution: either Normal Saline or Ringer's Lactate.

O   **What is the preferred method of rehydration in infants and children?**

The preferred method is oral rehydration with standardized electrolyte solutions assuming the patient is not in shock, vomiting, or unable to take oral fluids adequately. In those situations I.V. rehydration is the preferred method.

○   **21 Hydroxylase deficiency accounts for 95% of all cases of congenital adrenal hyperplasia. 75% of these cases are the salt losing variety and the other 25% are the classic virilizing form. What are the electrolyte abnormalities associated with the salt losing variety?**

Hyponatremia and hyperkalemia.

○   **What are the sodium concentrations of the most common commercially available IV fluids?**

0.9 normal saline = 154 meq/l
0.45 normal saline = 77 meq/l
0.3 normal saline = 54 meq/l
0.2 normal saline = 33 meq/l

○   **What are the most common conditions in pediatrics associated with metabolic alkalosis?**

Chronic vomiting- pyloric stenosis and anorexia/bulimia.
Nasogastric suctioning - post-op usually.
Chronic diuretic treatment - infants with Bronchopulmonary Dysplasia (BPD).

FETUS, NEONATAL AND INFANT

○ **What are the Wessel criteria for the diagnosis of infantile colic?**

33333! Crying or irritability lasting longer than 3 hours a day, 3 days a week, or 3 weeks total, all in an infant under 3 months old. Colic usually subsides after the age of 3 months.

○ **What percentage of infants have colic?**

25%. The etiology is unknown.

○ **When does physiological jaundice of the newborn occur?**

2–4 days after birth. Bilirubin levels may rise up to 6-9 mg/dl.

○ **A neonate presents with a history of poor feeding, vomiting, respiratory distress, has abdominal distention, and is found to have hyperbilirubinemia. What is the likely cause of this complex?**

This neonate is septic.

○ **Name some causes of jaundice occurring in the first day of life.**

Sepsis, congenital infections, ABO/Rh incompatibility.

○ **Outline the Apgar scoring system.**

Index	0 points	1 point	2 points
Pulse	Ø	< 100	> 100
Resp. effort	Ø	Weak cry	Strong cry
Color	Cyanotic	Extremities cyanotic	Pink
Tone	Flaccid	Weak tone	Strong
Response	Ø	Motion	Cry

○ **Sudden Infant Death Syndrome (SIDS) is the <u>most</u> <u>common</u> cause of death for infants in the first year of life. It occurs at a rate of 2/1000, or 10,000/year. What are 6 risk factors associated with SIDS?**

1. Prematurity with low birth weight.
2. Previous episode of apnea or apparent life-threatening event (ALTE).
3. Mother is a substance abuser.
4. Family history of SIDS.
5. Male gender.
6. Low socioeconomic status.

○ **What is the normal pulse rate of a newborn?**

120–160 bpm. Though many newborns have a pulse of just over 100.

○   **External chest compressions should be initiated for a newborn with assisted ventilation when the heart rate is less than how many beats per minute?**

60 bpm or 60-80 bpm and not increasing.

○   **SIDS has a bimodal distribution. At what ages do the peaks occur?**

2.5 and 4 months.

○   **Define failure to thrive (FTT).**

FTT is defined as infants who are below the third percentile in height or weight or whose weight is less than 80% of the ideal weight for their age. Almost all patients with FTT are under 5 years old, while the majority of children are 6–12 months old.

○   **What is the <u>most</u> <u>common</u> cause of FTT?**

Poor intake is responsible for 70% of FTT cases. One third of these cases are educational problems, ranging from inaccurate knowledge of what to feed a child to over-diluting formula to "make it stretch further."

○   **What is the prognosis for patients with FTT?**

Only 1/3 of patients with FTT due to environmental factors have a normal life. The remainder grow up small for their size, and the majority also have developmental, psychological, and educational deficiencies.

○   **Do term babies have functioning sweat glands?**

Yes, but they are hyporesponsive compared with that of adults.

○   **How do infants generate heat?**

Metabolism of brown fat and muscular activity.

○   **What induces the lipolysis of brown fat stores?**

Norepinephrine and thyroid hormones.

○   **What abnormalities should be considered if the umbilical cord has not fallen off after 30 days?**

Neutropenia or a functioning abnormality of the neutrophils.

○   **What is a good rule of thumb in estimating the necessary size of an umbilical catheter?**

The measured distance from the umbilicus to the shoulder.

○   **How common is discordant growth in twin pregnancies?**

Very, as it is seen in almost one-third of twin pregnancies.

○   **Is the first or second born twin at greater risk of developing respiratory distress syndrome (RDS)?**

The second born.

○   **What is funisitis?**

The sense of urgency a child feels in an amusement park. Alternately, it also means inflammation of the umbilical cord vessels.

❍   **Preterm infants of what age should be evaluated for retinopathy of prematurity (ROP)?**

<32 weeks. They should be evaluated if they have a birthweight <1250 gm or have supplemtsal O_2>4 hrs.

❍   **What specimen from the newborn is most apt to confirm the suspicion of maternal drug abuse?**

Meconium.

❍   **What is the most common type of clavicular fracture during delivery?**

Greenstick fracture.

❍   **What are the two most common causes of fetal death?**

Congenital malformations and chromosomal abnormalities.

❍   **What equipment needs to be ready for resuscitation of a newborn?**

Suction bulb, towels for drying, suctioning, laryngoscope with a 0-00 Miller blade, umbilical clip, appropriate oxygen mask and small ventilating bad and a 3.0 uncuffed ET tube. This should suffice for the majority of resuscitations. Rarely is IV access or medications needed, though these should be nearby.

❍   **What is the best way to position the newborn prior to intubation or meconium suctioning?**

With the head facing you and a small towel roll placed underneath the shoulders. The large cranium will cause excess flexion, and the towel will help equilibrate the height.

❍   **What is the normal heart rate and systolic blood pressure of a newborn? A 1 month old?**

HR 125 and SBP 60+/-10 mmHg, and HR 120 with SBP 80+/-, respectively.

❍   **What is the appropriate endotracheal tube size and laryngoscope size for a 1 year old child? 5 year old?**

ETT 3.5-4.0 with Miller 1, and ETT 5.0 with Miller 2 or Macintosh 2.

❍   **What is the most common cause of infant arrhythmias (esp. bradycardia)?**

Hypoxia.

❍   **What are the three methods of estimating the size of the ETT needed in a child?**

Memorize all the sizes, 2) the diameter of the tube should be approximately the same as the child's pinky, or 3) calculate as follows: size (mm)= [16 +age in years] / 4.

❍   **What is the definition of apnea in an infant?**

Apnea is either cessation of breathing for more than 20 seconds, or a shorter period associated with cyanosis or bradycardia.

❍   **What is the definition of ALTE?**

An Apparent Life Threatening Event is apnea associated with color change (cyanosis or redness), a loss of muscle tone, and choking or gagging.

❍   **Compared to an otherwise healthy infant, how much more likely is a child with a history of ALTE to go on to have SIDS?**

About 3-5 times more likely.

❍   **What percentage of infants who have SIDS had a prior ALTE?**

About 5%.

❍   **A newly delivered infant has respiratory movement, a closed mouth, but no air audible in the lungs. What is the most likely diagnosis?**

Choanal Atresia.

❍   **What is the correct workup for an infant of 16 days with a temperature of 38C, but appears well?**

Don't let looks deceive you at this age. A full septic workup, antibiotics and admission are in this child's future.

ADOLESCENCE

❍ **A female with breast budding and a small amount of pubic hair near the labia is in what Tanner stage of development?**

Stage II (ages 8–15).

❍ **At what Tanner stage of development do males have facial hair development?**

Stage IV (ages 12–17).

❍ **How much does the average teenager grow during adolescence?**

Teenagers generally double their weight and increase their height by 15–20%.

❍ **What are the <u>most</u> <u>common</u> causes of delayed puberty?**

Constitutional growth delay, familial short stature, and chronic illness.

❍ **What percentage of teenage girls have eating disorders?**

20%.

❍ **When is the female growth spurt in respect to menarche?**

Females have menarche just after their peak growth spurt. This is just the opposite in males, who are well on their way through puberty before they hit their peak growth spurt.

❍ **What is the first sign of puberty in the male?**

Their amazingly mature personality (just teasing, of course). Puberty in the male begins with the growth of the testes followed by thinning and pigmentation of the scrotum, growth of the penis, and lastly the development of pubic hair.

❍ **By what age will a child reach half his/her adult height?**

2 years; however, by 2 years, a children are only 20% of their adult weight.

❍ **How can you distinguish between short stature in a child due to heredity and short stature due to a constitutional delay in growth?**

Bone age determination. In children with familial short stature, bone ages will be normal. In children with constitutional growth delay, the bone ages will also be delayed, as will sexual maturation.

❍ **A 15-year-old adolescent male has developed small breasts. The parents want this situation surgically corrected. What do you recommend?**

Surgery is a consideration if the physical abnormality is causing severe psychological pain or if the breasts have persisted for a long time. Otherwise, surgery is not a commonly recommended treatment as gynecomastia in adolescence generally lasts only 1–2 years. It has been reported that gynecomastia occurs in 36–64% of pubertal males.

○   **What drugs can cause gynecomastia?**

Marijuana, hormones, digitalis, spironolactone, cimetidine, ketoconazole, antihypertensives, antidepressants, and amphetamines.

○   **According to Erikson, what is the main psychosocial task of adolescence?**

Establishing a sense of identity.

○   **What is the difference between adolescence and puberty?**

Adolescence is a time of psychosocial transition from being a child to being an adult. Puberty is the spectrum of physical changes that happen in the body. The two commonly occur at nearly the same time.

○   **What percentage of deaths in the 15-19-year-old range is due to injury?**

75-85%.

○   **What percentage of all adolescent deaths are due to alcohol related automobile accidents?**

25%.

○   **What percentage of fatalities in African American teenagers are due to firearms?**

About 50%.

○   **Who are more likely to develop chronic fatigue syndrome, females or males?**

Females.

○   **A 13-year-old girl just started menarche. Is she capable of having children at this time?**

Generally not. Most girls do not ovulate for 1-2 years after menarche.

○   **What is the most common breast tumor in adolescence?**

Fibroadenoma (>90%).

○   **How useful is mammography in identifying lesions in adolescents?**

Not very as the breast tissue is too dense.

○   **What endocrine abnormalities can lead to galactorrhea in a teenage girl?**

Hypothyroidism and an increase prolactin (i.e. from a pituitary adenoma).

○   **Which is most common, primary or secondary dysmenorrhea?**

Primary. This is due to increased levels of PGF_2 and PGE_2 produced from the arachidonic acid released from sloughing endometrium.

○   **In an adolescent female without a history of PID, what is the most common cause of chronic pelvic discomfort?**

Endometriosis.

○   **When is the pain of endometriosis most severe?**

Right before menses.

O   **What are the most common etiologies of secondary amenorrhea?**

Structural abnormalities, foreign bodies (i.e. IUD), endometriosis and endometritis.

O   **What are the four components, according to the DMS-IV criteria, that are necessary for the diagnosis of anorexia nervosa?**

1.   Fear of becoming obese (not diminished by weight loss)
2.   Dysmorphia-disturbance in way body is perceived
3.   Refusal to keep weight over age/height minimum
4.   Absence of 3 or more menstrual cycles in post-menarchal females

O   **What are the two subclassifications of anorexia nervosa?**

Restricts (limit intake) and Bulimia (binge eating followed by countermeasures).

O   **What changes can you see in a thyroid panel in a teenager with anorexia nervosa?**

Decreased T3 and increased rT3.

O   **How do you diagnose bulimia nervosa?**

A history of overeating followed by forged purging is all that is needed. Erosion of the tooth enamel and back of fingers second and third fingers in the dominant hand should lead you to suspect the diagnosis.

O   **What electrolyte abnormalities are commonly seen in bulimia nervosa?**

Hypokalemia, hypochloremia and metabolic alkalosis.

O   **What are the main causes of death in patients with anorexia nervosa?**

About 10% of these patients end up dying from complications (i.e. electrolyte imbalances, arrhythmias, or congestive heart failure).

O   **What is the Female Athlete Triad?**

Amenorrhea, disordered eating and osteoporosis.

O   **What is the treatment for the Female Athlete Triad?**

Calcium supplements and oral contraceptives.

O   **What is the most common structural anomaly that causes primary amenorrhea?**

Imperforate hymen.

O   **How do you diagnose primary amenorrhea?**

By one of three criteria: 1) No menses by the age of 16; 2) No menses within one year of breast or pubic hair development having reached Tanner stage V; or 3) No menses within 3 years of the development of secondary sex characteristics.

O   **Assuming your patient with primary amenorrhea is not pregnant, what are the next tests of choice?**

Karyotype analysis to rule out the presence of a Y chromosome (Testicular Feminization), TSH, TFT's and prolactin levels, as indicated after a thorough history and physical.

O   **What is secondary amenorrhea?**

A history of no periods for 6 months in a previously menstruating female or a history oligomenorrhea followed by no periods in 12 months.

O   **A 17-year-old female comes to your office complaining that she has had no period for over a year. What should be the next step in defining the cause of her amenorrhea?**

Serum Prolactin and TSH, to rule out hyperprolactinemia and hypothyroidism, respectively. If these are both normal, proceed with a progesterone challenge to rule out anovulation.

O   **What is the most common cause of chronic anovulation?**

Polycystic Ovary Syndrome (PCO).

O   **How common is a varicocele?**

Dilation of the veins of the spermatic cords occurs in about 15% of adolescents (usually on the left side).

O   **What is the most common solid tumor in adolescent males?**

Testicular seminoma.

O   **What is the cure rate of testicular seminoma if the tumor is confined to the testicle?**

95% with orchiectomy and radiation.

O   **Of epididymitis and testicular torsion, which will present with a positive Prehn sign?**

Testicular torsion (pain persists with elevation of the testes).

O   **How long after the onset of testicular torsion do irreversible changes develop?**

About 4.5-5 hours.

O   **During a routine examination of a 12-year-oldmale you encounter, in the upper scrotum, a boggy enlargement. Should you(and he) be concerned?**

No. This is most likely a varicocele, which is very common. About 15-17% of adolescent males have an asymptomatic varicocele.

O   **How soon after conception is the average home pregnancy kit able to detect the HCG and register as positive?**

Depending on sensitivity, anywhere from 1 to 3 weeks.

O   **In a normal uterine pregnancy, what is the doubling time of the HCG levels?**

48 hours. This can be used as one of several screening measures to rule out a hydatiform mole.

O   **How effective are condoms in pregnancy prevention as used by adolescents?**

Not very, with up to 15% failure rate.

❍   **How effective are birth controls pills (BCPs) in pregnancy prevention as used by adolescents?**

Very, with a pregnancy rate of about 0.8% per year.

❍   **A vaginal smear of an adolescent with primary amenorrhea shows a positive estrogen effect. What can you give to induce menses?**

Medroxyprogesterone 10mg po QD for 5 days every 6-12 weeks.

❍   **A 17-year-old females comes to the ED complaining of excessive uterine bleeding. What hormonal adjunct can you give to stop the flow?**

Norethynodrel (25 mg) usually stops blood flow within 24 hrs.

❍   **Describe the developmental findings in a 12-year-old girl with breast development at Tanner stage 4 and pubic hair at tanner stage 3?**

Secondary mounds formed from areola and papilla. Increased amount of pubic hair, which is darker and starting to curl.

❍   **At what Tanned development stage do girls achieve menarche?**

SMR stage 3 (30%) or stage 4 (90%).

❍   **At what point in the menstrual cycle is a gonorrhea infection most likely to present?**

In the first 7 days of menses (80-90%).

❍   **A 17-year-old female complains of vaginal irritation. She has a whitish discharge with a "fishy" odor on exam. Smear reveals clue cells. What is your diagnosis and treatment?**

Gardnerella vaginitis. Treatment is with metronidazole cream or tablets.

❍   **How do you treat the first episode of genital herpes?**

Oral acyclovir (200 mg 5 times/day for 10 days).

❍   **What is the most common STD in sexually active teenage males?**

Non-gonococcal urethritis due to *Chlamydia trachomatis*.

❍   **How long after intake can marijuana still be detected in the urine?**

From 3 days after one episode to 28 days in a frequent user.

❍   **How much more likely to become an alcoholic is the son of the town alcoholic as compared to the son of the town priest?**

Four times.

❍   **The anesthetic drug Ketamine is related chemically to what illicit drug?**

Phencyclidine (PCP, Angel Dust).

❍   **A fifteen-year-old teenager has his first cigarette at a party. What is the risk that he will become a regular smoker by the age of 18?**

About 65-75%.

O   **How soon after the last cigarette can nicotine withdrawal effects begin?**

Within two hours, with a peak around 24 hrs.

GROWTH AND DEVELOPMENT

○ **Child development: At what age are infants able to perform the following motor skills?**

1. Sit up by themselves.
2. Walk.
3. Crawl.
4. Walk up stairs.
5. Smile.
6. Hold their head up.
7. Roll over.

Answers: (1) 5–7 months, (2) 11–16 months, (3) 9–10 months, (4) 14–22 months, (5) 2 months, (6) 2–4 months, and 7) 2–6 months.

○ **At what age are infants capable of the following language skills?**

1. "Mama/Dada" sounds.
2. One word.
3. Naming body parts.
4. Combine words.
5. Understandable speech.

Answers: (1) 6–10 months, (2) 9–15 months, (3) 19–25 months, 4) 17–25 months, and (5) 2 years–4 years.

○ **At what age will a child be able to uncover a toy that is hidden by a scarf?**

9–10 months. This is called object permanence—the understanding that "out of sight" is not "out of existence."

○ **Joe Montana (the greatest quarterback of all time) comes to you with his 3-year-old son distressed that he can't catch a ball to save his life. You reassure Joe that children are not expected to perform that motor skill until they are what age?**

5–6 years old.

○ **How many times a day should a healthy infant feed in the first 3 months of life?**

Infants should average 6–8 feedings a day. The schedule should be dictated by the infant (i.e., when he/she is hungry). By 8 months, feedings are generally only 3–4 times a day.

○ **What, if any, nutritional value does cow's milk have over breast milk?**

Cow's milk has a higher protein content than breast milk. Both have the same caloric content (20 kcal/oz). Breast milk has a higher carbohydrate concentration, a greater amount of polyunsaturated fat, and is easier for the infant to digest. And for the obvious immunological advantage, "breast is best.".

○ **A mother of a 2 month old breast fed infant comes to you complaining of breast pain, swelling, fever, and a red coloration just above her left nipple. She is a strong believer in the axiom "Breast is Best" and wants to know if she can continue to breast feed her infant. What do you tell her?**

She most likely has bacterial mastitis, which is most common in the first 2 months of breast feeding. This is most frequently caused by *Staphylococcus aureus*. The mother should take antibiotics and may continue breast feeding if she chooses.

○ **At what age should solid foods be introduced?**

4–6 months. One food should be introduced at a time with 1–2 week intervals between the introduction of a new food. This way potential allergies can be defined.

○ **How much weight should an infant gain per day in the first 2 months of life?**

15–30 gm/day. Newborns commonly lose 10% of their body weight during the first week of life due to a loss of extracellular water and a decrease in caloric intake. Healthy infants soon double their birth weight in 5 months and triple their weight in a year.

○ **When do infants begin teething?**

By 6 months. They may become irritable with a decreased appetite and excessive drooling. Acetaminophen can be used to control the pain, but "Jack Daniel's on the gum kills the pain and is more fun!"

○ **When should toilet training be started?**

Not until at least 18 months (though this is very dependent on society norms).

○ **Short stature with normal weight should make you think of what general categories for investigation?**

Familial height history (constitutional delay, familial short stature), chondrodysplasias, endocrinopathies (hypothyroidism, GH deficiency, cortisol excess).

○ **The mother of an 8-year-old boy is worried that her child has attention deficit hyperactivity disorder. She states that for the last 4 months he has been fidgety, unable to stay seated, and talks incessantly and out of turn in school. At home, however, he seems relatively calm. What do you tell her?**

Although the symptoms are suspicious for ADHD, it is too early to make this diagnosis. In order to meet the DSM-IV criteria, the symptoms have to last at least 6 months and occur in more than one setting.

○ **What neurological condition may mimic some of the symptoms of ADHD?**

Petit mal epilepsy can present as concentration and attention problems.

○ **What is the treatment for ADHD?**

Behavioral and psychosocial therapy along with stimulant medications.

○ **What is the most commonly used stimulant in the treatment of ADHD and how effective is it?**

Methylphenidate (Ritalin), given at 0.3-1.0 mg/kg, is efficacious in 75-80% of children.

○ **What is the "parachute reflex" and when does it usually develop?**

At about 8 months of age, the infant will extend the arms and legs as a protective gesture when lowered head first in a prone position.

○ **When do the Moro, rooting, and palmar grasp reflexes usually disappear?**

At about 5-6 months of age.

○ **What age group is the Wechsler Intelligence Scale (WISC) used for?**

It measure the IQ's of 5-15-year-olds.

○ **At what age do most children stop sucking their thumbs?**

4-years-old.

○ **At what age do most children achieve bladder control?**

About half of all American children achieve bladder control at 2.5 years of age. Girls showing toilet-training earlier than boys.

○ **When does the anterior fontanelle usually close?**

Between 9-14 months of age.

○ **What should you be concerned about in a child with early closure of the fontanelles?**

Premature cranial synostosis.

○ **A 20-month-old child still has a palpable anterior fontanelle. What conditions could cause this?**

Rickets, hypothyroidism, hydrocephalus, hypophosphatemia, or Trisomy 18.

○ **How do you calculate the size of a fontanelle?**

Take the length (which is the anterior-posterior dimension) plus the width (which is the transverse dimension) and divide by 2.

○ **What is craniosynostosis?**

Early fusion of cranial suture lines. This can lead to asymmetric growth, bridging of the sutures and deforming of the skull.

○ **What is Crouzon syndrome?**

The type of craniosynostosis with midface hyperplasia, most commonly presenting with exophthalmos.

○ **What four conditions can give you craniotabes?**

Rickets (in infancy), hypervitaminosis A, syphilis, and hydrocephalus.

○ **Which are the first teeth to erupt? When does that happen?**

At 5-9 months the central incisors appear, after which there is about 1 new tooth per month. At 6-7 years, the first permanent teeth erupt (also central incisors).

○ **What is the treatment for a ranula?**

Most of these sub-lingual mucoceles self-resolve. If large, surgical marsupialization can be performed.

O   **You push a sitting infant sideways, and it reflexively holds its hand out to protect its fall. What is this called?**

Lateral propping reflex.

O   **At what age can a child copy a circle?**

3 years.

O   **At what age can a child copy a "Red Cross" symbol?**

8 years.

O   **At what age can a child copy a vertical diamond?**

7 years.

O   **At what age can a child copy a cube?**

11 years.

O   **What are the first four of Ericsson's life-cycle crises?**

Trust vs. mistrust (infancy), autonomy vs. shame and doubt (early childhood), initiative vs. guilt (early childhood), and industry vs. inferiority (school age).

O   **In regards to acquisition of verbal skills, who develop faster-twins, or single birth infants?**

Single birth infants.

O   **A 10 month old infant is showing preference for his right hand. Should this be a cause of concern?**

Yes, children usually develop hand dominance by 18-24 months. Anytime hand dominance develops prior to this, you should be alert for possible cerebral palsy.

O   **At what age can a child follow a simple, two-step command?**

24 months.

O   **What are the 2 most common causes of death in 1-6 month olds?**

SIDS and abuse.

O   **T/F: Full-term infants and preterm infants have comparable risk of child abuse?**

False, preterm is much higher (3 times as much).

O   **What are the most common reasons for foster home placement? How has this changed over the years?**

Abuse, neglect and AIDS are currently the most common reasons. In the past, poverty, mental retardation, disease, and absence/death of parent were the most common reasons.

❍   **T/F: IQ's and school performance of adopted children are equal to non-adopted children?**

True.

❍   **What is the most reliable early sign of a hearing problem?**

When the parents express concern that the child is not hearing properly.

❍   **Hearing loss of how many decibels (dB) are necessary for a classification of mild hearing loss? Moderate? Severe? Profound?**

Mild is 20-40 dB loss, moderate is 40-60 dB loss, severe is 60-80 dB loss, and profound is anything greater than 80 dB loss.

❍   **A 4-year-old child present with increased hearing impairment and asymptomatic hematuria. What is your diagnosis?**

Alport syndrome (aka hereditary nephritis). This is an autosomal dominant disease that more commonly afflicts males.

❍   **What is Rumination Syndrome?**

This is a relatively rare disorder characterized by repetitive gagging, regurgitation, mouthing, and re-swallowing of food, often with repetitive head movements. Children often present with accompanying FTT. This is most commonly seen in infants between 2-12 months of age. Look for clues of unstable family environment.

❍   **At what age should a child with stuttering have your concern?**

5-6 years, as most children have outgrown stuttering by this age.

❍   **T/F: Most children with autism are mentally retarded?**

True. About 75% have an IQ less than 70.

❍   **At what age do most autistic children exhibit signs and symptoms of their disease?**

Usually before 3 years of age.

❍   **What is Asperger syndrome?**

Autism but without intellectual deficits or delays in language.

❍   **What is Rett syndrome?**

A neurodegenerative disorder only affecting girls. It is presumed to be inherited in an X-linked dominant fashion and is lethal to the male fetus. It is characterized by a normal development until 1 year of age, at which time symptoms appear (autistic behavior, repetitive hand-wringing, sighing respirations with periods of apnea, tonic-clonic seizures, and ataxia).

❍   **What are common predisposing factors for pica?**

Mental retardation and lack of parental nurturing.

❍   **When should you be concerned over a 1-year-old child who constantly ingests non-nutritional items?**

As pica usually starts at 1-2 years of age, this should be high in your differential. However, mouthing objects is extremely common at this age, so a look at the family structure and signs of other disorders (i.e. schizophrenia, autism) can be investigated, and arrange for follow-up visits.

O   **How successful is positive reinforcement alone in eliminating enuresis?**

80-90%.

O   **If positive reinforcement is insufficient in eliminating enuresis in a child, what else can be done?**

Imipramine or Desmopressin nasal spray (DDAVP).

O   **What is the formula for calculating the Intelligence Quotient (IQ)?**

Mental Age divided by chronological age times 100.

O   **What is range of IQ is considered average?**

90-109.

O   **What range of IQ is considered mild mental retardation?**

50-69.

O   **What is the most common preventable cause of mental retardation worldwide?**

Iodine deficiency. This leads to maternal and fetal hypothyroxinemia.

O   **What are the 2 most common childhood psychiatric disorders?**

Attention Deficit Hyperactivity Disorder (ADHD), and Oppositional Disorder.

O   **Are children of parents with an affective disorders more likely to have psychiatric problems?**

Yes, 25% will have a major affective disorder and 45% will have a psychiatric disorder themselves.

O   **How is skeletal age determined?**

By comparing the presence or absence of certain ossification centers to known standards. This is useful in the evaluation of short stature.

O   **The parents of a 3-year-oldboy is concerned about an episode where he held his breath until he lost consciousness and actually had a small seizure. What do you tell them?**

This is fairly common and there is no risk of the child developing a seizure disorder. Advise them to ignore the child when he holds his breath and leave the room. Without any reinforcement the child will soon discontinue the behavior.

O   **Which children have more nightmares?**

Girls > boys, usually starting at < 10 years old. More common in children with anxiety and affective disorders.

O   **How do you treat Obsessive-Compulsive Disorder in children?**

SSRI's (such as Fluoxetine, Sertraline, and Paroxetine) and counseling.

❍   **Children with what psychological disorder are at relatively high risk of developing antisocial personality disorder as adults?**

Conduct disorder.

❍   **With regards to hallucinations, can you distinguish organic psychosis from psychiatrically based psychosis?**

Yes. Psychiatrically based psychosis is more likely to induce auditory hallucinations, whereas organic psychosis induces more visual, tactile, or olfactory hallucinations..

❍   **What is the average time that an American child watches TV per day?**

3-4 hours.

❍   **A mother calls you distraught and tells you her 12-year-old son skipped school and stole a yo-yo from a local store. What should you be concerned about?**

Almost all children steal at some point, so this is not as much of a concern. Truancy, however, is never an appropriate behavior and usually is the result of disorganization at home and/or a developing personality disorder. This needs to be investigated and resolved.

❍   **Who are more likely to have learning disabilities, boys or girls?**

Boys are two times more commonly diagnosed with learning disabilities in comparison with their female counterparts.

❍   **What percentage of school-age children are diagnosed with a learning disability?**

5%.

❍   **How is dyslexia diagnosed?**

By finding a significant difference between the IQ scores as tested and reading achievement test scores.

❍   **A mother comes to you complaining that her child is failing in school. What tests would you perform initially?**

Hearing and vision tests should be done routinely. Evaluation for learning disabilities and IQ deficits should be performed as well.

❍   **Which infants tend to sleep for shorter periods and awaken more frequently at night - breast-fed or non breast fed?**

Breast fed infants.

❍   **What sleeping position is best for infants?**

The supine position has been found to drastically decrease the incidence of SIDS.

❍   **The mother of a 6 week old infant complains that her child cries almost 3 hours a day. Does she have cause for concern?**

No. This is normal in that age group. This should decline to about 1 hour a day at 12 weeks.

❍   **What is the definition of infantile colic?**

Fits of crying for over 3 hours a day more than 3 days a week in an otherwise healthy infant.

○ **When do infants sleep through the night?**

70% will sleep through the night without waking at 3 months of age. This increases to about 90% by 6 months of age.

○ **By what age do infants generally no longer need night feedings?**

About 6 months old.

○ **At what stage of sleep do children experience pavor nocturnus (night terrors) and somnambulism (sleepwalking)?**

Stage 4 (non-REM).

○ **The mother of an eight-year-old child is worried about her child's occasional episodes of sleep walking. What do you tell her?**

This is fairly common in this age group, and it usually disappears by age 15. Counseling is commonly recommended.

○ **How long does an episode of pavus nocturnus usually last?**

Night terrors last between 30 seconds to 5 minutes. The child does not remember the episode in the morning.

○ **A child is born deaf, has different colored irises, is partly albino and has a white forelock. What is the diagnosis?**

Waardenburg syndrome.

○ **What percentage of newborns have pseudostrabismus?**

30%.

○ **By what age are 90% of children walking?**

15 months.

○ **For an apparently normal appearing child who is saying no words at 18 months, what is the first thing to assess?**

Hearing .

○ **What percent of children still wet the bed at night at school entry?**

10% (up to 30% of boys still wet the bed 1-6 times per year and up to 15% of girls at school entry; however more frequent bedwetting or never been dry for > 3 months involves about 10% of children, boys more than girls).

○ **A child is sitting well, is saying "dadada" and has a neat pincer grasp. How old is he?**

9 months.

○ **What is the difference between jargon and babbling?**

Infants babble, as the first nonspecific words, they are combinations of consonant and vowel sounds; jargon is advanced (1-3 year old) talking in which many of the words are not "real", but the sounds and cadence resembles mature conversation.

○ **Describe premature thelarche.**

Breast buds without other signs of pubertal development and later onset with normal cadence and timing of pubertal development.

○ **By what age should term infants should regain their birth-weight by what age if bottle fed? ...If breast fed?**

Bottle: 1 week
Breast: 2 weeks

○ **Colic, (a.k.a. paroxysmal fussing) usually begins and ends between what ages?**

2 weeks to 3-4 months.

○ **What is the most common time of the day for colic to occur?**

Late afternoon and evening.

○ **What helps colic?**

Holding, correct positioning, gentle rocking.

○ **What is the normal range of infant crying in the first 3 months of life?**

2 weeks: 2 hours per day
1 month: 3 hours per day
3 months: 1 hour per day

○ **How many stools per day do breast fed infants have from 1 week to 2 months of life?**

4-10.

○ **What is the average and range of total daily sleep time in infants at 1 month, 12 months, 24 months of age?**

1 Month: 14-22 hours
12 Months: 12-18
24 Months: 13-15

○ **Open vowel sounds (ows and ahs) are usually made by what age?**

3-4 months.

○ **By what age should an infant begin to swipe (bat) intentionally at objects?**

4 months.

○ **By what age does the automatic/involuntary grasp response disappear?**

5 months.

❍   **At what age is a mature pincer grasp usually attained?**

9-11 months.

❍   **A 9 month old begins to scream and cry whenever anyone besides his mother approaches. What is your diagnosis, and is this something to be concerned about?**

Stranger anxiety. This is a normal developmental stage that generally occurs in the second half of an infant's first year. The child's temperament, along with his developmental age, will determine the severity of the reaction. The parent(s) should be reassured that the child is developing normally. This stage may last weeks to months. In very shy children, this may last longer.

❍   **Separation anxiety also develops late in the first year of life. What is it and how should parents be advised?**

This realization that a parent is not present occurs because the infant has developed object permanence. The child can remember the parents, even in their absence. Short leaves, with open statements of return, should be offered to reassure the infant (even if he/she understands little of the discussion).

❍   **At what temperature should hot water be set and why?**

120-130 degrees F is safe. Water temperatures of 140 degrees F will cause full thickness burns at 5 second exposure.

❍   **By what age is a child generally begin to demand that he feed himself?**

12 months. By this time, a child has a well developed pincer grasp, is beginning use of spoon, and decreased energy needs; the child is quite determined to feed his/her self.

❍   **A child is eating alone, enjoys helping with table chores and food preparation and is helpful with younger children. He can use a knife. How old is he?**

This is generally the case by 5-6 years.

❍   **Dropping food over the side of a highchair and looking for it on the floor is typical activity for a child of what age?**

9 months. However, he may continue this activity for months.

❍   **A child loves to be carried in a back carrier pack - about how old is he?**

3-4 months, when head control is good. By 12 months of age, however, he may not like to be confined, and may begin to be too heavy for parents to carry.

❍   **Object permanence is well developed by what age?**

9-10 months.

❍   **When do most children begin to climb stairs?**

Between 15-18 months.

❍   **By what age can children walk up stairs?**

18-20 months.

❍   **when can children alternate feet on the stairs?**

2 1/2 to 3 years.

○   **What is the average age children jump with both feet off the floor at the same time?**

24 months.

○   **What is the average age children can stand on one foot?**

2 years.

○   **What is the average age a child jumps off the bottom step?**

2 years.

○   **A child is beginning to read competently, understands simple addition and subtraction, and can count easily to 100+. He cannot ride a bike. What is his developmental age?**

Likely 6-7 cognitively, however may have motor delays or no exposure.

○   **Broad jump, balancing on one leg, and hoping occur at what ages, on average?**

3, 4, and 5 respectively.

○   **A toddler is bouncing to music, babbling and has a few understandable words, and demands to feed himself. How old is this child?**

About 15-18 months.

○   **How many children use a transitional object? What is its purpose?**

About 2/3 of toddlers have an inanimate object for comfort. This security object is most often used for falling asleep or in times of stress. Use continues through the 4th birthday and even later by some.

○   **How do you counsel a parent who is interested in potty training a 2-year-old?**

Toilet training is an exciting and key development stage for a child. Parents should realize that the child wants to imitate and please parents, that this is a time when the child will take control of his environment and achieve a sense of mastery. Child must be able to complete a series of motor tasks, but must also be able to respond to a bodily feeling. Children may be ready when they can walk well, undress/take pants off easily, get to the bathroom, sit on the potty chair. Children who identify and dislike wet/dirty diapers may be nearing but not necessarily ready for training. The child must be able to understand feeling offullness in bladder or bowel and anticipate viding, he must have voluntary control of sphincters.

○   **What is the peak age for tantrums?**

2-4 years, however the peak in anger outbursts is at 18 months in both girls and boys.

○   **A 12-month-old is saying "baba" and has no other words. He points at objects all the time and gestures his understanding of what things are used for (phone to ear, cap to head). His mother notes that he understands simple commands. His motor development is normal – he is walking. She is worried because many other 1-year-olds that they know are saying 5-10 words. What do you tell her?**

Because of his "rich gesturing" which is highly predictive of language development, he is likely to develop good language and communication skill, and may just be a "late bloomer" with respect to verbal skills.

❍   **Is there a relationship between early language disorders and later school and learning difficulties?**

Early language disorders are highly predictive for later learning difficulties: 40% of children with language problems early in life will have school and learning problems later.

❍   **Do children who are exposed to 2 languages (e.g. live in bilingual households) have delayed onset of language skill?**

No, there is no evidence that being exposed to a bilingual household delays language, although it may appear that children have temporary delays in expressive abilities. Delayed language may be a manifestation of a broad variety of social/familial conflicts or developmental delays.

❍   **Fears are common throughout childhood. List typical fears at age 1, 3, 6, 8, 10, and 13-17 years of age.**

1-year-olds: Separation, strangers, crowds, sudden movements;
3-year-olds: Masks, old people, distortions and deformities, dark, animals;
6-year-olds: Supernatural, hidden people (robbers in room), bodily injury, being left alone;
8-year-olds: School and personal failure, mockery by friends/peers;
10-year-olds: Wild animals, criminals, older children, loss of possessions, world catastrophes;
Teens: Body changes, sexuality and other sexual fears, loss of face, world events.

❍   **A child can walk with alternating feet on steps, catches a large ball, knows her colors, knows her full name, age and sex, and can be understood by strangers. How old is she?**

About 4 years.

❍   **A lack of understanding of cause and effect, despite rather mature language skills is typical in what age child?**

4-5-year-old has thought patterns exemplified by juxtapositions (does not understand cause and effect, just closeness in time - I took a bath because I was clean), egocentrism (things evolve around the child - why does it snow? so I can go sledding), animism (belief that inanimate objects are alive; why is the sun shining? because he is awake), and artificialis (thinking that things/events are caused by humans - what made you sick? because I was bad).

❍   **Dysfluency in speech are common at what age?**

3-4 years.

❍   **During grade school children are in the concrete operational stage of development according to Piaget. What does this mean?**

1.   Ability to consider multiple variables at the same time
2.   Perform operations relating to objects (addition, map creation)
3.   Understand serial relationships
4.   Appreciate classification systems

❍   **What are the 3 broad areas of difficulty in patients with Attention Deficit Disorders?**

Impulse control, inattentiveness, hyperactivity.

❍   **How long must difficulty with impulse control, inattentiveness or hyperactivity be present to consider ADHD?**

It generally begins before age 7, and lasts at least 6 months.

❍ **At what age does empathy for another's distress usually begin?**

2 years.

❍ **Do 2-year-old have the ability to cognitively consider another's viewpoint?**

No, egocentrism reigns at this age and throughout the preschool years.

❍ **Approximately how long should attention span be for a 3rd grader?**

45 minutes.

❍ **What is the difference between Tanner stage III and IV breast development?**

Stage IV - distinct nipple from areola and areola forms a mound above breast tissue.

❍ **T/F: All young adolescents are concerned about their body image and bodily changes.**

True.

❍ **A young girl is able to skip and dresses and undresses. How old is she?**

5 years.

❍ **What does the ELMS test?**

Early Language Milestones is a test of receptive, expressive, and visual language for 0-36month olds.

❍ **At what age do the first teeth erupt**

5-7 months (range 0-13 months).

❍ **At what age do the secondary teeth, first molars erupt?**

6-7 years.

❍ **What is the average amount of sleep required by a 12-year-old?**

9-10 hours.

❍ **How much sleep does a 5-year-old require?**

11 hours.

❍ **Why is it important to distinguish between mastitis and a breast abscess, aside from the initial treatment?**

A breastfeeding mother with a breast abscess should not continue to breast feed until the abscess is gone, as opposed to mastitis, which is not a contraindication to breast feeding.

NEUROLOGY

○ **A 14-year-old female with hearing loss over the last 6 months presents at 2 am with vertigo that has progressively become worse over the last 2 months. On exam, she is mildly ataxic. What is the diagnosis?**

Eighth nerve lesion, possibly an acoustic schwannoma or meningioma.

○ **What is a vestibular schwannoma?**

An acoustic neuroma or a tumor of the eighth cranial nerve. In addition to hearing loss and vertigo, patients also present with tinnitus. Surgical removal is the treatment of choice because this tumor may spread to the cerebellum and the brainstem.

○ **Where are congenital berry aneurysms located?**

In the circle of Willis.

○ **What three bacterial illnesses present with peripheral neurologic findings?**

Botulism, tetanus, and diphtheria.

○ **Which type of bacteria is most commonly cultured from brain abscesses: aerobic or anaerobic?**

Anaerobic.

○ **A child complains of blurry vision. On exam she has an abnormal pupil reflex and a white reflex on funduscopic examination. What is the treatment?**

Surgical removal of the eye. This is a retinoblastoma that can grow to other sites in the brain or body. This is an inheritable condition, and she should be counseled on the dangers when she is ready for children.

○ **What area of the brain is dysfunctional when a patient has Cheyne-Stokes respirations?**

The cortex. The nervous system is relying on diencephalic control.

○ **What causes cerebral palsy?**

70% of the cases are idiopathic. Other causes are in utero infections, chromosomal abnormalities, or strokes. Cerebral palsy is a defect in the central nervous system that occurs prenatally, perinatally, or before the age of 3.

○ **Which subtypes of cerebral palsy are also associated with mental retardation?**

Spastic and sometimes athetotic cerebral palsy. Mental retardation occurs in 25% of patients with cerebral palsy.

○ **What is the most common cause of floppy baby syndrome?**

Cerebral palsy.

❍   **A 16-year-old presents with progressively severe intermittent vertigo for 6 months and progressive unilateral hearing loss for 3 months. What is the diagnosis?**

Cerebellopontine angle tumor. Confirm diagnosis with a MRI scan.

❍   **A 15-year-old presents with a history of being knocked unconscious for 10 seconds while playing touch football one week ago. Since then, he has had intermittent vertigo, nausea, vomiting, blurred vision, a headache, and malaise. His neuro exam and CT are normal. What is the diagnosis?**

Post concussive syndrome. Most individuals recover fully over a 2 to 6 week time span. However, a few of these cases have persistent deficits.

❍   **Differentiate between decerebrate and decorticate posturing.**

<u>Decerebrate</u> <u>posturing</u> is when the elbows and legs are extended which is indicative of a midbrain lesion.

<u>Decorticate</u> <u>posturing</u> is when the elbows are flexed and the legs are extended. This suggests a lesion in the thalamic region. Remember: De<u>COR</u>ticate = hands by the heart (cor).

❍   **When is the onset of epilepsy <u>most</u> <u>common</u>?**

Before the age of 20. In acquired epilepsy, onset usually occurs in patients younger than 20 or older than 60.

❍   **How long must a generalized tonic-clonic seizure last without a period of consciousness to be considered status epilepticus?**

20 minutes. Status epilepticus may result from grand mal seizures or anticonvulsant therapy withdrawal.

❍   **A patient opens his eyes to voice, makes incomprehensible sounds, and withdraws to painful stimulus. What is his GCS?**

9.

<u>Glascow coma scale:</u>

<u>Eye</u> opening Eye opening	Best verbal response	Best motor response
4 spontaneously	5 oriented x 3	5 obeys command
3 on request	4 confused conversation	4 localizes pain stimulus
2 to pain	3 words spoken	3 flexes either arm
1 no opening	2 groans to pain	2 extends arm to pain
	1 no response	1 no response

❍   **Differentiate between partial seizures and generalized seizures.**

Partial seizures arise from a single focus and may spread out, whereas generalized seizures involve the whole cerebral cortex. Absence and grand mal seizures are examples of generalized seizures. Generalized and complex partial seizures involve a loss of consciousness.

❍   **Recurrent seizures in patients with a history of febrile seizures generally occur in what time frame?**

About 85% occur within the first 2 years. The younger the child, the more likely recurrence will happen. If a patient has a febrile seizure in the first year of life the recurrence rate is 50%. If it occurs in the second year, the recurrence is only 25%.

❍   **What will happen if you shine a light in the eyes of a patient who is in a diabetic coma?**

The pupils will constrict.

○ **Distinguish between the gait of a patient with a cerebellar lesion and the gait of a patient with an extrapyramidal lesion.**

The patient with a cerebellar lesion will have truncal ataxia, which is an unsteady, irregular gait with broad steps. A patient with extrapyramidal lesion will have a festinating gait. In the latter case, the patient takes several small, shuffling steps without swinging his/her arms.

○ **The Weber's test is performed on a patient complaining of hearing loss. This patient hears the sound more loudly in his right ear. Which type of hearing loss does this patient have?**

Conductive hearing loss on the right or sensory hearing loss on the left.

○ **What are the expected results when the Rinne's test is conducted on this patient?**

The Rinne's test is performed by placing the tip of the tuning fork on the mastoid process until the patient can no longer hear the tone. The fork is then relocated to just in front of the pinna until the patient can no longer hear the tone. In normal patients, the ratio is 1:2. This patient may not hear the tone any longer when the fork is placed adjacent to the pinna.

○ **Which is more common, a subdural hemorrhage or an epidural hemorrhage?**

A subdural. Subdurals can result from the tearing of the bridging veins. Bleeding occurs less rapidly because the veins, not arteries, are damaged.

○ **A 16-year-old woman complains of a throbbing, dull, unilateral headache that lasts for hours then goes away with sleep. She also has been nauseous and has vomited twice. She reports small areas of visual loss plus strange zigzag lines in her vision. What is the diagnosis?**

A classic migraine headache. This title is a misnomer because the classic migraine is in fact rare, accounting for only 1% of migraines. It can be differentiated from the common migraine, the most frequently occurring migraine, because visual disturbances of scotomata and fortification spectra arise in addition to all the other migraine symptoms.

○ **What factors may precipitate migraine headaches?**

Bright lights, cheese, hot-dogs and other foods containing tyramine or nitrates, menstruation, monosodium glutamate, and stress.

○ **Describe the key signs and symptoms of a classic, a common, an ophthalmoplegic, and a hemiplegic migraine headache.**

1) Common: This headache is indeed the most common. It is a slow evolving headache that lasts for hours to days. A positive family history as well as two of the following are prevalent: Nausea or vomiting, throbbing quality, photophobia, unilateral pain, and increase with menses. Distinguishing feature from "Classic" migraine is the lack of visual symptoms.

2) Classic: Prodrome lasts up to 60 minutes. Most common symptom is visual disturbance, such as homonymous hemianopsia, scintillating scotoma, fortification spectra, and photophobia. Lip, face, and hand tingling, as well as aphasia and extremity weakness may occur. Nausea and vomiting may also result.

3) Ophthalmoplegic: Most frequently manifests in young adults. Patient has an outwardly deviated, dilated eye, with ptosis. The third, sixth, and fourth nerves are typically involved.

4) Hemiplegic: Unilateral motor and sensory symptoms, mild hemiparesis to hemiplegia are exhibited with this type of headache.

O   **What elements in a patients history suggest an intracranial tumor?**

(1) wake patients from their sleep, although cluster headaches may do this, (2) are worse in the morning, (3) increase in severity with postural changes or Valsalva maneuvers, (4) are associated with nausea and vomiting even though migraines have similar symptoms, (5) are associated with focal defects or mental status changes, and (6) occur with a new onset of seizures.

O   **A baby girl was born to a man who developed Huntington's chorea at the age of 44. What are her chances of developing the same disease?**

50%. Huntington's chorea is an autosomal dominant disorder that first manifests itself between the ages of 30-50. Unfortunately, this little girl can expect to become demented, amnesiac, delusional, emotionally unstable, depressed, paranoid, antisocial, and irritable if she inherits the disease. She will also develop chorea, bradykinesia, hypertonia, hyperkinesia, clonus, schizophrenia, intellectual impairment, and bowel incontinence. She will eventually die a premature death 15 years after the onset of her symptoms.

O   **Which chromosome carries the genetic defect in patients with Huntington's chorea?**

The short arm of chromosome #4.

O   **A 17-year-old woman with a history of flu like symptoms (URI) one week ago now presents with vertigo, nausea, and vomiting. No auditory impairment or focal deficits are noted. What is the most likely cause of her problem?**

Labyrinthitis or vestibular neuronitis.

O   **At what age is bacterial meningitis most common?**

Infants under 1.

O   **Which bacteria is the most common cause of meningitis in infants under 1?**

Group B *Streptococci* and *E. coli*.

O   **How does bacterial meningitis differ from viral meningitis in terms of the corresponding CSF lab values?**

Bacterial meningitis will indicate low glucose and high protein levels, while viral meningitis will have normal glucose and a normal protein.

O   **On LP, opening pressure is markedly elevated. What should be done?**

Close the 3-way stopcock, remove only a small amount of fluid from the manometer, abort the LP, and initiate measures to decrease the intracranial pressure.

O   **A patient presents with acute meningitis. When should antibiotics be initiated?**

Immediately. Do not wait. Patients should receive a CT prior to LP only if papilledema or focal deficit is present.

O   **What is the most worrisome diagnosis of a purpuric, petechial rash in an infant?**

Meningococcemia. Other causes include *Hemophilus influenzae, Streptococcus pneumoniae,* and *Staphylococcus aureus*.

❍ **A 16-year-old female complains of weakness and tingling in her right arm and leg for 2 days. She reports an episode of right eye pain and blurred vision that resolved over one month, but the onset of that pain started 2 years ago. She also recalls a two week episode of intermittent blurred vision the previous year. What is the diagnosis?**

Presumptive multiple sclerosis. Confirm with MRI and CSF (look for oligoclonal bands).

❍ **What is the most common presenting symptom of MS?**

Optic neuritis (about 25%).

❍ **A patient with MS presents with a fever. The nurse asks, "Should I give the patient Tylenol?" What is your response?**

Yes! Lowering the temperature is important for MS patients because small increases in temperature can worsen existing signs and symptoms.

❍ **Which is the most common type of muscular dystrophy?**

Duchenne's muscular dystrophy.

❍ **Which forms of muscular dystrophy are autosomal dominant and which forms are X-linked?**

Myotonic dystrophy and Fascioscapulohumeral dystrophy are autosomal dominant. Duchenne's muscular dystrophy and Becker muscular dystrophy are X-linked.

❍ **Pseudohypertrophy of the calves is characteristic of which type of muscular dystrophy?**

Duchenne's muscular dystrophy. Hypertrophy is due to fatty infiltration of the muscles.

❍ **What neoplastic process is most commonly associated with myasthenia gravis?**

Thymoma.

❍ **Which is the most common medication associated with Neuroleptic Malignant Syndrome?**

Haloperidol. Other drugs, especially antipsychotic medications, are also causative.

❍ **What is the hallmark motor finding in Neuroleptic Malignant Syndrome?**

"Lead pipe" rigidity.

❍ **What is Shy-Drager syndrome?**

A rare, gradually progressive nerve disorder characterized by very low blood pressure, lack of coordination, muscle wasting, stiffness, and lack of bladder and/or bowel control. This syndrome occurs more often in young people.

❍ **What is the most common cause of syncope?**

Vasovagal or simple fainting (50%).

❍ **A child that you have been following since birth is brought to you at age 9 months because he is having frequent convulsions and cannot control his muscles enough to even hold his head up anymore. You noted a developmental road block at the age of 6 months, and now it seems the child**

is regressing in both motor and cognitive skills. On exam, the patient has a cherry-red macula.
What is the patient's prognosis?

This patient probably has Tay-Sachs disease and will go blind and become demented and paralyzed. He
will die before the age of 4.

O   What is the probable ethnic background of the patient described in the above case?

Eastern European Jewish or French Canadian.

O   For the following clinical presentations, identify if each is associated with peripheral vertigo or
with central vertigo.

1.   Intense spinning, nausea, hearing loss, diaphoresis.
2.   Swaying or impulsion, worse with movement, tinnitus, acute onset.
3.   Unidirectional nystagmus inhibited by ocular fixation, fatigable.
4.   Mild vertigo, diplopia, and ataxia.
5.   Multi-directional nystagmus not inhibited by ocular fixation, non-fatigable.

Answers: peripheral vertigo: (1), (2), and (3); central vertigo: (4) and (5).

O   What maneuver can be performed to determine whether vertigo is peripheral or central?

The Nylen-Bárány maneuver. It is performed as follows: The patient is rapidly brought from the sitting to
the supine position, and the head is then turned 45°.

O   What is the significance of bilateral nystagmus with cold caloric testing?

It signifies that an intact cortex, midbrain, and brainstem are present.

O   How are upper motor neuron (UMN) lesions of CN VII (facial nerve) distinguished from
peripheral lesions?

1.   UMN: A unilateral weakness of the lower half of the face.
2.   Peripheral: Involves the entire half of the face.

O   What are the main stages in brain development, when do they occur, and what are the clinical
abnormalities seen?

Neurulation occurs between 3-7 weeks gestational age and results in the formation of the primitive neural
tube. Failure of neurulation results in neural tube defects ranging from anacephaly to spina bifida. Neural
proliferation occurs between 2-4 months gestational age and defects can result in both macrocephaly and
microcephaly. Neuronal migration occurs between 3-5 months gestational age and abnormalities lead to
lissencephaly, pachy-and polymicrogyria, and neuronal heterotopias. Organization occurs from 5 months
gestational age to years post-natal and defects are likely causes of mental retardation. Finally, myelination
takes place from birth to years post-natal and these syndromes have not been well described.

O   What is the brain structure which is most likely to be involved in intraventricular hemorrhage
in a premature infant?

The germinal matrix.

O   What is the most common motor deficit seen in premature infants after a periventricular
hemorrhage?

Spastic diplegia. Since the axons that carry information from the motor neurons controlling the legs run the closest to the ventricles, these are the most often affected, resulting in a spastic diplegia. Upper extremities can also be involved but usually to a lesser degree.

O   **What symptoms form the classic tetrad seen in kernicterus?**

Choreoathetosis, supernuclear ophthalmoplegia, sensorineural hearing loss, and enamel hypoplasia.

O   **What are the two classic forms of brachial plexopathy seen after birth trauma?**

Erb's palsy results from damage to the upper plexus (C5 and C6 roots) due to stretching from traction on the shoulder. This is the most common and results in the 'waiter's tip' positioning of the arm. Klumpke's palsy results from traction on the abducted forearm causing injury to the lower plexus and an absent grasp.

O   **What is the most common type of neuropathology seen in Fetal Alcohol Syndrome?**

Excessive neuronal migration with leptomeningeal glioneuronal heterotopias.

O   **Which areas of the brain are most affected in hypoxic-ischemic encephalopathy in the full term infant?**

The cortex, especially the hippocampus, and basal ganglia.

O   **What term applies to the late post-asphyxial changes seen in the basal ganglia?**

Status marmoratus, which doesn't develop until the end of the first year although the injury occurs perinatally, consists of neuronal loss, gliosis and hypermyelination. This gives a marbled appearance to the basal ganglia.

O   **What are the three types of Arnold-Chiari malformations?**

Type I consist of downward displacement of the lower cerebellum may be associated with syringomyelia and presents mainly in adolescents with symptoms related to either hydrocephalus or syringomyelia. Type II is more severe and associated with a myelomeningocele. It presents in newborns with hydrocephalus and myelomeningocele. Type III is associated with encephalocele and is analogous to type I and II.

O   **What are the two types of lissencephaly?**

Type I lissencephaly or Bielschowsky type consists of a thick, 4-layered cortex. It is found in the Miller-Dieker syndrome, a chromosomal (17p-) abnormality characterized by a narrow forehead, long philtrum, upturned nares, retrognathism, digital anomalies and excess vascularization of the retinas. Type II lissencephaly or the Walker type, consists of a thin unlayered cortex. There is often muscle involvement in this form of lissencephaly (Fukuyama-type muscular dystrophy).

O   **What are the two main forms of neurofibromatosis?**

Type 1 (NF1), von Recklinghausen disease or peripheral neurofibromatosis, consists of cafe-au-lait spots, neurofibromas, plexiform neuromas, iris hamartomas (Lisch nodules), optic gliomas, and osseous lesions. It is caused by a mutation in the gene on chromosome 17, and accounts for 85% of all neurofibromatosis. Type 2 (Nf2), central neurofibromatosis, involves tumors of cranial nerve viii and the gene is linked to chromosome 18.

O   **What are the main intracranial lesions of tuberous sclerosis (TS)?**

Tubers, subependymal nodules and subependymal giant cell astrocytomas.

O   **What cardiac abnormality is associated with TS?**

Rhabdomyomas appear in infancy and can be large enough to cause heart failure and death in as many as one quarter of the patients. They often resolve spontaneously.

O   **What are the renal lesions associated with TS?**

These include angiomyolipomas and renal cysts.

O   **How is Prader-Willi syndrome and Angelman syndrome related?**

Both syndromes are caused by deletions of chromosome 15q11q13. If the deletion is on the paternal chromosome, the Prader-Willi syndrome consisting of hypotonia, hyperphagia, hypogenitalism and mild to moderate retardation is seen. If the deletion is on the maternal chromosome then the 'happy puppet' syndrome of Angelman is seen. This consists of severe mental retardation, ataxia with jerking of the limbs and trunk and a happy demeanor.

O   **What is the most common cranial suture involved in craniosynostosis and what is the shape of the head that results?**

The sagittal suture. The head is long and narrow (scaphocephaly).

O   **What is the bobble-headed doll syndrome?**

This is seen in infants with dilatation of the third ventricle from an obstructive lesion and consists of a 2-4 HZ oscillatory movement of the head. The patient is usually developmentally delayed.

O   **What is the most common form of gangliosidosis?**

Tay-Sachs disease affects 1 in 2000 persons among the Ashkenazi Jewish population. It may present first with excessive startle disease in infancy, followed by hypotonia which is replaced by spastic tetraplegia. By the first year of age, the infants are helpless, blind and unresponsive. The cherry- red spot seen on retinal exam is classic but can also be seen in other forms of gangliosidosis. THE enzyme involved is b-hexosaminidase A.

O   **Niemann-Pick disease results from the accumulation of what?**

There are three forms of Niemann-Pick disease which all result from accumulation of sphingomyelin in the reticuloendothelial system. Only types A and B are caused by a deficiency of sphingomyelinase. Type C is relatively restricted to the nervous system.

O   **Metachromatic leukodystrophy is caused by a deficiency of which enzyme?**

Arylsulphatase A.

O   **Which of the mucopolysaccharidoses is X-linked?**

Hunter disease involving deficiency of the iduronate-2-sulphatase.

O   **Which disease is associated with curvilinear bodies on skin or conjunctival biopsy?**

Neuronal Ceroid-lipofuscinosis.

O   **What is the phenotype of the majority of patients with phenylketonuria (PKU)?**

Blonde, blue eyes.

O   **What area of the brain is primarily involved in glutaric aciduria type I?**

NEUROLOGY

181

Glutaric aciduria type I, which results from the deficiency of glutaryl-CoA dehydrogenase, results in striatal degeneration. This leads to the clinical syndrome of dystonia and choreoathetosis.

❍   **Intrauterine seizures can be seen with which vitamin deficiency?**

Pyridoxine (vitamin B6).

❍   **Which leukodystrophy has been associated with an abnormal proteolipid protein (PLP)?**

Pelizaeus-Merzbacher disease.

❍   **Which leukodystrophy is associated with Rosenthal fibers?**

Alexander's disease. Rosenthal fibers contain glial fibrillary acidic protein.

❍   **Which neurons are spared in Huntington disease?**

Cholinergic interneurons whose axons terminate in the striatum and interneurons expressing somatostatin and neuropeptide Y.

❍   **What is Segawa dystonia?**

Segawa dystonia is also known as hereditary progressive dystonia with marked diurnal fluctuations. Patients are not dystonic when they first awaken but become so about 30 minutes after awakening. It is exquisitely sensitive to levodopa treatment and is also called dopa-responsive dystonia. It is often misdiagnosed as cerebral palsy (CP). However, Segawa disease is progressive while CP, by definition, is static.

❍   **What is the pathology associated with Rett syndrome?**

Rett syndrome is a neurodevelopmental disorder only seen in females. It presents with acquired microcephaly, psychomotor retardation, spasticity, seizures and characteristic hand-wringing movements. The brains at autopsy are found to be small and the neurons have decreased numbers of dendrites.

❍   **What are the three most common predisposing factors in the formation of a brain abscess?**

Cyanotic heart disease, otitis and sinusitis.

❍   **What is the most common cranial neuropathy seen in Borreliosis (Lyme disease)?**

Unilateral or bilateral facial palsy. Less frequently, The VIII nerve can also be affected.

❍   **What is Rasmussen's encephalitis?**

This is a inflammatory encephalitis that usually involves the frontal or temporal lobes in a unilateral distribution. The major clinical manifestation includes dementia and epilepsia partialis continua. It is treated with anti-immune therapy such as steroids and IVIG with hemispherectomies as a last resort.

❍   **What is the most common paraneoplastic syndrome seen in children?**

Opsoclonus-myoclonus ('dancing eyes-dancing feet') is seen with neuroblastoma. Unlike most paraneoplastic syndromes seen in adulthood, it is responsive to anti-immune therapy.

❍   **What are growing skull fractures?**

These are seen as a complication of skull fracture in children under three years of age. They are caused by the presence of leptomeningeal cyst that is formed by an unrecognized dural laceration. It prevents the two sides of the bone from aligning together during recovery.

O   **What is the most common type of head injury in children under the age of two?**

Non-accidental trauma causes significant brain injury in this age group and should always be considered when seeing a young child with an intracranial hemorrhage (shaken-baby syndrome). These are often severe and the risk of reoccurrence, if not recognized, is high.

O   **What is the Russell syndrome seen with hypothalamic gliomas?**

This is a diencephalic syndrome seen in infants under two years of age characterized by gastrointestinal abnormalities, euphoria, hyperkinesis, cachexia and nystagmus. It can also be seen with craniopharyngiomas and posterior fossa tumors.

O   **What is the usual presentation of choroid plexus papillomas in infants?**

Extreme hydrocephalus because of the over-production of CSF by the tumor.

O   **When should steroids be used in the treatment of increased intracranial pressure (ICP)?**

Steroids are beneficial in the treatment of vasogenic edema, so should be used to treat increased ICP associated with tumors, abscesses and brain trauma.

O   **What cutaneous manifestation is seen in patients with Sturge-Weber disease?**

A Port-wine stain, or angiomatous naevus, is seen in the distribution of cranial nerve V. This may be associated with pial angiomas. Seizures are the main clinical manifestation but hemiparesis can also be seen.

O   **What systemic diseases can be associated with MoyaMoya disease?**

MoyaMoya disease ('puff of smoke') refers to the generous fragile collaterals which form due to slowly progressive stenosis and obliteration of the large vessels of the brain. It can be seen in association with sickle cell disease, neurofibromatosis, tuberous sclerosis, chronic basilar meningitis, X-ray irradiation and homocystinuria.

O   **What is the typical EEG findings of absence seizures?**

Typically, absence seizures are preceded by a run of 3 Hz spike and wave. This can almost always be brought out by hyperventilation during the EEG.

O   **What is the West syndrome?**

Infantile spasms, hypsarrhythmia on EEG, and developmental delay.

O   **What are the 'core' seizures seen in LGS?**

Myotonic and tonic, atypical absences, atonic, and myoclonic seizures.

O   **What is the drug of choice in juvenile myoclonic epilepsy?**

Valproate.

O   **What is the main difference in the history obtained between seizures and breath-holding spells?**

Breath-holding spells are always provoked. Cyanotic breath-holding spells are provoked by crying precipitated by fright, anger, pain, or frustration. Pallid breath-holding spells are provoked by pain, especially a minor bump to the head.

○   **What is Sandifer syndrome?**

Opisthotonic posturing which occurs because of GE reflux due to hiatal hernias may be mistaken for seizures, spasticity or other movement disorders.

○   **What percent of migraine patients have their onset of headaches prior to age 5 years of age?**

20%.

○   **Ophthalmoplegic migraine affects which cranial nerve?**

Cranial nerve III.

○   **In which stage(s) of sleep does night terrors (parvor nocturnus) occur?**

They occur during stage III and IV of sleep, distinguishing them from nightmares which occur during REM sleep.

○   **What are the clinical findings of Klein-Levin syndrome?**

This syndrome occurs in adolescent males and presents with episodes of hypersomnia, hyperphagia and frontal lobe-type personality changes.

○   **Which metabolic peripheral neuropathy can be clinically misdiagnosed as Friedreich's ataxia?**

Vitamin E deficiency.

○   **Which toxic neuropathy can be clinically misdiagnosed in infants as Guillain-Barré syndrome?**

Botulism. Unlike in older patients that ingest the toxin, infants are usually colonized by the bacteria. A risk factor seems to be feeding the infant honey.

○   **Is congenital myotonic dystrophy inherited from the mother or the father?**

Myotonic dystrophy is an autosomal dominant disorder that normally presents in adolescence or adulthood. The congenital form is usually inherited from the mother.

○   **What is the difference between neonatal myasthenia and congenital myasthenia?**

Neonatal myasthenia is transiently seen in newborns of mothers with myasthenia gravis. The symptoms begin a few hours after birth, can last for up to three days, and are due to circulating maternal antibodies. Congenital myasthenia presents at birth with ophthalmoplegia and is caused by the lack of various proteins important to the transduction of the signal across the synaptic cleft.

○   **What components of the history are the most important in evaluating a child with neurological problems?**

Developmental, perinatal, birth and family.

○   **What is the significance of a mildly depressed and pulsatile fontanelle in an infant?**

Nothing. This is normal.

❍ **What does the clasp-knife phenomenon indicate?**

That the child has some spasticity, indicating upper motor neuron (CNS) dysfunction. This is elicited by sensing resistance to passive movement followed by sudden release of resistance.

❍ **What would you expect to find in a child with rigidity?**

Cogwheel sensation, or constant resistance to passive movement.

❍ **What are the inheritance patterns for Duchenne's muscular dystrophy and Becker muscular dystrophy?**

Both are inherited in an x-linked fashion.

❍ **What is Gower's sign?**

A specific way to rise to standing from the supine position that is seen in certain forms of muscular dystrophy. The child first rolls over onto hands and knees. Then the child stands up by "walking" his/her hands up the leg.

❍ **Two days after surgery, an adolescent complains of left lower leg weakness. CSF analysis shows elevated protein but normal WBC count. What idiopathic disease might be at work here?**

Guillain-Barré syndrome.

❍ **What is the most useful test to diagnose multiple sclerosis in children?**

MRI showing multiple white matter plaques in the periventricular regions.

❍ **In a child in a coma you elicit positive doll's eyes reflex. Does this mean the eyes move with the head, or away from the head?**

Away from the movement of the head. This sign determines viability of the brainstem. A positive sign means the brainstem is working properly.

❍ **Which way do the eyes move in normal caloric testing?**

Remember the mnemonic COWS- Cold Opposite, Warm Same. Absence of the nystagmus occurs with eighth nerve damage.

❍ **What is the most common cause of acute onset, painless monocular blindness in patients between 15-45?**

Optic neuritis. 60% of these patients eventually develop multiple sclerosis.

❍ **Patients diagnosed with pseudotumor cerebri should be periodically tested for what development?**

Loss of visual fields.

❍ **What is the most effective way to reduce the incidence of post lumbar puncture headaches?**

Use the smallest gauge possible (in the original studies that describe this phenomenon, 16 gauge needles were used and up to 12 cc of fluid was removed!).

❍ **How do older children with stroke present?**

Acute hemiplegia.

O   **A Babinski sign is indicative of an abnormality of what tract?**

Corticospinal. It is indicative of an upper motor neuron lesion.

O   **In an extremely ticklish patient that will not let you perform the Babinski maneuver, or makes it difficult to interpret, what other maneuver could be used?**

The Chaddock maneuver. In this maneuver, the outer part of the dorsum of the foot is stroked. Extension of the toe is a positive sign.

O   **What is the incidence of a child with a history of febrile seizures developing a convulsive disorder compared with a child who has never had a febrile seizure?**

It is the same.

O   **What is the drug of choice for febrile seizures?**

Trick question, no treatment is usually given, aside from reducing the fever. However, if treatment must be used, the drug of choice is Phenobarbital.

O   **What type of movement disorder is associated with rheumatic fever?**

Sydenham chorea.

O   **What is the treatment for Sydenham chorea?**

Prednisone (1-2 mg/kg/day).

O   **A child is brought in with a new onset "tic". What is your treatment?**

None at this time. Simple clonic motor tics usually resolve spontaneously in less than a year.

O   **How do you diagnose Tourette's syndrome?**

Clinically. The patient must have complex tics for > 6 months, usually with vocal components (such as coprolalia), in the absence of any other medical etiology.

O   **What other problems are commonly seen in patients with Gilles de la Tourette's syndrome?**

ADHD, learning difficulties, emotional problems, or social problems.

O   **What is the drug of choice in the treatment of Tourette's syndrome?**

Haloperidol or pimozide.

O   **What can you give to ameliorate the dystonic reactions sometimes seen in a patient taking haloperidol?**

Benztropine (Cogentin).

O   **What metabolic abnormalities can cause neonatal seizures?**

Hypoxemia, hypoglycemia, hypocalcemia, hypomagnesemia and hyponatremia.

O   **Why should you look in the eyes of a patient with neurofibromatosis (Von Recklinghausen's disease)?**

To look for Lisch nodules and optic glioma.

O   **What are these Lisch nodules you are looking for?**

Pigmented iris hamartomas.

O   **On a routine newborn examination of a full term black infant you notice a large cafe-au-lait spot on the thigh. What is the most likely diagnosis?**

Normal examination.

O   **A 5-year-old is brought to the ED for a new onset seizure. On examination you notice a rash on the face and a large, rough lesion in the lumbosacral area. What is the most likely diagnosis?**

Tuberous sclerosis. The skin lesion on the back is a Shagreen patch.

O   **What disease classically presents with a port wine stain on the face?**

Sturge-Weber syndrome.

O   **What is the treatment for infant botulism?**

Trivalent immune serum as well as respiratory support.

O   **What is the definition of ataxia?**

Ataxia is an impairment in the coordination of movement without the loss of muscle strength.

O   **What is the most common posterior fossa tumor ?**

Astrocytoma.

O   **What clinical features are found in patients with ataxia-telangiectasia?**

Clinical features include: 1) neurologic dysfunction, which primarily manifests as ataxia, choreoathetosis, involuntary myoclonus and abnormalities of oculomotor function; 2) telangiectasias of the bulbar conjunctiva, which appear between the ages of 2-5; 3) endocrine dysfunction, such as abnormal glucose tolerance; 4) agenesis of the ovaries; 5) predisposition to cancers, such as Non-Hodgkin lymphoma. Some patients may have immunodeficiency as well.

O   **Can ataxia be a manifestation of Guillain-Barré syndrome?**

Yes- if there is a significant sensory neuropathy present, there may be an impairment of afferent sensory input to the cerebellum, causing a "sensory ataxia", in addition to the muscle weakness and areflexia seen in these patients.

O   **What clinical features define a simple febrile seizure?**

1. Brief duration, usually less than 15 minutes
2. Generalized seizure
3. Occur within the first 24 hours of a febrile illness
4. Occur in children between 1-4 years of age, who have
5. Normal neurologic development
6. Normal neurologic examination after the seizure

○   **Will a child with simple febrile seizures have a normal electroencephalogram (EEG)?**

Yes-an interictal EEG will be normal except for possible post-ictal generalized background slowing.

○   **What is the likelihood of a second febrile seizure in a child with a normal neurologic exam and normal psychomotor development?**

The recurrence rate after the first simple febrile seizure is approximately 30%.

○   **What clinical features characterize children with benign paroxysmal vertigo?**

Clinical features include : 1) age less than 4 years; 2) sudden onset of vertigo, which manifests as sudden imbalance, where the child will cry out, appear frightened and try to hold onto a stabilizing object; 3) autonomic symptoms, such as nausea, vomiting and sweating; 4) nystagmus, which will be present during the episode and often helps diagnose this condition. There is no loss of consciousness during these episodes.

○   **What tests or maneuvers may help distinguish breath-holding spells from seizures?**

Distinction may be made by an electroencephalogram (EEG), because during a provocative maneuver as ocular compression, patients with breath-holding spells will have an exaggerated vagal response, leading to bradycardia coincident with EEG slowing.

○   **Which patients who present with prolonged generalized seizures would benefit from the administration of pyridoxine?**

Infants without a prior history of seizures.

○   **What side effects of valproic acid limit its usefulness in young children with generalized seizures?**

Though valproic acid is very effective in treating generalized seizures, it has been shown to cause irreversible hepatic dysfunction and bone marrow failure, leading to death, in children less than 2 years of age.

○   **What side effects limit the long term use of phenytoin to treat generalized seizures in young children?**

Though gingival hyperplasia can be managed with good dental hygiene, phenytoin can cause problematic cosmetic effects, such as hirsutism and coarsening of the facial features, which limit its usefulness in treating young children with generalized epilepsy.

○   **What type(s) of seizures are well controlled with carbamazepine?**

Generalized tonic-clonic, partial and complex partial seizures.

○   **What type(s) of seizures are well controlled with ethosuximide?**

Absence (petit mal) seizures.

○   **Clonazepam is a useful adjunct therapy to treat what type(s) of seizures?**

Akinetic and generalized motor seizures.

○   **What clinical features are seen in children with cluster headaches?**

Cluster headaches are unilateral and are associated with autonomic nervous system symptoms as tearing and rhinorrhea. Episodes occur close together, or in "clusters".

○ **What criteria must be met before the diagnosis of migraine headache can be made?**

In addition to repeated episodes of headache, at least three of the following symptoms must be present: 1) family history of migraine headache; 2) visual, sensory, motor or vertiginous aura prior to the onset of the headache; 3) nausea/vomiting or recurrent abdominal pain accompanying the headache; 4) unilateral head pain that is throbbing or pounding; 5) relief of pain by a brief period of sleep.

○ **What symptoms and signs distinguish transverse myelitis from Guillain-Barré syndrome?**

Both transverse myelitis and acute polyneuritis share the acute onset of lower extremity weakness and paresthesias as presenting symptoms and signs. Patients with transverse myelitis will initially complain of back pain (in the absence of trauma) and urinary retention. Patients with acute polyneuritis will have bowel and bladder dysfunction later in the course. On physical examination of patients with transverse myelitis, a distinct "sensory level" will also be elicited; impairment of touch, pain and temperature sensation will be seen, but proprioception will remain intact.

○ **What is the pathophysiology of Guillain-Barré syndrome?**

The pathologic hallmark of acute polyneuritis is demyelination of motor and sensory nerves, thought to be due to an autoimmune process, causing the classic ascending paralysis, areflexia and paresthesias seen in these patients.

○ **What is the "Fisher variant" of Guillain-Barré syndrome?**

Patients with the Fisher variant of acute polyneuritis will have areflexia, oculomotor palsies and ataxia as the predominant physical findings.

○ **How does one distinguish patients with poliomyelitis from those with Guillain-Barré syndrome?**

In contrast to patients with acute polyneuritis, who have symmetric ascending paralysis, patients with poliomyelitis will have asymmetric ascending paralysis. In patients with poliomyelitis, the deep tendon reflexes will be variably depressed; patients with Guillain-Barré syndrome are areflexic. In addition, the prodrome of poliomyelitis is explosive, with fever and meningismus.

○ **What is the pathophysiology of myasthenia gravis?**

Antibodies against the acetylcholine receptor of the post-synaptic neuromuscular junction-this results in failure of neuromuscular transmission, with consequent fluctuating muscle weakness.

○ **What are the presenting signs and symptoms of juvenile myasthenia gravis?**

The juvenile form of myasthenia gravis accounts for 25% of all cases and is the predominant form seen in the pediatric population, usually in school-age children. Most patients will have ptosis, oculomotor palsies and truncal or limb weakness that becomes progressively worse with continued muscle activity.

○ **What is the "Tensilon test"?**

The Tensilon test secures the diagnosis of myasthenia gravis. Edrophonium (Tensilon), which is an anticholinesterase drug, is given slowly by the intravenous route. Patients with myasthenia gravis will have a brief, but dramatic, resolution of their muscle weakness.

❍   **A 4-year-old presents with the acute onset of unsteadiness of gait. He has otherwise been well, except for a recent upper respiratory infection. Examination reveals ataxia, tremor and bilateral dysmetria. What is the most likely diagnosis?**

Acute cerebellar ataxia, which is characterized by the acute onset of ataxia in an otherwise healthy child, usually between the ages of 1 and 4 years. Antecedent viral infections precede the onset of symptoms in over half of patients. Resolution of symptoms usually occurs within 2 weeks of the onset of symptoms.

❍   **What must be excluded in the above patient before the diagnosis of acute cerebellar ataxia?**

A posterior fossa mass or tumor.

❍   **What is the natural progression of spinal muscular atrophy in patients who present in infancy?**

Rapid degeneration of anterior horn cells, which leads to marked progressive muscular weakness, leading to respiratory failure and death.

❍   **What other organ systems are involved in patients with Duchenne muscular dystrophy?**

Cardiomyopathy, to varying degrees, is found in nearly every patient, as well as intellectual impairment, most often in the form of learning disabilities.

❍   **Is Lyme disease a common cause of seventh nerve palsy?**

Yes-there is a subset of patients with Lyme disease who present solely with an isolated seventh nerve palsy.

❍   **What is the likelihood that a patient with Bell's Palsy will completely recover?**

Complete recovery is seen in up to 80% of patients, usually within three weeks of the onset of symptoms.

❍   **In what region of the central nervous system do the majority of encephaloceles present?**

Up to 80% of encephaloceles occur in the occipital region.

❍   **What is the developmental defect that results in an encephalocele?**

Defective closure of the rostral portion of the neural tube in association with a defect in the bones of the skull-this occurs between the third and fourth weeks of gestation.

❍   **What other clinical findings are associated with encephaloceles?**

Severe mental retardation, seizures and motor deficits.

❍   **What are other clinical findings that may be present in patients with myelomeningoceles?**

Deficits in lower extremity motor function; disturbances in bowel and bladder function; hydrocephalus, which is seen in up to 75% of cases; and arthrogryposis, which are contractures of the lower extremities due to lack of lower extremity movement in utero.

❍   **What CNS malformation may be seen in patients who have myelomeningocele and hydrocephalus?**

Arnold-Chiari malformations.

❍   **What is the defect responsible for spina bifida occulta?**

Spina bifida occulta occurs because of a vertebral defect, usually in the lumbosacral region, that does not lead to a herniation of the contents of the spinal canal.

O   **What are the cutaneous manifestations that may be seen in patients with spina bifida occulta?**

Some patients may have a hairy tuft or a "birth mark" at the base of the spine. Occasionally, there may be a sinus tract that leads to an intraspinal cyst. Most patients, however, are asymptomatic.

O   **What is the definition of " non-communicating" hydrocephalus?**

If the obstruction to the flow of cerebrospinal fluid occurs within the ventricular system, then non-communicating hydrocephalus results.

O   **What is the definition of "communicating" hydrocephalus?**

If the obstruction to the flow of cerebrospinal fluid occurs outside the ventricular system at the level of any of the exit foramina or if there is an excessive production of cerebrospinal fluid, then communicating hydrocephalus results.

O   **What clinical features make up the Dandy-Walker syndrome?**

The clinical features making up the Dandy-Walker syndrome include: 1) failed formation of the cerebellar vermis; 2) cyst in the floor of the fourth ventricle; 3) anterior compression of the aqueduct of Sylvius; 4) obstruction of the exit foramen of the fourth ventricle.

O   **How do neonatal seizures differ from seizures in older children?**

In contrast to older children, in whom idiopathic epilepsy is common, seizures in neonates are usually secondary phenomena of underlying disease.

O   **What are some of the underlying disease states that may lead to neonatal seizures?**

1. Metabolic disturbances, such as hypoglycemia, hypocalcemia, hypomagnesemia, hyponatremia;
2. Hypoxic ischemic encephalopathy;
3. Intracranial hemorrhage;
4. CNS infections, both bacterial and viral;
5. Pyridoxine dependent seizures;
6. Maternal drug abuse in the third trimester, such as methadone addiction or passive exposure ex-utero, such as that from crack cocaine;
7. Local anesthetic intoxication;
8. Familial neonatal convulsions.

O   **What is the most common cause of neonatal seizures?**

Hypoxic-ischemic encephalopathy, which accounts for nearly 60% of cases.

O   **What is the treatment for infantile botulism?**

Therapy is supportive, such as nasogastric feeding and support of respiration. Antibiotics do not halt the progression of the disease.

O   **What are the three characteristic findings of Klippel-Feil syndrome?**

1. Low occipital hairline;
2. Short neck;
3. Limited neck motion, often due to fusion of the cervical vertebrae. Malformations of other organs , such as the brain, extra-ocular muscles, musculoskeletal system, are common.

○   **What is the definition of macrocephaly?**

Macrocephaly is defined as a head circumference two standard deviations above the mean.

○   **What is the definition of microcephaly?**

Microcephaly is defined as a head circumference two standard deviations below the mean.

○   **What agents are useful to decrease the production of cerebrospinal fluid (CSF) in patients with hydrocephalus?**

Acetazolamide, furosemide and glycerol have all been used to decrease CSF production.

○   **What central nervous system abnormalities are seen in patients with Arnold-Chiari malformations?**

There are three types of Arnold-Chiari malformations. In type I, the medulla and parts of the cerebellum are displaced downward into the spinal canal. In type II, the fourth ventricle is elongated and descends into the spinal canal; features of type I are also present. Type III, which is rare, involves a defect in the cervical vertebrae through which neural tissue herniates.

○   **What is "benign intracranial hypertension" (pseudotumor cerebri)?**

Benign intracranial hypertension is a syndrome in which patients have symptoms and signs (headache, papilledema) of increased intracranial pressure; however, physical examination shows no focal neurologic deficits or encephalopathy and there is no evidence of an intracranial mass or obstruction to the flow of CSF. CSF analysis will be normal except for increased opening pressure.

○   **What drugs are thought to be associated with the development of benign intracranial hypertension (pseudotumor cerebri)?**

Antibiotics, such as tetracycline, minocycline, penicillin, gentamicin; oral contraceptives; steroids; NSAIDS such as indomethacin; thyroid; lithium carbonate.

○   **Deficiency of what vitamin may cause benign intracranial hypertension (pseudotumor cerebri)?**

Vitamin A.

○   **What is the most common cause of intracranial bleeding in children?**

Congenital malformations of cerebral blood vessels, such as arteriovenous malformations (AVM's).

○   **What are the two most common presentations of arteriovenous malformations (AVM's) in children?**

50-75% of patients with AVM's will present with intracranial hemorrhage (usually subarachnoid hemorrhage), while 25-40% will present with seizures.

○   **What is the most common complication from a linear skull fracture?**

A subgaleal hematoma is the most common complication. These hematomas can become very large, especially if they liquefy and dissect through the subgaleal space.

○   **A 10-year-old presents with a large scalp laceration with an underlying depressed skull fracture that needs to be elevated in the OR; however, this will not occur for several hours. The child is otherwise stable. Should the overlying laceration be repaired before the child goes to the OR?**

Yes: rarely is the site of the laceration the site of incision to repair the depressed skull fracture. Meticulous wound care and closure will prevent hemorrhage and prolonged exposure of the fracture site to skin organisms, especially if there is a delay in definitive operative treatment. Antibiotic treatment to cover skin flora is also recommended.

○   **A 5-month-old child presents with coma. There is no history of reported trauma or viral prodrome. On examination the child is afebrile, comatose, with decerebrate posturing and fixed, dilated pupils and a bulging fontanel. What other physical examination finding would help to confirm the diagnosis?**

Funduscopic examination-if retinal hemorrhages are present, then this is most likely a case of a shaking-impact injury. A CT scan may show subdural or intracranial hemorrhage.

○   **What is the immediate treatment of the patient in the question above?**

1. Intubation and hyperventilation;
2. Establish IV access;
3. Vigorous resuscitation of shock, if present;
4. Elevation of the head of the bed to 30 degrees;
5. Management of increased intracranial pressure, either by an ICP monitor and/or infusion of a hyperosmotic agent, such as mannitol. Once the patient is stable, a definitive radiologic procedure, such as a CT scan, should be performed to confirm the diagnosis.

○   **Can significant head trauma, causing intracranial bleeding, lead to hypovolemic shock in a child?**

As a general rule, closed head trauma, not matter how significant, rarely causes hypovolemic shock in children. However, children less than 12 months of age who have large epidural hematomas with overlying skull fractures may decompress the hematoma into the scalp to a degree that significant blood loss can occur. This is the one rare exception to the rule.

○   **A child with a significant closed head injury develops generalized seizures. Which (intravenous) anticonvulsant should be administered?**

Phenytoin, as it will not cloud the sensorium or cause sedation, so that subsequent neurologic examinations can be done easily.

○   **What is the first cranial nerve abnormality seen in the early stages of transtentorial herniation?**

Because of its course along the parahippocampal gyrus of the temporal lobe, which is that portion of the brain that herniates through the tentorium, the third cranial nerve is compressed, leading to a unilateral fixed, dilated pupil.

○   **A child presents with severe somnolence and a two week history of gradually worsening headache. On examination he is somnolent and responsive only to pain. He also has bilateral sixth nerve palsies. What is the cause of his symptoms?**

A diffuse increase in intracranial pressure, probably the result of an intracranial mass.

○   **An otherwise healthy child presents with high fever, headache, stiff neck and somnolence. On examination he has a left hemiparesis. What is the cause of these signs and symptoms?**

This child most likely has a subdural empyema, which can occur alone or with meningitis.

○   **What is the mechanism for the development of a subdural empyema?**

Subdural empyemas occur most often as a sequelae of chronic sinusitis; there may be direct extension of bacterial pathogens from sinus cavities that are contiguous with the CNS or from septic venous thromboses. Subdural empyemas may also occur on first presentation, or after several days of therapy, in patients with bacterial meningitis.

○   **What are the four major groups of signs and symptoms seen in children with brain tumors?**

1) severe, recurrent headaches, with/without vomiting; 2) cerebellar ataxia; 3) acute deterioration in level of consciousness; 4) acute onset of cranial nerve palsies.

○   **What signs and symptoms are suggestive of a mass lesion/tumor in the infratentorial region?**

Patients with infratentorial mass lesions will more often present with cerebellar dysmetria, gait ataxia, vomiting and cranial nerve palsies.

○   **What signs and symptoms are suggestive of a mass lesion/tumor in the supratentorial region?**

Patients with supratentorial mass lesions will more often present with intellectual disturbances, speech difficulties, visual field cuts, seizures and hemiparesis.

○   **What is "lissencephaly"?**

Lissencephaly is an unusual disorder that is characterized by the absence of cerebral gyri and poorly formed sylvian fissures, leading to a smooth appearance of the surface of the brain. This defect is caused by faulty migration of neuroblasts during embryogenesis.

○   **What clinical features are found in infants with lissencephaly?**

These infants present with failure to thrive, microcephaly, marked developmental delay, hypoplasia of the optic nerve, microphthalmia and severe seizures.

○   **What clinical features are found in patients with Aicardi syndrome?**

Aicardi syndrome, which is thought to be due to a defect in the X chromosome and therefore is seen exclusively in females, is associated with defects in several organ systems. Patients will have agenesis of the corpus callosum, intractable seizures, mental retardation, hemivertebrae and abnormalities of the retina, including coloboma of the optic disc.

○   **What clinical features are found in patients with Möbius syndrome?**

Infants with Möbius syndrome initially present with bilateral facial weakness, poor feeding/sucking and strabismus, due to absence of the motor nuclei or nerve fibers of the sixth and seventh cranial nerves. Other brainstem nuclei may be involved as well.

○   **What infectious agents may cause myositis?**

Infectious causes of myositis are usually viral in origin and include Influenza A and Coxsackie virus, types A and B. Multiple abscesses of muscle from *Staphylococcus aureus* and trichinosis are unusual causes of myositis.

○   **What type of breathing pattern is seen in patients with "Cheyne-Stokes" respirations?**

Patients with Cheyne-Stokes respirations will have periods of hyperpnea followed by shorter periods of apnea.

O   **Where is the dysfunction in the CNS in patients who have Cheyne-Stokes respirations?**

Patients with Cheyne-Stokes respirations have bilateral cerebral hemisphere dysfunction with normal brainstem function.

O   **In patients with true vertigo, at what levels of the CNS may the defect occur?**

Patients who have true vertigo have a vestibular defect that may be peripheral (involving the labyrinth in the inner ear or the vestibular nerve) or central (involving the vestibular nuclei and its central pathways).

O   **Can otitis media be a cause of vertigo in children?**

Yes; children with acute otitis media may often complain of decreased hearing and impaired balance, but occasionally purulent otitis media may lead to a serous labyrinthitis, resulting in vertiginous symptoms and temporary hearing loss.

O   **What is the most common cause of labyrinthitis in children?**

Labyrinthitis in children is most often due to viral causes, such as influenza, measles and mumps.

O   **Which symptoms help to distinguish vestibular neuronitis from labyrinthitis in children?**

Both labyrinthitis and vestibular neuronitis are causes of vertigo in children and often are associated with coexisting viral infection. However, children with labyrinthitis will have hearing loss, while those with vestibular neuronitis will not.

O   **What clinical features characterize children with cyclic vomiting?**

Cyclic vomiting is a migraine variant that maybe present in young children. These patients will have cyclic, or even monthly, episodes of vomiting with abdominal pain that are alleviated by periods of deep sleep. Later in life, these children often develop migraine headaches.

O   **What clinical features characterize children with acute confusional states?**

Acute confusional states are migraine variants that have unusual presentations, such as the onset of headache that is followed by a period of vomiting, lethargy and confusion, disorientation and unresponsiveness. These episodes of "acute confusion" may last for several hours, after which the patient may have no memory of the event. There will be a family history of migraine headache.

O   **How does one make the diagnosis of acute confusional state?**

The diagnosis is often made by a history of headache followed by a period on confusion or unresponsiveness that is not due to any other organic cause and a family history or migraine headache. An EEG may reveal localized areas of slowing during and shortly after the attack, after which the EEG will be normal.

O   **What skin manifestation is seen in nearly every patient with neurofibromatosis?**

Cafe-au-lait spots -> than 5 that are 5 mm in diameter in prepubertal patients, > than 6 that are 15 mm in diameter in postpubertal patients.

O   **What two skin manifestations may be present in patients with neurofibromatosis?**

Axillary or inguinal freckling; and cutaneous neurofibromas, which appear during adolescence or pregnancy and are small, rubbery purplish masses.

○ **What other clinical features are seen in patients with neurofibromatosis, type 1?**

In addition to cafe-au-lait spots, axillary freckling and neurofibromas, patients may have Lisch nodules, which are hamartomas of the iris; osseous lesions, such as dysplasia of the sphenoid wing and bowing of the tibia and fibula; and optic gliomas. Patients may also have CNS abnormalities, such as seizures, learning disabilities, and difficulty paying attention.

○ **What clinical feature distinguishes patients with neurofibromatosis, type 2?**

Bilateral acoustic neuromas, which are a cause of hearing loss. Problems with balance and facial weakness are most characteristic of patients with neurofibromatosis, type 2.

○ **What neurocutaneous syndrome may be seen in patients with infantile spasms?**

Tuberous sclerosus.

○ **What characteristic skin lesions are present in the majority of patients with tuberous sclerosus?**

Hypopigmented patches, occasionally resembling an "ash leaf", are seen in nearly 90% of patients with tuberous sclerosus.

○ **What instrument may aid in the identification of the hypopigmented patches in patients suspected of having tuberous sclerosus?**

A Wood's lamp, which provides an ultraviolet light source, will aid in the identification of patients with tuberous sclerosus.

○ **What are the characteristic brain lesions seen in patients with tuberous sclerosus?**

Tubers, which are often found in the convolutions of the cerebrum, in the foramen of Munro, periventricular area and in the subependymal region.

○ **What two skin manifestations may be seen in patients with tuberous sclerosus?**

1. "Shagreen patches", which are raised lesions with an "orange peel" consistency, often found in the lumbosacral region;
2. Sebaceous adenomas, which are red nodules of the nose and cheeks that are seen in children over 4 years of age.

○ **What cardiac lesions are seen in some patients with tuberous sclerosus?**

Cardiac rhabdomyomas, which can be present in up to 50% of patients with tuberous sclerosus, are often found in the left ventricle .

○ **Are patients with tuberous sclerosus at an increased risk of malignancy?**

Yes-tubers of the CNS can occasionally progress to malignant astrocytomas.

○ **Which clinical features characterize patients with Sturge-Weber syndrome?**

1. Facial nevus, or port wine stain;
2. Seizures;
3. Mental retardation;

4.   Intracerebral calcifications;
5.   Hemiparesis.

O   **Do all infants with facial port wine stains need an evaluation for Sturge-Weber syndrome?**

No. Only those patients with port wine stains that involve the distribution of the trigeminal nerve require evaluation.

O   **What ophthalmologic complications may be found in patients with Sturge-Weber syndrome?**

The following complications involving the eye ipsilateral to the facial nevus may occur: enlargement of the eye, buphthalmos, and glaucoma.

O   **What type of seizures are seen in patients with Sturge-Weber syndrome?**

Most often, focal tonic-clonic seizures that involve the side of the body contralateral to the facial nevus.

O   **A healthy 5-month-old infant presents with episodes of sudden flexion of the neck and upper extremities, occurring upon awakening. The child has been developing normally, the pregnancy and delivery were uneventful. The child has a normal neurologic exam, as well as a CT of the head which shows no abnormalities. An EEG shows a hypsarrhythmic pattern, confirming your suspicion of infantile spasms. What is the prognosis for this child?**

This patient has "cryptogenic" infantile spasms, which often has an excellent prognosis for normal neuro-development.

O   **What drug(s) is(are) preferred for the management of infantile spasms?**

Adrenocorticotrophic hormone (ACTH) or prednisone-the dosage and length of therapy are controversial.

O   **What is the most common movement disorder in childhood?**

Transient tic disorder, which presents most often in boys. The movements consist of eye-blinking, throat clearing or other repetitive facial movements. These "tics" usually regress after one year and do not require drug treatment. Family history is often positive for "tics".

O   **How does one distinguish patients with transient tic disorder from those with *Gilles de la Tourette* syndrome?**

In contrast to patients with transient tic disorder, patients with *Gilles de la Tourette* syndrome will sometimes have coprolalia (repetitive use of obscene words), echolalia (repetition of words addressed to the patient), palilalia (repetition of one's own already spoken words) and echokinesis (imitation of others' movement). These tics are lifelong.

O   **When is drug therapy needed for patients with *Gilles de la Tourette* syndrome?**

When the motor or verbal tics significantly impair daily activities of living.

O   **What other neurologic conditions may be associated with *Gilles de la Tourette* syndrome?**

Attention deficit-hyperactivity disorder may be seen in up to 50% of patients with *Gilles de la Tourette* syndrome.

O   **What drug therapy is most often successful in treating patients with *Gilles de la Tourette* syndrome?**

Haloperidol.

❍   **A 6-month-old infant presents with a progressively enlarging, pulsating mass on his skull. He had fallen off the changing table and hit his head on the floor one month earlier, but did not seek medical care at the time. What is the most likely diagnosis?**

A leptomeningeal cyst, which is an unusual complication of linear skull fractures. The cyst is caused by interposition of the leptomeninges and occasionally, traumatized brain, through the interrupted dura and edges of the fracture. The mass will then expand because of communication with the CSF space and the cyst.

❍   **A 7-year-old presents with a generalized seizure. His mother also mentions that she has noted a deteriorating performance in school, as well as difficulty controlling his temper and clumsy gait. On physical examination his skin seems darkly pigmented, even in the perineal region. He also has hyperreflexia and clonus. What test would help with your diagnosis?**

This is a common presentation of adrenoleukodystrophy. A CT scan or MRI of the brain may demonstrate periventricular demyelination.

❍   **How do you explain his darkly pigmented skin?**

Up to 50% of patients with adrenoleukodystrophy will have primary adrenal insufficiency.

❍   **What is the prognosis for this patient?**

Most patients with adrenoleukodystrophy will die within 10 years of the onset of symptoms.

❍   **A 6-year-old child falls 5 feet, hitting his head on concrete and then has a generalized seizure lasting less than 1 minute. His neurological exam is completely normal. What is the most likely diagnosis?**

Post-traumatic seizure.

❍   **His parents want to know the likelihood of another seizure. What do you tell them?**

Approximately 25% of children with post-traumatic seizure will have additional seizures beyond one week after the injury.

❍   **A child has a severe closed head injury with increased intracranial pressure, which has not been well managed with intubation/hyperventilation, sedation and osmotic agents. His vital signs have otherwise been stable. Which agent would you next use to try to reduce the intracranial pressure?**

Induction of coma with pentobarbital.

❍   **How does pentobarbital lower raised intracranial pressure?**

Pentobarbital decreases cerebral blood flow by causing vasoconstriction of the cerebral vasculature and by reducing cerebral metabolism.

❍   **A 3-year-old child presents with coma. He had intractable, non-bilious vomiting for 24 hours prior to the onset of coma. There is no history of trauma. SGOT and SGPT are elevated but the serum bilirubin is normal. What is the most likely diagnosis?**

Reye's syndrome.

❍   **What is Horner's syndrome?**

Miosis, ptosis, and anhydrosis (lack of sweat).

O   **A 16-year-old obese girl with a history of irregular menses presents with a severe headache and blurry vision. Your physical exam is unremarkable except for papilledema. Her head CT is negative. An LP is done and opening pressure is 380 mm H_2O. What is the diagnosis and treatment?**

Pseudotumor cerebri. Draining some fluid is therapeutic. Also, start her on a course of steroids.

RHEUMATOLOGY, IMMUNOLOGY AND ALLERGY

○ **Which class of immunoglobulins is responsible for urticaria (hives) and angioedema?**

Both are mediated by IgE.

○ **Which class of immunoglobulins is responsible for food allergies?**

IgE.

○ **What are the <u>most</u> <u>common</u> food allergies?**

Dairy products, eggs, and nuts.

○ **When do the clinical manifestations of a new drug allergy usually become apparent?**

1-2 weeks after starting the drug.

○ **Which drug is the <u>most</u> <u>common</u> pharmaceutical cause of true allergic reactions?**

Penicillin accounts for approximately 90% of true allergic drug reactions and for more than 95% of fatal anaphylactic drug reactions. Parenterally administered penicillin is more than twice as likely to cause a fatal anaphylactic reaction than orally administered penicillin.

○ **How long after exposure to an allergen does anaphylaxis occur?**

The symptoms of anaphylaxis may occur within seconds or may be delayed up to 1 hour.

○ **A patient who is on Σ-blockers and who develops anaphylactic cardiovascular collapse may not respond to epinephrine or dopamine infusions. Which drug can be used in this setting?**

Glucagon may be useful for refractory hypotension associated with Σ-blocking agents.

○ **Anaphylaxis-related deaths are primarily caused by penicillin. What is the second <u>most</u> <u>common</u> cause?**

Insect stings. Approximately 100 deaths in the US occur annually because of anaphylaxis that is induced by insect stings.

○ **Most children with mucocutaneous lymph node syndrome (MLNS) are below what age?**

MLNS, or Kawasaki disease, is predominantly found in children under 9 years of age.

○ **Are the nodules of erythema nodosum most often symmetrically or asymmetrically distributed?**

Erythema nodosum produces distinctive bilateral tender nodules with underlying red or purple shiny patches of skin that develop in a symmetric distribution along the shins, arms, thighs, calves, and buttocks.

O   **What therapy is effective for treating erythema nodosum?**

There is no therapy known to alter the course of the disease. The disease usually lasts several weeks but the pain associated with the tender lesions can be relieved with non-steroidal anti-inflammatory agents.

O   **What percentage of patients with MLNS also develop acute carditis?**

Fifty percent will develop carditis, usually myocarditis with mild to moderate congestive heart failure. Pericarditis, conduction abnormalities, and valvular disturbances may occur but are less common.

O   **A patient presents with fever, acute polyarthritis, or migratory arthritis a few weeks after a bout of Streptococcal pharyngitis. What disease should be suspected?**

Acute rheumatic fever. Although the early symptoms may be nonspecific, a physical exam eventually reveals signs of arthritis (60-75%), carditis (30%), choreiform movements (10%), erythema marginatum, or subcutaneous nodules.

O   **What treatment should be started after the diagnosis of acute rheumatic fever has been made?**

Penicillin or erythromycin should be given even if cultures for Group A *Streptococcus* are negative. High-dose aspirin therapy is used at an initial dose of 75-100 mg/kg/day. Carditis or congestive heart failure is treated with prednisone, 1-2 mg/kg/day.

O   **What is Lhermitte sign in ankylosing spondylitis?**

A sensation of electric shock that radiates down the back when the neck is flexed. This is a sign that atlantoaxial subluxation and cervical spine instability may be present.

O   **Cite an example of each of the 4 major types of allergic reactions: type I—immediate hypersensitivity; type II—cytotoxic, type III—Arthus reaction; and type IV—delayed hypersensitivity.**

Type I: Asthma, food allergies (IgE).
Type II: Transfusion reaction (IgG and IgM).
Type III: Serum sickness, post streptococcal glomerulonephritis (complex activates complement).
Type IV: Skin testing (activated T-lymphocytes).

O   **Which of the four types of allergic reactions can be caused by a drug allergy?**

A drug allergy can produce all four types of allergic reactions.

O   **Myocardial infarction can occur with which two rheumatic diseases?**

Kawasaki disease and polyarteritis nodosa (PAN).

O   **What is the <u>most</u> <u>common</u> cause of anaphylactoid reactions?**

Intravenous iodinized radiographic contrast media.

O   **A bacterial infection and an allergic phenomenon can both cause a generalized confluent exfoliation of skin. What are the two diseases, and what test should be performed to distinguish between the two?**

Ritter's disease, or dermatitis exfoliativa neonatorium, is caused by infection by *Staphylococcus* and thus is also known as Staphylococcal Scalded skin syndrome (SSSS). This condition causes exfoliation at the superficial granular layer of the epidermis. Toxic epidermal necrolysis (TEN) appears very similar, but is an allergic phenomenon. A skin biopsy distinguishes the two conditions because the exfoliative cleavage plane is deeper at the dermal-epidermal junction with TEN.

○ **What is required to make a diagnosis of mucocutaneous lymph node syndrome, or Kawasaki disease, in a young patient with a prolonged fever?**

The diagnosis requires four of these five common clinical findings:

1. Conjunctival inflammation.
2. Rash.
3. Adenopathy.
4. Strawberry tongue and injection of the lips and pharynx.
5. Erythema and edema of extremities.

Desquamation of the fingers and the toes may be striking, but it is a late finding and is not one of the key clinical features of the disease.

○ **What is the probable diagnosis in an adolescent girl with unexplained pain and tenderness at the head of the second metatarsal? What clinical and x-ray findings are expected?**

Frieberg's infarction is an avascular necrosis of a metatarsal head, most often the second metatarsal, but occasionally occurring bilaterally. Typical findings include local swelling and tenderness, restricted range of motion at the MTP joint, evidence of sclerosis on x-ray, and flattening or irregularity of the metatarsal head.

○ **What is the treatment of choice for the patient in anaphylactic shock?**

Epinephrine, 0.3-0.5 mg intravenously.

○ **How long should a patient with a generalized anaphylactic reaction be observed?**

Because recurrence of hemodynamic collapse and airway compromise is common within the first 24 hours, patients should be observed for at least that period of time. Treatment with antihistamines and steroids should be continued for 72 hours.

○ **How does relapsing polychondritis affect the airway?**

Approximately 50% of patients with relapsing polychondritis have airway involvement and may present with pain and tenderness over the cartilaginous structures of the larynx. Dyspnea, stridor, cough, hoarseness, and erythema and edema of the oropharynx and nose may also be exhibited.

○ **How should a patient with airway involvement from relapsing polychondritis be managed?**

Admit these patients for high-dose steroids and for close observation. Repeated exacerbations may lead to severe airway compromise and asphyxiation.

○ **A patient who is on chronic steroids presents with weakness, depression, fatigue, and postural dizziness. What pathological process should be suspected? What is the treatment?**

Adrenal insufficiency. The treatment is to administer large "stress doses" of steroids.

○ **If adrenal insufficiency is suspected, what test should be performed? Which drug should be prescribed?**

A serum cortisol level should be drawn before administering a large dose of steroids. Dexamethasone is the preferred agent because it does not interfere with subsequent tests that may be indicated.

❍   **What cardiac complication commonly occurs with SLE as well as with juvenile rheumatoid arthritis and rheumatoid arthritis?**

Pericarditis.

❍   **What are the articular symptoms of late, Stage III, Lyme disease?**

Chronic arthritis, especially in the knee, periostitis, and tendonitis.

❍   **What are the articular symptoms of late, Stage III, Lyme disease?**

Chronic arthritis, especially in the knee, periostitis, and tendonitis.

❍   **A 10-year-old child presents limping and complaining of several weeks of groin, hip, and knee pain that worsens with activity. What diseases should be considered?**

Transient tenosynovitis of the hip, slipped capital femoral epiphysis, Legg-Calvé-Perthes, suppurative arthritis, rheumatic fever, juvenile rheumatoid arthritis, and tuberculosis of the hip.

❍   **What disease is suspected in an adolescent with a tender, purpuric dependent rash, colicky abdominal pain, migratory polyarthritis, and microscopic hematuria?**

Henoch-Schönlein purpura, a leukoblastic vasculitis. Intestinal or pulmonary hemorrhage may occur, and 7–9% percent of the cases will develop chronic renal sequelae. Salicylates are effective for the arthritis. Other treatment is directed at the symptoms. Steroids are not particularly effective.

❍   **A child has painful swollen joints along with a spiking high fever, shaking chills, signs of pericarditis, and a pale erythematous coalescing rash on the trunk, palms, and soles. Hepatosplenomegaly is found. What is the diagnosis?**

Systemic juvenile rheumatoid arthritis. Arthrocentesis is necessary to eliminate the possibility of septic arthritis. The rheumatoid factor and the antinuclear antibody usually are negative; one-fourth of patients will proceed to have joint destruction. This is the least common of the three types of JRA.

❍   **What treatment besides aspirin is effective in preventing the complications of Kawasaki disease?**

Intravenous immunoglobulins can reduce the incidence of coronary artery aneurysms to less than 5%.

❍   **Which joint is typically involved in the <u>most</u> <u>common</u> form of juvenile rheumatoid arthritis?**

The most common of the three forms of JRA usually involves the knee and does not lead to joint destruction. Reiter's syndrome, iridocyclitis, and inflammatory bowel disease all may be associated with this particular form of the disease.

❍   **A child has posttraumatic tenderness at the end of a long bone. A joint effusion is the only radiographic finding. What is the appropriate management?**

Immobilization and subsequent orthopedic evaluation for possible separation of the epiphysis from the metaphysis (i.e., Salter-Harris type I fracture).

❍   **A patient presents with pain along the radial aspect of the wrist extending into the forearm. What is the diagnostic test of choice?**

Finkelstein's test confirms the diagnosis of deQuervain's tenosynovitis, an overuse inflammation of the extensor pollicis brevis and the abductor pollicis where they pass along the groove of the radial styloid. The test is performed by instructing the patient to make a fist with the thumb tucked inside the other fingers. The test is positive for this condition if pain is reproduced when the examiner gently deviates the fist in the ulnar direction.

❍   **In carpal tunnel syndrome, Tinel's sign is produced by tapping the volar wrist over the median nerve. If the test is positive, what does the patient experience?**

Paresthesias extending into the index and long fingers.

❍   **What autoimmune disease produces lesions that are sometimes urticarial in appearance yet are not pruritic?**

Erythema multiforme.

❍   **What disease classically produces erythematous plaques with dusky centers and red borders resembling a bulls-eye target?**

Erythema multiforme. This disease can also produce non-pruritic urticarial lesions, petechiae, vesicles, and bullae.

❍   **Which drugs are <u>most</u> <u>commonly</u> implicated in toxic epidermal necrolysis?**

Sulfonamides and sulfones, phenylbutazone and related drugs, barbiturates, other antiepileptic drugs, and antibiotics.

❍   **What is the appropriate management for TEN?**

Admit for management similar to that required for extensive second-degree burns. The mortality of TEN can be as high as 50% because of fluid loss and secondary infections.

❍   **What can cause erythema multiforme?**

EM can be triggered by viral or bacterial infections, by drugs of nearly all classes, and by malignancy.

❍   **What is the <u>most</u> <u>common</u> cause of allergic contact dermatitis?**

Toxicodendron species, such as poison oak, poison ivy, and poison sumac are responsible for more cases of contact dermatitis than all the other allergens combined.

❍   **Why does scratching spread poison oak and poison ivy?**

The antigenic resin contaminates the hands and fingernails and is thereby spread by rubbing or scratching. A single contaminated finger can produce more than 500 reactive groups of lesions.

❍   **How is the antigen of poison oak or poison ivy inactivated?**

Careful washing with soap and water destroys the antigen. Special attention must be paid to the fingernails, otherwise the antigenic resin can be carried for weeks.

❍   **What underlying illnesses should be considered in a patient with nontraumatic uveitis?**

Collagen vascular diseases, sarcoid, ankylosing spondylitis, Reiter's syndrome, tuberculosis, syphilis, toxoplasmosis, juvenile rheumatoid arthritis, and Lyme disease.

❍   **What is the difference between episcleritis and scleritis?**

Both are associated with collagen vascular disorders; however, episcleritis is a benign superficial inflammation of the tissues between the sclera and the conjunctive. Conversely, scleritis is a more severe and more painful inflammation of the deep sclera which can result in visual loss.

O   **What is the probable diagnosis of a patient with myalgias, arthralgias, headache, and an annular erythematous lesion accompanied by central clearing?**

Stage I Lyme disease with the classic lesion of Erythema Chronicum Migrans (ECM). The primary lesion occurs at the site of the tick bite.

O   **What rheumatologic ailments produce pulmonary hemorrhage?**

Goodpasture's disease, systemic lupus erythematosus, Wegener's granulomatosis, and nonspecific vasculitides.

O   **What rheumatologic ailments can produce acute airway obstruction?**

Relapsing polychondritis and rheumatoid arthritis.

O   **What infectious agents may produce a chronic smoldering arthritis with sterile aspiration cultures?**

Tuberculosis and fungal infections. A synovial biopsy may be required to confirm the diagnosis.

O   **How is septic bursitis contracted?**

A puncture wound or an overlying cellulitis are the typical sources for septic bursitis.

O   **What rheumatologic ailments produce valvular heart disease?**

Ankylosing spondylitis, relapsing polychondritis, and rheumatic fever.

O   **Which immune cells are responsible for adaptive immunity?**

Antigen specific immunity is the responsibility of the B and T lymphocytes.

O   **What lymphocyte surface molecule is responsible for HLA class II antigens?**

CD4.

O   **What lymphocyte surface molecule is responsible for HLA class I antigens?**

CD8.

O   **Which are the only complement fixing immunoglobulins?**

IgG and IgM.

O   **Which is the major protective Ig of external secretions?**

IgA.

O   **Which Ig is the major host defense against parasites?**

IgE.

O   **What are the two main functions of T cells?**

To signal B cell to make antibody and kill virally infected or tumor cells

○   **T/F: CD4 to CD8 ratio in infants is 1.5 : 2.1.**

False. T cells are actually present in a higher numbers in infants due to the higher absolute lymphocyte counts, therefore the ratio is 3.5 : 4.1, rather than 1.5 : 2.1 ratio seen in children.

○   **What type of infections are newborns most susceptible to and why?**

Gram negative organisms. Since there is <u>no</u> passive transfer of IgM, which are heat stable opsonins, the opsonization process is impaired.

○   **So then, why aren't infants more susceptible to gram positive organisms?**

Passively transferred IgG serves as effective opsonins.

○   **Why is the vaccine containing HiB polysaccharide ineffective in children under 2 years of age?**

It is not immunogenic! Infants cannot produce antibody to polysaccharide antigen unless it is conjugated to a protein carrier.

○   **Peak mass of the thymus is reached at what time during development?**

Just before puberty.

○   **Early infectious complications of recurrent pneumonia, chronic mucocutaneous candidiasis, otitis media, diarrhea, and chronic rhinitis would alert you to what congenital immune defect ?**

Cell mediated defects of T and/or B cell lymphocyte immunodeficiencies.

○   **What are the <u>most reliable</u> and <u>cost effective</u> tests for assessing T, B, and, NK cell function?**

CBC and Sedimentation rate. If the sedimentation rate is normal a chronic bacterial infection is unlikely. If the absolute lymphocyte count is normal the patient is not likely to have a severe T cell defect. If the RBC's are without Howell-Jolly bodies congenital splenism is excluded. If the platelet count is normal, then Wiskott-Aldrich syndrome is excluded.

○   **What test would you order to exclude and/or diagnose the most common hypoglobulinemia?**

Quantification of Serum IgA.

○   **Write an order for the most cost effective test to evaluate T cell function in a child less than six years old.**

0.1 ml of 1:100 Candidia protein antigen intradermally.

○   **What prenatal diagnostic test would confirm either Adenosine Deaminase (ADA) or purine nucleoside phosphorylase (PNP) diseases?**

Enzymatic analysis of an amnion cell prior to 20 weeks gestation.

○   **What prenatal diagnostic test would confirm either X-linked agammaglobulinemia or X-linked SCID?**

Restriction Fragment Length Polymorphism (RFLP) at 18-22 weeks gestation.

○   **What prenatal diagnostic test would confirm Wiskott-Aldrich Syndrome?**

Fetal platelet size at 18-22 weeks gestation.

○   **12 month old infant with repeated pneumococcal pneumonia is found to have an immunoglobulin concentration of IgA, IgM, and IgE of <100 mg/dl and a lymph node biopsy demonstrating hypoplasia with absent germinal centers and rare plasma cells. Which viral vaccine would you be most cautious with administration?**

Hepatitis and polio vaccine. In children with Bruton's agammaglobulinemia, viral infections such as hepatitis, polio, and echovirus can be fatal.

○   **In contrast to infectious diseases associated with Bruton's Agammaglobulinemia what infection is rarely seen in Common Variable Immunodeficiency (CVID)?**

Echovirus Meningoencephalitis.

○   **Blood products given to an individual with selective IgA deficiency must be prepared in what way?**

Washed (5x in normal saline) normal donor erythrocytes or blood products. 44% of IgA deficient patients have auto IgA antibody, which when present may precipitate anaphylaxis and death with transfusion of unprepared donor cells.

○   **Is immune serum globulin (IVIG) therapy indicated for Transient Hypogammaglobulinemia of Infancy (THI)?**

No.

○   **Is immune serum globulin (IVIG) therapy indicated for Selective IgA deficiency?**

No.

○   **75% of children with X-linked lymphoproliferative disorder (XLD or Duncan's Disease) present with what disease manifestation?**

Epstein Barr infection which precipitates a fatal liver necrosis caused by polyclonal activated alloreactive cytotoxic T Cells against EBV infected autologous B cells.

○   **All newly diagnosed patients with Common Variable Immunodeficiency (CVID) should be screened for what prior to administration of IVIG?**

Anti IgA antibodies.

○   **X-linked agammaglobulinemia and CVID are most susceptible to which infections?**

Pyogenic bacterial infections most notably *S. aureus, H. influenzae, and S. pneumoniae.*

○   **Patients with Hyper IgM syndrome like those with agammaglobulinemias are at an increased risk for sinopulmonary infections, but unlike agammaglobulinemia patients they are at additional risk for?**

P. cranii pneumonitis.

○   **What four infectious agents are most commonly associated with asplenic individuals?**

S. pneumoniae, Neisseria sp., H. influenzae and, Salmonella sp.

○ **DiGeorge's Syndrome is a result of dysmorphogenesis of the 3rd and 4th pharyngeal pouch. What other anomalies might you expect?**

Right sided aortic arch, esophageal atresia, bifid uvula, atrial and ventricular septal defects, short philtrum of upper lip, hypertelorism, epicanthal folds, mandibular hypoplasia, low set notched ears, and hypoplasia of the parathyroid and thyroid glands.

○ **Which B cell deficient syndrome has the highest incidence of concomitant autoimmune disorders?**

X-linked immunodeficiency with Hyper IgM.

○ **What is the defect in X-linked Hyper IgM syndrome?**

Failure of B cells to terminally differentiated into isotype specific plasma cells.

○ **What is the population frequency of Severe combined immunodeficiency syndrome (SCID)?**

1 in 100,000 or 1 in 500,000 live births.

○ **Which disorder is considered the most severe of the recognized immunodeficiencies?**

SCID

○ **X-linked agammaglobulinemia (Bruton's) and C3 complement deficiency share what common clinical feature?**

Susceptibility to pyogenic infections.

○ **Fatality of hereditary angioedema can occur due to what condition?**

Edema of the larynx.

○ **What is the functional defect of Paroxysmal nocturnal hemoglobinuria (PNH)?**

A hemolytic anemia disorder that occurs as a result of DAF, CD59, C8bp not being expressed on the erythrocyte surface resulting in inappropriate anchoring of cell membrane proteins.

○ **Patients with Systemic Lupus Erythematosus (SLE) and their asymptomatic family members often have a partial deficiency of which complement component?**

Deficiency of CR1 which increases risk of developing immune complex disease.

○ **Patients which suffer from Familial Mediterranean Fever (FMF) have a genetic deficiency in a protease whose function is to inactivate chemotactic factor C5a and IL-8. How would the disease manifest clinically?**

Patients with this rare disorder suffer from recurrent episodes of fever with associated painful inflammation of joints, pleural, and peritoneal cavities.

○ **Acute neutrophilia occurs during what physiologic events?**

Physical exercise and epinephrine-induced reactions, such as a panic response.

○ **Reactive leukocytosis resembling a leukemia-like picture can occur in what clinical scenarios?**

Sepsis, systemic mycotic or protozoan, hepatic failure, diabetic acidosis, and azotemia.

○   **What is the definition of neutropenia?**

Absolute Neutrophil Count (ANC) < 1500 cell/ml.

○   **What percent neonates born to eclamptic mothers have transient neutropenia?**

50%.

○   **Aside from chemotherapeutics which suppress bone marrow, what other agents are most commonly implicated?**

Phenothiazine, semisynthetic penicillin, NSAID's, aminopyrine derivatives, antithyroid medications.

○   **What is the most common cause of transient neutropenia?**

Viral infections which most commonly include Hepatitis A, Hepatitis B, Influenza A and B, measles, rubella, and varicella.

○   **How long would you expect the neutropenia to persist?**

It may persist the first three to six days of the acute viral syndrome.

○   **What nutritional deficiencies may precipitate neutropenia?**

Vitamin B12, Folic Acid, and Copper.

○   **Neutropenia and bacterial infection may herald the onset of what clinical entity?**

Overwhelming sepsis.

○   **What is the most common form of benign chronic neutropenia?**

Autoimmune neutropenia of infancy.

○   **When is Benign Chronic Neutropenia disorder usually diagnosed?**

It is usually detected as an incidental finding during workup of child with fever.

○   **At what age do patients recover from Benign chronic neutropenia?**

By 4-years-old.

○   **What congenital enzymatic deficiency can mimic a primary neutropenic syndrome with presentation of neutropenia, chronic recurrent infections, hepatomegaly, and mental retardation?**

Both glycogen storage disease type 1a (Von Geirke's) and Type 1b.

○   **Which autosomal recessive disorder is characterized by pancreatic insufficiency and neutropenia?**

Schwachman-Diamond Syndrome.

○   **These rare autosomal recessive diseases are characterized by absence of adhesion glycoproteins or carbohydrate ligands on the cellular surface. Subsequently patients present with recurrent** necrotic acellular skin and soft tissue ulcers, cellulitis, gingivitis, ulcerative stomatitis, and otitis media despite high (50,000-100,000) blood granulocyte counts. What is the type of disorder?

Leucocyte adhesion deficiencies of which two subtypes exist, Type 1 LAD and Type 2 LAD.

○   **What is the mechanistic basis for Type 1 LAD or Type 2 LAD?**

Absence or diminished expression of adhesion molecules on the cell surface prevents proper adhesion and extravasation of neutrophils to endothelium at active sites of infection and inflammation.

○   **What is the likely symptomology of individuals with Hereditary myeloperoxidase deficiency?**

A majority of individuals remain asymptomatic. Remarkably, the incidence of disease is quite high with 1 in 2,000 individuals affected in the United States.

○   **What is the prognosis of Chediak-Higashi syndrome?**

Affected persons may die at any time as illness frequently progresses to an accelerated phase characterized by lymphadenopathy, hepatosplenomegaly, pancytopenia, hemorrhage of GI and brain. This accelerated phase if often precipitated by lymphotrophic viral infections such as Epstein-Barr.

○   **Would prophylactic antibiotics be indicative in this condition?**

No. Prevention with antibiotics has not been shown to be useful in this condition.

○   **What is the <u>most</u> <u>common</u> inherited disorder of phagocyte function?**

Chronic Granulomatosus Disease (CGD).

○   **Name the typical organisms isolated in culture of infected sites in patients with CGD .**

S. aureus, Klebsiella, Aerobacter, E. coli, Shigella, Salmonella, Pseudomonas, S. marcescens, C. albicans, and *Aspergillus.*

○   **What is a convenient screening test for CGD?**

The reduction of nitroblue tetrazolium (NBT) is used to screen for adequate superoxide anion during phagocytic activation.

○   **What percent of children would be expected to have an abnormal chest x-ray?**

90%.

○   **What long term prophylaxis is useful for these patients?**

Trimethoprim-sulfamethoxazole (TMP-SMZ) appears to increase disease-free intervals.

○   **Patients with CGD should undergo what type of testing prior to transfusions?**

Some patients have the McLeod phenotype in which they lack the Kell antigen. Serious transfusion reactions can occur in these people if they receive Kell antigen positive blood.

○   **Briefly explain the cellular basis for the Type I hypersensitivity reaction (Wheal and flare). Give a clinical example.**

This immediate type or anaphylactic hypersensitivity is mediated by circulating basophils and mast cells which become activated by cross-linking of IgE on their membrane surface. The prototypic IgE mediated disease is ragweed hay fever. Other, sometimes fatal, anaphylactic reactions are the classic insect venom, and food induced allergies.

○   **Briefly explain the cellular basis for the Type II hypersensitivity reaction (cytotoxic) Give a clinical example.**

These immune interactions involve integral cellular antigen components and IgG and IgM antibody formation to these "foreign" antigen determinants. The classic example is immune mediated hemolysis such as that seen in transfusion reactions or Hemolytic disease of the newborn.

○   **Which hypersensitivity reaction is responsible for a majority of the glomerulopathies?**

90% of glomerulonephritis is Type III or immune complex disease.

○   **What is a prototypic DTH type IV reaction?**

Contact allergy such as chemical induced contact dermatitis or poison ivy.

○   **In taking a history when one suspects allergy, what are some of the most important components to include?**

History of exposure to potential allergens, frequency, duration, location, and progression of symptoms, seasonal symptoms, onset of symptoms, relieving factors(medication, diurnal variation, change in location), and nature of symptoms (dry vs. productive cough, clear vs. purulent sputum).

○   **What test is most cost effective, sensitive, and specific in the diagnosis of allergy?**

In vivo skin testing.

○   **What in vitro tests may be useful in the diagnosis of allergic conditions?**

WBC with differential, Ig serum content, RAST, leukocyte histamine release test.

○   **A patient has a 5 mm "wheal and flare" reaction to ragweed, but denies seasonal allergic symptoms. What does this indicate?**

The patient has been exposed to the allergen, but may not be allergic.

○   **What are the signs and symptoms of theophylline toxicity?**

Nausea, insomnia, irritability, tremors, headache, seizure, tachycardia, cardiac rhythm disturbances, hypotension, ataxia, hallucinations, hypokalemia, and hyperglycemia.

○   **What effects of corticosteroids are likely after two hours?**

Fall in peripheral eosinophils and lymphocytes.

○   **What effects of corticosteroids are likely after six to eight hours?**

Improvement in pulmonary function in asthmatics and hyperglycemia.

○   **What are the clinical effects of phenobarbital and phenytoin on corticosteroids?**

Increased steroid clearance and hence decreased plasma concentration.

○   **What is the most common adverse effect on chronic systemic corticosteroid use?**

Suppression of linear growth.

○   **What infections are children receiving chronic steroids particularly susceptible to?**

Disseminated varicella and *Pneumocystis carinii* pneumonia

○   **What is the preferred dosing regimen of prednisone or prednisolone to lessen the hypothalamic-pituitary-adrenal axis suppressive effect?**

It is recommended that alternate day regimen given as a single dose between 6:00 and 8:00 am. If daily dosing is required, then administer a single dose between 6:00 and 8:00 am.

○   **What patients are not good candidates for immunotherapy desensitization?**

Patients with atopic dermatitis and food allergy.

○   **What is the prognosis of allergic rhinitis?**

90% of children will still have persistent symptoms 8 to 11 years later.
19% of children will develop asthma or wheezing.

○   **What constitutes triad asthma or Samter's Triad?**

The syndrome of nasal polyps, asthma, and aspirin intolerance comprise triad asthma.

○   **The most likely cause of foul-smelling, unilateral, blood-tinged, purulent discharge from a child's nose?**

Foreign body.

○   **The most effective treatment of allergic rhinitis?**

Topical use of corticosteroid such as beclomethasone nasal spray.

○   **What is the prognosis of childhood asthma?**

50% of all asthmatic children are symptom free within 10-20 years. In mild asthma, the remission rate is 50%, with only 5% experiencing severe disease. 95% of children with severe childhood asthma, however, become asthmatic adults.

○   **Is cor pulmonale resulting from sustained pulmonary hypertension a common complication of asthma?**

No.

○   **Define extrinsic asthma.**

Asthmatic exacerbation following environmental exposure to allergens such as dust, pollens, and dander.

○   **Define intrinsic asthma.**

Asthmatic exacerbation not associated with an increase in IgE or a positive skin.

○   **What is Harrison's sulci?**

An anterolateral depression of the thorax at the insertion of the diaphragm, which is sometimes present in children with recurrent sever retractions.

❍   **Does a child with asthma requires a chest x-ray?**

Every child with an exacerbation does not require a chest x-ray. However, it may be necessary to rule out other respiratory diagnosis.

❍   **When administering epinephrine in the treatment of asthma, how might the side effects of epinephrine be minimized?**

Side effects such as pallor, tremor, anxiety, palpitations, and headache can be minimized if doses of no more than 0.3 ml are given.

❍   **If the response to epinephrine and bronchodilators are unsatisfactory, what might be administered next – and at what dose?**

Aminophylline may be given IV at a dose of 5mg/kg for 5-15 minutes at a rate no greater than 25 mg/min. Steroids should also be administered at this time, though the effects won't be seen for about 6 hours.

❍   **What are the historical risk factors for status asthmaticus?**

Chronic steroid-dependent asthma, prior ICU admission, prior intubation, recurrent ER visits in past 48 hours, sudden onset of severe respiratory compromise, poor therapy compliance, poor clinical recognition of attack severity, and hypoxic seizures.

❍   **What percent of patients with atopic dermatitis have elevated serum IgE levels?**

80%.

❍   **Describe the diagnostic criteria of atopic dermatitis in infants?**

Must have three major features: 1) family history, 2) extensor eczematous or lichenified dermatitis, and 3) evidence of puritus. Patients must also have three minor features: chronic scaling of scalp, postauricular fissures, ichthyosis, xerosis, or hyperlinear palms.

❍   **Describe the clinical manifestation of urticaria?**

Well-circumscribed, erythematous raised skin lesions.

❍   **What is most common form of urticaria caused by physical factors?**

Cold urticaria.

❍   **What is the most effective treatment for control of urticaria?**

0.5 mg/kg Hydroxyzine (Atarax).

❍   **What substances can induce pseudoallergic anaphylaxis?**

Iodinated radiocontrast media, opiates, D-tubocurarine, thiamine, aspirin, and captopril.

❍   **When do most anaphylactic reactions occur?**

Within the first 30 minutes after initial exposure.

❍   **What are typical initial symptoms of an anaphylactic reaction?**

A tingling sensation around the mouth, followed by a warm feeling and tightness in the chest or throat.

❍   **What is standard treatment of anaphylactic reaction?**

Aqueous epinephrine 1:1000 at 0.1 ml/kg with maximum dosage of 0.3 ml for a child.

❍   **Which vaccines must be avoided by patients who have a severe allergy to eggs?**

Influenza and yellow fever vaccines.

❍   **Which antitoxoids are still prepared with horse serum, and thus may precipitate serum sickness?**

Crotalid envenomation and clostridia antitoxin.

❍   **What is the major cause of serum sickness?**

Drug allergy, particularly to penicillin.

❍   **Are atopic individuals at an increased risk for developing adverse drug reactions?**

No. However, they may suffer a more severe reaction if they do acquire a drug allergy.

❍   **What is the most common manifestation of an adverse drug reaction?**

Cutaneous eruption with urticarial, exanthematous, and eczematoid types occurring predominantly.

❍   **What text may be used to identify an anaphylactic hypersensitivity to penicillin?**

Skin testing with benzylpenicilloyl-polylysine (BPL PrePen) identifies a majority of children who are at risk.

❍   **What cell wall inhibitor does not cross react in patients who are allergic to penicillin?**

Aztreonam.

❍   **When treatment with penicillin is absolutely necessary, which route of desensitization is the safest?**

Oral.

❍   **What infectious agent is implicated in chronic blepharitis infection?**

Staphylococcal.

❍   **An 8-year-old boy is complaining of lacrimation, itching, and burning of both eyes, with significant photophobia. The patient has a past medical history significant for asthma. What is your diagnosis?**

Vernal conjunctivitis.

❍   **If you decide to treat the vernal conjunctivitis with topical steroids, what must be monitored?**

Intraocular pressure.

❍   **When treating idiopathic aplastic anemia, the curative treatment of choice is?**

Bone marrow transplantation (BMT) with an HLA matched donor.

○ **Which AML is treated by pharmacological means only, with BMT usually <u>not</u> being considered unless a relapse occurs?**

M3, or promyelocytic leukemia.

○ **What percentage of children with acute lymphoblastic leukemia are cured by conventional chemotherapy?**

70%.

○ **What is the disease-free survival rate of patients with ALL after BMT?**

15%-65%, with relapse rates of 30%-70%.

○ **In general, which patients have the best disease-free prognosis after BMT?**

Those which have been transplanted in remission, or those who went into an earlier remission.

○ **What is the incidence of infection with autologous BMT?**

5-10%.

○ **When is BMT recommended for patients with either Non-Hodgkin's or Hodgkin's lymphoma?**

Early after relapse, when there is little bulky disease and a greater chance of BMT tolerance.

○ **What blood dyscrasias are currently being considered for treatment through BMT?**

Fanconi's anemia, thalassemias, sickle cell disease, Diamond-Blackfan syndrome, congenital sideroblastic anemia.

○ **Define Graft Versus Host Disease (GVHD)?**

Engraftment of immunocompetent donor cells into an immunocompromised host, resulting in cell mediated cytotoxic destruction of host cells if an immunologic incompatibility exists.

○ **What is the <u>most</u> important variable considered to account for BMT rejections?**

HLA disparity.

○ **When does acute GVHD present and what are the typical manifestations?**

Acute GVHD typically occurs about day 19 (median) just as the patient begins to engraft and is characterized by erythroderma, cholestatic hepatitis, and enteritis.

○ **What is the clinical definition of chronic GVHD (cGVHD)?**

As early as 60-70 days past engraftment, patients exhibit signs of a systemic autoimmune process, manifesting as Sjögren syndrome, systemic lupus erthrematosus, scleroderma, primary biliary cirrhosis, and recurrent infections with encapsulated bacteria, fungus, or viruses.

○ **What are the risk factors for development of cGVHD?**

Increasing age, prior acute GVHD, buffy-coat transfusions, parity of female donor.

○ **How long is immunosuppressive treatment required for BMT recipients?**

Usually 6-12 months or until a state of tolerance is attained.

O   **What treatment may be an alternative for patients at high risk for or with refractory chronic GVHD?**

Thalidomide has been shown to have a 59% response rate with a 76% survival for those with refractory and 48% survival for those with high risk cGVHD.

O   **What are the potential risks for treatment of GVHD with T-cell depletion techniques?**

By depleting the T-cell population, the success of engraftment decreases as well as the ability to defend against potential malignancies.

O   **What is the typical dosing regimen of methotrexate given to prevent GVHD?**

Given on days 1, 3, 6, and 11 post-transplantation and weekly thereafter.

O   **Treatment with methotrexate may result in what complications and how is it treated?**

Methotrexate may worsen renal impairment, resulting in fluid retention and may aggravate existing mucositis. In these situations, rescue of the dihydrofolate reductase system with leucovorin is indicated.

O   **What is the mechanism of action of cyclosporine?**

It selectively inhibits the translation of IL-2 mRNA by helper T-cells, thus attenuating the T-cell activation pathways.

O   **What are the significant categories of toxic side effects of cyclosporine therapy?**

<u>Neurotoxic</u>: Tremors, paraesthesia, headache, confusion, somnolence, seizures, and coma.
<u>Hepatotoxic</u>: Cholestasis, cholelithiasis, and hemorrhagic necrosis.
<u>Endocrine</u>: Ketosis, hyperprolactinemia, hypertestosteronemia, gynecomastia, and impaired spermatogenesis.
<u>Metabolic</u>: Hypomagnesemia, hyperuricemia, hyperglycemia, hyperkalemia, and hypocholesterolemia.
<u>Vascular</u>: Hypertension, vasculitic hemolytic-uremic syndrome, and atherogenesis.
<u>Nephrotoxic</u>: Oliguria, acute tubular damage, fluid retention, interstitial fibrosis, and tubular atrophy.

O   **Which drugs should be used to treat children who suffer from headaches associated with cyclosporine administration?**

Propranolol.

O   **What is the incidence of cataracts with patients who have received single dose, total body irradiation (TBI), fractionated TBI, and chemotherapeutics alone?**

The incidence of cataracts with signal dose TBI is 80%, fractionated TBI is 20%-50%, and 20% after chemotherapy alone.

O   **What are the long-term effects of corticosteroid treatment?**

Growth failure, cushingoid appearance, hypertension, cataracts, GI bleeding, pancreatitis, psychosis, hyperglycemia, osteoporosis, aseptic necrosis of the femoral head, and suppression of the pituitary-adrenal axis.

O   **What annual hormone evaluation is essential in post transplant patients?**

Growth hormone and gonadal hormones, as patients approach puberty.

○   **How long does immune-cell function recovery take in post transplant patients?**

B cells respond to mitogenic stimulation in 2 to 3 months, however adequate serum IgG levels may take as long as 7 to 9 months, and IgA levels lagging up to two years. CD8 T cells – 4 months. CD4 T cells – 6 to 9 months.

○   **Name the most common types of infections seen in post-transplant, engraftment patients?**

Oral thrush, bacterial sepsis, catheter infections, fungal infections, pneumonia, and sinusitis.

○   **Name the most common types of infections seen post-transplant and post-engraftment (Days 1-100)?**

CMV and EBV infection, viral hepatitis, toxoplasmosis, diffuse interstitial pneumonia, and cystitis.

○   **Name the most common types of infections seen post-transplant and post-engraftment (Days 100-365)?**

Varicella, Herpes, CMV, toxoplasmosis, Pneumocystis canrii pneumonia, viral hepatitis, and common bacterial infections.

○   **With BMT recipients 30-100 days post-transplant, what percentage of patients will be infected with cytomegalovirus, if prophylaxis is not used?**

50-60%.

○   **When should re-immunization be instituted with patients who have no evidence of chronic GVHD?**

Diptheria and tetanus toxoid: 3 to 6 months status post transplant
Inactivated (Salk) polio: 6 to 12 months
Measles, mumps, and rubella (MMR): 1 to 2 years

○   **What cardiac condition accounts for the highest percentage of heart transplants?**

Cardiomyopathies, which account for 66% of pediatric heart transplants.

○   **What precludes a child from eligibility for cardiac transplantation?**

Pulmonary vascular disease, and pulmonary hypertension.

○   **How are cardiac allografts matched for transplant recipients?**

ABO blood group, and body weight (HLA matching is not currently used).

○   **In what time period, post-operatively, is a transplant patient at greatest risk for acute rejection?**

During the first 3 months.

○   **T/F: Most clinical cardiac transplant rejections occur without detectable clinical symptoms.**

True. Cyclosporine has significantly modified the clinical course of rejection.

○   **What is the five-year survival rate of pediatric heart transplant recipients?**
72%.

O   **What neoplastic disease is most commonly associated with post-transplantation patients?**

Lymphoproliferative disease (LPD), which is associated with the Epstein-Barr virus.

O   **What infectious agent accounts for 25% of infectious episodes of allograft heart recipients?**

Cytomegalovirus.

O   **What is the most common site of bacterial infection seen in transplant patients?**

Lung (35%).

O   **What side effect is most commonly seen with cyclosporine therapy?**

Hypertension resulting from plasma volume expansion and defective renal sodium excretion.

O   **Name the three most frequent causes of mortality in pediatric heart transplant patients.**

Infection (32%), refection (23%), and graft coronary artery disease (20%).

O   **What condition indicates a chronic form of rejections in heart-lung transplant recipients, and is the major limitation in long term survival for these patients?**

Obliterative bronchiolitis.

O   **What commonly used immunosuppressive agent would be contraindicated in heart-lung transplant patients?**

Steroids. Their use may affect airway healing.

O   **What is the leading cause of death for these patients?**

Infection.

O   **What is the five-year survival rate of pediatric heart-lung transplant recipients?**

40%.

O   **What is the most sensitive and specific sign of an infectious disease in an immunocompromised host?**

Fever.

O   **What is the most common indication for pediatric liver transplantation?**

Hepatic biliary atresia, after a failed portoenterostomy (Kasai procedure).

O   **What is the most important pre-liver transplantation management for a patient?**

Ensure adequate nutritional status, with regard to caloric intake, vitamins, and mineral supplementation.

O   **What percent of liver transplant patients will become infected with cytomegalovirus if prophylaxis is not given?**

50%.

O   **What are some common types of early infection in liver transplant patients?**

Gram negative enteric pneumonia, cholangitis, soft tissue wound infections, intraabdominal abscess, peritonitis, disseminated candidiasis.

O   **During the first six months, post liver transplant patients have a 15% chance of developing what type of hepatitis?**

CMV Hepatitis.

O   **Why is chronic dialysis therapy to be avoided in children?**

Dialysis for end stage renal disease (ERSD) in children is associated with failure to thrive, social maladaption, lack of sexual maturity, and chronic encephalopathy.

O   **Name two causes of ESRD with patients less than 5 years old.**

Congenital and obstructive uropathy.

O   **What is the most common cause of ESRD in children 13-17 years old?**

Glomerulopathies.

O   **What tissue typing studies are necessary on a patient prior to renal transplantation?**

HLA-A, B, C D/DR, and ABO.

O   **One month after renal transplant, what infectious agent most commonly causes a urinary tract infection?**

Pseudomonas aeruginosa.

O   **What percent of patients have recurrence of original disease?**

7%.

O   **What type of glomerulopathy is mot likely to recur?**

Focal segmental glomerulosclerosis.

O   **A renal transplant patient thirty days post-transplant presents with fever, oliguria, hypertension, and elevated serum creatinine. What two diagnostic tests would you perform next?**

Renal ultrasound and renal scan to evaluate renal blood flow.

O   **What diagnostic study is necessary to differentiate between rejection reaction, acute tubular necrosis, cyclosporine A toxicity, or recurrence of renal disease?**

Renal biopsy.

O   **What percentage of renal transplant patients will have at least one episode of rejection reaction?**

100%.

❍   **Of patients experiencing rejection reactions, what percent are successfully treated during the first episode?**

62%.

❍   **What is the major cause of death in renal transplant recipients who are one year post-transplantation?**

Infection.

❍   **Name the post-transplantation complications in pediatric renal patients.**

Acute tubular necrosis, refection reaction, vascular or urological block, recurrence of original disease, drug toxicity, infection, bleeding, pancreatitis, lymphocele, uroma, and bowel obstruction.

❍   **In transplant patients receiving immunosuppressive therapy, how does one evaluate abdominal pain?**

Chronic steroid use often masks abdominal catastrophes therefore, abdominal pain in a transplant patient is a surgical emergency until otherwise indicated.

❍   **A pediatric renal transplant patient is exposed to a child in an enclosed room with chicken pox for >1 hour. What do you do?**

Patient should receive one vial/kg body weight of varicella-zoster immunoglobulin (VZIG) to be given within 72 hours of the exposure.

❍   **What immunosuppressive agents have the highest risk of reactivating CMV infection?**

Azathioprine, and OKT3/antilymphocyte globulin.

❍   **What complication will develop in 33% of patients with clinically diagnosed CMV?**

Pulmonary involvement, which may rapidly progress to respiratory failure and death.

❍   **EBV infection is linked with what late complication (years)?**

Post-transplant lymphoproliferative disorder.

❍   **Transplant patient on chronic immunosuppressive agents presents with two week history of persistent, severe headache without fever. What is your diagnostic management?**

Neurological exam, CT scan, MRI, and an lumbar puncture unless contraindicated by evidence increased intracranial pressure.

❍   **A liver transplant patient presents with increase liver aminotransferase and direct bilirubin without pain or fever. Which diagnostic text would be useful?**

Doppler flow study, to rule out arterial thrombosis.

❍   **What would you suspect if a liver transplant patient presented with rapidly increasing ascites and liver dysfunction?**

Protein vein thrombosis.

❍   **What is the mechanism of immunosuppression with treatment modality hydroxychloroquine?**

Alkalinization of proteolytic vesicles.

O   **Anti dsDNA antibodies are most indicative of what disease?**

Systemic lupus erythematosus.

O   **Anti Ro(SSA) and La(SSB) are associated with what disease?**

Neonatal lupus syndrome.

O   **The presence of antineutrophil cytoplasmic antibodies (c-ANCA) with a diffuse staining pattern in serum immunofluorescence is most commonly associated with what disease?**

Wegener's Granulomatosus. It is also seen in Kawasaki Disease and HIV.

O   **The presence of anti phospholipid antibodies with patients who have either primary or secondary antiphospholipid syndromes are at increased risk for what pathological events?**

Risk of thrombic events, thrombocytopenia, hemolytic anemia, stroke, chorea, transverse myelitis, and vascular heart disease.

O   **What are the HLA allele associations for the following types of Juvenile Rheumatoid Arthritis (JRA): Pauciarticular Type I, Type II, and polyarticular rheumatoid factor positive?**

JRA Pauciarticular Type I: HLA-DR5, -DR6, and –DR8
JRA Pauciarticular Type II: HLA-B27
Polyarticular RA positive: HLA-DR4

O   **In which two subgroups of JRA is joint destruction more likely?**

RA factor positive polyarticular, and systemic-onset JRA.

O   **What percent of the above patients develop severe arthritis?**

>50%.

O   **What are the most common manifestations of JRA?**

High intermittent fever, rheumatoid rash, arthralgia or myalgia (during febrile episodes), and persistent arthritis of greater than six weeks duration.

O   **What is the overall prognosis of JRA patients?**

At least 75% of patients with JRA will have long term remissions without significant residual deformity or loss of function.

O   **What pharmacological treatment is not indicated in the treatment of JRA?**

Corticosteroids.

O   **How does ankylosing spondylitis differ from rheumatoid arthritis?**

Ankylosing spondylitis is characterized by involvement of the sacroiliac joints and lumbodorsal spine, predilection for males, occurrence of aortitis, familial incidence, RF negative, and lack of rheumatoid nodules or incidence of acute iridocyclitis.

O   **Reiter's disease may occur following infection with which microbial agents?**

Shigella, Yersinia, Enterocolitica, Campylobacter, and Chlamydia.

○   **What percent of children with inflammatory bowel disease have articular manifestations of the disease?**

10%.

○   **Which therapies are most effective for children afflicted with rheumatological disease?**

Physical and occupational therapies.

○   **What are the most frequent early symptoms of SLE in children?**

Fever, malaise, arthritis or arthralgia, and rash.

○   **Is discoid lupus common in children?**

No.

○   **What is the best screening test for SLE?**

A positive ANA titer should be demonstrable in all patients with active SLE.

○   **What hematologic conditions are seen with patients who have SLE?**

Anemia, thrombocytopenia, and leukopenia occur frequently.

○   **What neurologic disorders, if present, serve as diagnostic criteria for SLE?**

Seizures and psychosis.

○   **What pharmacologic agents are most commonly associated with drug induced lupus?**

Anticonvulsants, antihypertensive, and isoniazid.

○   **List the major causes of SLE mortality.**

Nephritis, central nervous system complications, infection, pulmonary lupus, and myocardial infarction.

○   **When is anticoagulation therapy indicated in SLE?**

Patients with the persistent presence of antiphospholipid antibodies (because of the risk of venous or arterial thrombosis), migraine, recurrent fetal loss, TIA, stroke, avascular necrosis, transverse myelitis, pulmonary hypertension or embolus, livedo reticularis, leg ulcers, or thrombocytopenia.

○   **What is the potentially irreversible sequelae of neonatal lupus?**

Congenital heart block.

○   **What is the most effective means of diagnosing vasculitis in children?**

Clinical diagnosis is most reliable.

○   **List the potentially fatal manifestations of Henoch-Schönlein syndrome.**

Acute renal failure; GI complications, such as hemorrhage, intussusception, and bowel infarction; and CNS involvement, which may precipitate seizures, paresis, or coma.

O   **What clinical manifestations are seen in all patients with Henoch-Schönlein syndrome?**

Dermatological manifestations, which will be present in all patients. However, skin lesions are extremely varied. The classic lesion begins as a small wheal or erythematous maculopapule, which becomes petechial or pupuritic. The palpable purpural lesions will progress from red to purple to rusty color as they age.

O   **Aside from the skin rash, what are the three most common manifestations of Henoch-Schönlein syndrome?**

Arthritis, 67%; GI complaints, 50%; and renal involvement, 25-50%.

O   **What syndrome is the leading cause of acquired heart disease in the US, and what percent of cases are fatal?**

Kawasaki's disease. 1-2% or cases are fatal.

O   **What test is most useful for recognizing coronary vascular disease, dilation, or aneurysmal formation?**

Two dimensional echocardiogram.

O   **List the possible complications of Kawasaki's disease during the acute phase of the illness?**

Arthritis, myocarditis, pericarditis, mitral insufficiency, CHF, iridocyclitis, meningitis, and sterile pyuria.

O   **Which form of vasculitis may be seen after infection with Hepatitis B?**

Polyarteritis nodosa.

O   **What side effects might one see only rarely with the administration of IV gamma globulin?**

Anaphylaxis, chills, fever, headache, and myalgia.

O   **Which tissue biopsy is most helpful for diagnosing Polyarteritis nodosa, but is rarely employed?**

Testicular biopsy.

O   **T/F: Erythema nodosum is most common in children less than six years old.**

False. This disease is rarely seen before the age of six. It progressively increases in frequency up to the third decade in life.

O   **Behçet syndrome is characterized by recurrent oral and genital ulcers and ocular inflammation. What additional symptoms are associated with a particularly poor prognosis?**

CNS abnormalities, such as cranial nerve palsies and psychosis.

O   **The combination of pain, tenderness, and swelling of the costosternal junction is referred to as what syndrome?**

Tietze syndrome, or costochondritis.

O   **What is the clinical scenario of Familial Mediterranean Fever, and what is the attributed cause?**

Amyloid deposition is the cause of this condition, which manifests with a proteinuria that progresses to nephrotic syndrome and renal failure.

❍   **What is the treatment for Familial Mediterranean Fever?**

Colchicine, which may greatly lessen the occurrence of the amyloid deposition.

❍   **What inflammatory conditions might one expect with secondary amyloidosis?**

JRA, cystic fibrosis, inflammatory bowel disease, and chronic infections such as tuberculosis.

TRANSPLANTATION

○ **In idiopathic aplastic anemia the curative treatment of choice is?**

Bone marrow transplantation (BMT) with an HLA matched donor.

○ **What may be administered as part of the preparative regime to lessen the likelihood of rejection in patients with aplastic anemia who have received transfusions ?**

Anti-thymocyte globulin (ATG) with cyclophosphamide.

○ **Which AML is treated by pharmacological means only, with BMT usually <u>not</u> being considered unless a relapse occurs?**

M3 or promyelocytic leukemia is usually quite responsive to all *trans*-retinoic acid and consolidation chemotherapy.

○ **What percent of children with Acute lymphoblastic leukemia are cured by conventional chemotherapy?**

70%.

○ **What is the disease free survival of patients with ALL after BMT?**

15% to 65% with relapse rates of 30%-70%.

○ **In general which patients have the best prognosis after BMT for disease free survival?**

Those which have been transplanted in remission or those that went into an earlier remission.

○ **What is the incidence of infection with autologous BMT?**

5-10%.

○ **When is BMT recommended for those with Chronic myelogenous leukemia?**

Within one year of diagnosis.

○ **When is BMT recommended for patients with either Non-Hodgkin or Hodgkin's lymphoma?**

Early after relapse when there is little bulky disease and a greater chance to tolerate the BMT regimen.

○ **What blood dyscrasias are currently being considered for treatment through BMT?**

Fanconi's Anemia, Thalassemias, Sickle cell disease, Diamond-Blackfan syndrome, and Congenital sideroblastic anemia.

○ **Define Graft versus host disease (GVHD)?**

Engraftment of immunocompetent donor cells into an immunocompromised host results in cell mediated cytotoxic destruction of host cells if a immunologic incompatibility exists.

O   **What is the <u>most</u> important variable considered to account for BMT rejection?**

HLA disparity.

O   **When does acute GVHD present and what are the typical manifestations?**

Acute GVHD typically occurs about day 19(median) just as the patient begins to engraft and is characterized by erythroderma, cholestatic hepatitis, and enteritis .

O   **10-year-old girl is 21 days status-post BMT and presents with a fever, maculopapular rash over 30% of her body, >1,000 ml diarrhea/ day, and rising LFT's with a total bilirubin of 4 mg/100ml. What is the clinical stage of GVHD?**

Stage ++.

O   **What is the clinical definition of chronic GVHD (cGVHD)?**

As early as 60-70 days status post engraftment patient exhibit signs of a systemic autoimmune process manifesting as Sjögren syndrome, Systemic lupus erythematosus, scleroderma, primary biliary cirrhosis, and commonly experience recurrent infection with encapsulated bacteria, fungus, or viruses.

O   **What are the risk factors for development of cGVHD?**

Increasing age, prior acute GVHD, buffy coat transfusions, parity of female donor.

O   **What agent may be a treatment alternative for patients at high risk for or with refractory chronic GVHD?**

Thalidomide has been shown to have a 59% response rate with a 76% survival for those with refractory and a 48% survival for those with high risk cGVHD.

O   **What are significant toxic side effects of cyclosporine therapy?**

<u>Neurotoxic</u>; tremors, paraesthesia, headache, confusion, somnolence, seizures, coma.
<u>Hepatotoxic</u>; cholestasis, cholelithiasis, hemorrhagic necrosis.
<u>Endocrine</u>; ketosis, hyperprolactinemia, hypertestosteronemia, gynecomastia, impaired spermatogenesis.
<u>Metabolic</u>; Hypomagnesemia, hyperuricemia, hyperglycemia, hyperkalemia, hypocholesterolemia.
<u>Vascular</u>: Hypertension, vasculitic hemolytic-uremic syndrome, and atherogenesis. Nephrotoxic; oliguria, acute tubular damage, fluid retention, interstitial fibrosis, tubular atrophy.

O   **Which drugs may exacerbated the nephrotoxicity of cyclosporine?**

Aminoglycoside, amphotericin B, acyclovir, digoxin, furosemide, indomethacin, or trimethoprim.

GENITOURINARY AND RENAL

○ **What is the <u>most</u> <u>common</u> cause of acute renal failure?**

Acute tubular necrosis. Acute tubular necrosis occurs after a toxic or an ischemic injury to the kidneys caused from shock, surgery, or rhabdomyolysis.

○ **Why is surgical correction of cryptorchidism important?**

Cryptorchidism is when a testae does not descend into the scrotum and is retained either in the abdominal cavity or in the inguinal canal. This condition can cause infertility in the affected testae and will increase the risk of cancer in that testae. Surgical correction is required to inhibit infertility, but the procedure has no bearing on the future development of testicular cancer. Surgery must be performed before the age of 5 to preserve fertility.

○ **What is the most important feature for distinguishing between testicular torsion and epididymitis?**

The rate of the onset of pain. Torsional pain begins instantaneously at maximum intensity, whereas epididymal pain grows steadily over hours or days. Clinically, elevation of the scrotum will relieve pain related to epididymitis, but is not effective with torsional pain.

○ **What is the <u>most</u> <u>common</u> cause of epididymitis?**

1. Prepubertal boys: Coliform bacteria
2. In men younger than 35: Chlamydia or Neisseria gonorrhea.
3. Older than 35: Coliform bacteria
4. Epididymitis is frequently caused by urinary reflux, prostatitis, or urethral instrumentation.

○ **What does epididymitis in childhood suggest?**

Obstructive or fistulous urinary defects. Epididymitis is rare in children.

○ **What is the significance of the "blue dot" sign?**

This is pathognomonic of torsion of the appendix testis or epididymis. With transillumination of the testis, a blue reflection occurs. When detected early, a patient with torsion of the appendages will experience intense pain near the head of the epididymis or testis that is frequently associated with a palpable tender nodule. If normal flow to the affected testis can be confirmed by a testicular ultrasound, immediate surgery can be avoided. Most appendages will calcify or degenerate within 10 to 14 day without harm to the patient.

○ **How does the pain associated with epididymitis differ from that produced by prostatitis?**

1. Epididymitis: The pain begins in the scrotum or groin and radiates along the spermatic cord. It intensifies rapidly, is associated with dysuria, and is relieved with scrotal elevation (Prehn's sign).
2. Prostatitis: Patients will have frequency, dysuria, urgency, bladder outlet obstruction, and retention. They may have low back pain and perineal pain associated with fever, chills, arthralgias, and myalgias.

○ **What percentage of patients with epididymitis will also have pyuria?**

25%.

❍   **What is the eponym for idiopathic scrotal edema? How is this disease treated?**

Fournier's gangrene is a polymicrobial infection of the subcutaneous tissue that is characterized by widespread tissue necrosis. Treatment consists of broad-spectrum parenteral antibiotics and immediate surgical debridement.

❍   **What 4 clinical findings are indicative of acute glomerulonephritis (GN)?**

1. Oliguria.
2 Hypertension.
3. Pulmonary edema.
4. Urine sediment containing red blood cells, white blood cells, protein, and red blood cell casts.

❍   **What is the differential diagnosis for rapidly progressive GN?**

1. Systemic Lupus Erythematosus (SLE): An autoimmune disorder resulting, in part, from a necrotizing vasculitis of primarily small vessels which is complicated by direct immunoglobulin deposition in glomeruli. The mortality rate is 18-58%, depending on the histologic type.
2. Henoch-Schönlein Purpura: Another systemic necrotizing vasculitis of small vessels. Patients present with a nephritic syndrome without edema or hypertension or with hematuria.
3. Hemolytic Uremic Syndrome (HUS): Patients present with microangiopathic hemolytic anemia, thrombocytopenia, and renal dysfunction. The onset is rapid. It occurs in children about 1 week after a gastroenteritis or an URI. HUS may occur in adults, most commonly complicating pregnancy or the post partum period. Acute renal failure develops in 60% of children with HUS and usually resolves in weeks with only supportive therapy.
4. Thrombotic Thrombocytopenic Purpura: This condition is closely related to HUS with a higher occurrence in young adults. It is associated with fevers, more neurologic problems, and less renal involvement (i.e., usually with hematuria and proteinuria). The prognosis is much worse as compared to HUS with a 75% three-month mortality rate.
5. Polyarteritis Nodosa (PAN): A systemic necrotizing vasculitis affecting primarily medium and small caliber arteries that can occur from infancy to old age. The peak incidence occurs at approximately 60 years of age. Ninety percent of patients with PAN will have renal involvement.

❍   **Which syndrome is characterized by a rapidly progressive, antiglomerular basement membrane antibody-induced GN that is preceded by pulmonary hemorrhage and hemoptysis?**

Goodpasture's syndrome.

❍   **What is the _most_ _common_ cause of hematuria?**

Lesions of the bladder or lower urinary tract. When hematuria originates in a kidney, the probable causes are polycystic kidney disease and nephropathy.

❍   **What are some causes of false-positive hematuria?**

Food coloring, beets, paprika, rifampin, phenothiazine, Dilantin, myoglobin, or menstruation.

❍   **A urinalysis reveals red cell casts and dysmorphic RBCs in the urine. What is the probable origin of hematuria?**

Glomerulus.

❍   **A 4-year-old boy presents with a painless mass in his scrotum that fluctuates in size with palpation. The mass transilluminates. What is the diagnosis?**

This is probably a communicating hydrocele. An inguinal-scrotal ultrasound should distinguish hydrocele from bowel and a testicular nuclear scan should rule out the possibility of testicular torsion.

○ **What is the composition of the <u>most</u> <u>common</u> kidney stones?**

Calcium oxalate (65%), followed by magnesium ammonium phosphate (struvite) (20%), calcium phosphate (7.5%), uric acid (5%), and crystine (1%).

○ **What percent of urinary calculi are radiopaque?**

90%.

○ **What are the admission criteria for patients with renal calculi?**

Patients should be admitted if they have infection with concurrent obstruction, a solitary kidney and complete obstruction, uncontrolled pain, intractable emesis, or large stones (because only 10% of stones > 6 mm pass spontaneously). Other indications for admission and urologic consultation include renal insufficiency and complete obstruction or urinary extravasation, as demonstrated by the IVP.

○ **What percent of patients with urinary calculi will not have hematuria?**

10%.

○ **A urinary pH of 7.3 is conducive to the formation of what kind of stones?**

Struvite and phosphate stones. Alkalotic urine actually inhibits the formation of uric acid and cystine stones. Conversely, struvite and phosphate stones are inhibited by a more acidic urine.

○ **Which type of stone formation is caused by a genetic error?**

Cysteine stones. These stones are produced because there is an error in the transport of amino acids that results in cystinuria.

○ **Where is kidney stone formation most likely to occur?**

In the proximal portion of the collecting system.

○ **What is the five year recurrence rate for kidney stones?**

50%. The ten year recurrence rate is 70%.

○ **What percent of patients spontaneously pass kidney stones?**

80%. This is largely dependent on size. 75% of stones less than 4 mm pass spontaneously, while only 10% of those larger than 6 mm pass spontaneously. Analgesics and increased fluid intake aid in outpatient management of kidney stones.

○ **What is the <u>most</u> <u>common</u> cause of nephrotic syndrome in children?**

Minimal change disease is the most common cause in children.

○ **Name some common nephrotoxic agents/substances.**

Aminoglycoside, NSAIDs, contrast dye, and myoglobin.

○ **What is the definition of oliguria? Of anuria?**

Oliguria is defined as a urine output of less than 500 mL/day. Anuria is associated with a urine output of less than 100 mL/day.

O   **What is the initial treatment for priapism?**

Terbutaline, 0.25–0.5 mg subcutaneously.

O   **What is the most common origin of proteinuria?**

Benign orthostatic proteinuria is the most common. Other entities include any that involve pathology of the glomerulus. Other origins are tubular pathology or over production of protein.

O   **What are the risk factors for subclinical pyelonephritis?**

Multiple prior UTIs, longer duration of symptoms, recent pyelonephritis, diabetes, anatomic abnormalities, immunocompromised patients, and in indigents.

O   **When are symptoms related to renal insufficiency displayed?**

When 90% of the nephrons have been destroyed. Hypertension, diabetes mellitus, glomerulonephritis, polycystic kidney disease, tubulointerstitial disease, and obstructive uropathy are all causes of chronic renal failure.

O   **What is the most common cause of intrinsic renal failure?**

Acute tubular necrosis (80-90%), resulting from an ischemic injury (the most common cause of ATN) or from a nephrotoxic agent.

Less frequent causes of intrinsic renal failure (10-20%) include vasculitis, malignant hypertension, acute GN, or allergic interstitial nephritis.

O   **If a urine dipstick is positive for blood yet the UA on the same urine is negative for RBCs, what is the probable disease?**

Rhabdomyolysis. Severe muscle damage can result in free myoglobin in the blood. Very high levels can lead to acute renal failure.

O   **What is the most common neoplasm in men under 30?**

Seminomas. This is also the most common type of testicular neoplasm. The peak incidence is between the ages of 20-40 with a smaller peak occurring below the age of 10. Ninety to ninety five percent of these cancers are germinal tumors. However, only 60-70% are germinal in children. Cryptorchidism is a significant risk factor for this cancer.

O   **What is the best tumor marker for testicular cancer?**

Placental alkaline phosphatase (PLAP). Seventy to ninety percent of patients with testicular cancer have elevated PLAP. Other tumor markers are Σ-fetoprotein and Σ-human chorionic gonadotropin.

O   **Testicular torsion is most common in which age group?**

14-year-olds. Two-thirds of the cases occur in the second decade. The next most common group is newborns.

O   **T/F: Testicular torsion frequently follows a history of strenuous physical activity or occurs during sleep.**

True.

○   **T/F: Forty percent of patients with testicular torsion have a history of similar pain in the past that resolved spontaneously.**

True.

○   **What is the definitive diagnostic test for testicular torsion?**

Emergent surgical exploration. Although radionuclide imaging and Doppler ultrasonography may be helpful, they are time-consuming, and their accuracy is operator-dependent. The warm ischemia time for testicular salvage may be as short as four hours. Therefore, after the diagnosis is made, immediate urologic consultation and surgical exploration are necessary.

○   **What is the definitive treatment for testicular torsion?**

Bilateral orchiopexy in which the testes are surgically attached to the scrotum.

○   **What is an important difference between testicular teratomas in children and adults?**

In children, teratomas are benign lesions. In adults, teratomas may metastasize.

○   **What is the most common cause of urinary tract infections (UTI)?**

E. coli (80%). *E. coli* is also the most common cause of pyelonephritis and pyelitis due to its ascension from the lower urinary tract. *Staphylococcus saprophyticus* accounts for 5-15% of the UTI cases.

○   **Varicoceles are most common in which part of the scrotum?**

The left. Varicoceles are a collection of veins in the scrotum. These patients have a higher incidence of infertility, presumably because of the increased temperature of the testes surrounded by the warm blood of the varicocele. Incidentally, the left testes is the first to descend and also hangs lower than the right in the majority of men. Hernias are also more common on the left side too.

○   **What is the most common renal tumor in children?**

Wilms tumor. This occurs in children under 5 years of age.

○   **One to two percent of the affected patients will have a recurrence of the Wilms tumor. Where is this recurrence most likely to be?**

In the chest.

○   **A second trimester ultrasound is performed on a pregnant female and it demonstrates oligohydramnios, nonvisualization of the bladder, and absent kidneys. What disorder should be suspected?**

Bilateral renal agenesis.

○   **What tumor in children is associated with horseshoe kidneys?**

Wilms tumor.

○   **What anatomic factors predispose a child to a urinary tract infection?**

Vesicoureteral reflux, obstruction, urinary stasis, and calculi.

O   **What is the most common cause of arterial hypertension in children?**

Chronic pyelonephritis.

O   **What is the gold standard laboratory test for diagnosing a urinary tract infection?**

Urine culture.

O   **When should a voiding cystourethrogram be used to assess reflux in a child?**

Approximately three weeks after treatment of an acute urinary tract infection in all males and females under five years of age. Reflux is found in 25% of all children under the age of 10 years who have had symptomatic or asymptomatic bacteria. It is more frequently observed in children under three years of age.

O   **If vesicoureteral reflux is present, what test should then be performed?**

Intravenous pyelography with nephrotomography to evaluate kidney size and detect possible calyceal blunting, ureteral dilatation, and renal scarring.

O   **What are the indications for long-term prophylaxis against urinary tract infection?**

Neurogenic bladder, urinary tract stasis with obstruction, calculi, recurrent cystitis, and persistent vesicoureteral reflux.

O   **How can reflux be harmful to the kidneys?**

It exposes the renal pelvis to much higher vesicle pressures produced during voiding and it facilitates a passage of bacteria from the bladder to the kidneys.

O   **How are grade I and grade II vesicoureteral reflux treated?**

The child should be given low doses of antimicrobial medications such as sulfamethoxazole-trimethoprim or nitrofurantoin. At the beginning of treatment, urine cultures should be obtained on a monthly basis until the efficacy of prophylaxis has been established, then cultures can be obtained at 3-month intervals. The likelihood of spontaneous resolution is high.

O   **What percent of children with grade III reflux may ultimately need surgical treatment?**

50%.

O   **What is the treatment for grade IV and V reflux?**

Early surgical treatment is indicated after a brief period of prophylaxis and confirmation of the persistence of reflux.

O   **A newborn presents with a palpable abdominal mass. What is the most common cause?**

A hydronephrotic kidney.

O   **What syndrome is associated with abdominal muscle deficiency, undescended testes, dilation of the bladder and ureters and occasionally with infravesical obstruction.**

Prune-belly syndrome, aka Eagle Barrett Syndrome.

O   **Were is the most common site of urinary tract obstruction in children?**

The ureteropelvic junction.

○ **What is the most common cause of obstruction of the ureteropelvic junction?**

Congenital stenosis of the ureteropelvic junction.

○ **A neonate presents with a renal mass, what is the differential diagnosis?**

Ureteropelvic junction obstruction, multicystic renal dysplasia, solid renal tumor, and renal vein thrombosis.

○ **What is a ureterocele?**

A congenital cystic dilatation of the distal ureter that protrudes into the bladder and has a pin point ureteral orifice.

○ **What is the most common cause of a urethral stricture in a male child?**

Urethral trauma due to either iatrogenic causes (catheterization, endoscopic procedures, previous urethral reconstruction) or accidental such as straddling injuries or pelvic fractures.

○ **What are the consequences of untreated bladder exstrophy?**

Total urinary incontinence and increased incidence of bladder cancer (usually adenocarcinoma).

○ **What is the initial treatment for a child born with bladder exstrophy?**

The bladder should be covered with a plastic dressing that will prevent desiccation of the bladder mucosa but allow urinary drainage and the infant should immediately be transferred to a center equipped for the treatment of such anomalies. Ideally, closure of the exstrophied bladder should be performed within the first 48 hours of life before permanent changes in the bladder wall are established.

○ **What are the causes of a neurogenic bladder in children?**

Myelomeningocele, lipomeningocele, and sacral agenesis. Acquired diseases and traumatic lesions of the spinal cord are less frequent.

○ **When should urodynamic studies be performed following repair of a myelomeningocele?**

Six months of age.

○ **What is the difference between primary and secondary nocturnal enuresis?**

Primary enuresis is when the child never has a period of nighttime continence, while secondary nocturnal enuresis is a developing condition in a formerly ìdryî child following a significant emotional event.

○ **How do you treat nocturnal enuresis?**

Reassure the parents that the problem is self-limiting and advise them not to invoke punitive measures that may adversely affect the psychological development of the child.

○ **What is the most common congenital anomaly of the penis?**

Hypospadias.

○ **What is hypospadias?**

A congenital penile deformity resulting from incomplete development of the distal or anterior urethra.

○   **What anomalies are associated with agenesis of the penis?**

Anal, rectal, and renal anomalies.

○   **What is phimosis?**

An inability to retract the prepuce at an age when it should normally be retracted.

○   **What is a paraphimosis?**

A condition where a phimotic prepuce is retracted behind the coronal sulcus and this retraction cannot be reduced.

○   **What are the complications of cryptorchidism?**

Infertility, tumor development in the undescended testes, hernias, and torsion of the cryptorchid testes.

○   **In a patient with cryptorchidism what is the risk of developing a malignant testicular tumor in the third to fourth decade of life?**

20-44%.

○   **What is the most common tumor which develops in an undescended testes?**

Seminoma (60%).

○   **What are the findings in a patient with testicular torsion?**

The scrotum is swollen, tender and difficult to examine. The cremasteric reflex is absent.

○   **What is the most common cause of acute scrotal pain and swelling in patients over 18 years of age?**

Epididymitis.

○   **What is the treatment for testicular torsion?**

Prompt surgical exploration. If the testes is explored within six hours of torsion, 90% of the gonads will survive after detorsion and fixation.

○   **What is a varicocele?**

Dilatation of the pampiniform venous plexus due to valvular incompetence of the spermatic vein.

○   **What are the complications of circumcision?**

Hemorrhage, infection, dehiscence, denudation of the shaft, glandular injury, and urinary retention.

○   **What is balanitis?**

Infection of the prepuce most often due to mixed flora.

○   **What is the most common composition of urinary calculi in children in the United States?**

Calcium oxalate.

❍ **Gross hematuria of renal origin has what characteristics?**

The color is generally brown or cola-colored and may contain red blood cells casts.

❍ **How should a child presenting with gross hematuria be managed initially?**

The patient should be hospitalized for evaluation because of the increased likelihood of finding hypertension and renal failure.

❍ **A 9-year-old male presents to your clinic with persistent microscopic hematuria detected on routine analysis brought on a febrile illness. Proteinuria is absent and the physical exam and laboratory evaluation are normal, what is the most likely diagnosis?**

Familial benign hematuria.

❍ **A 7-year-old male presents with sensorineural hearing loss, cataracts, and recurrent microscopic hematuria. What is the most likely diagnosis?**

Alport's syndrome.

❍ **A 5-year-old child presents with sudden onset of gross hematuria, edema, hypertension, and renal insufficiency two weeks after a sore throat, what is the most likely diagnosis?**

Acute post-streptococcal glomerulonephritis.

❍ **What are the indications for renal biopsy in a patient with suspected post-streptococcal glomerulonephritis?**

Development of acute renal failure or nephrotic syndrome, the absence of evidence of streptococcal infection, the absence of hypocomplementemia, the persistence of marked hematuria or proteinuria, diminished renal function or a low C-3 level for more than three months after onset.

❍ **What are the complications of acute post-streptococcal glomerulonephritis?**

Hyperkalemia, hypertension, hyperphosphatemia, hypocalcemia, acidosis, seizures, uremia, and volume overload.

❍ **What is the prognosis for a patient with post-streptococcal glomerulonephritis?**

95% of children will completely recover within one month.

❍ **Which syndrome consists of nephropathy, Wilms tumor, and genital abnormalities?**

Drash syndrome.

❍ **What are the causes of nephrotic syndrome during the first six months of life?**

Congenital infection, (syphilis toxoplasmosis cytomegalovirus), congenital nephrotic syndrome, and diffuse mesangial sclerosis of unknown etiology.

❍ **What are the most common causes of nephrotic syndrome between six months and one year of age?**

Idiopathic nephrotic syndrome or drug-induced nephrosis.

❍ **An 11-year-old female presents with a purpuric rash on the buttocks and lower extremities, arthralgias, and abdominal pain. What is the most likely diagnosis?**

Henoch-Schönlein purpura.

O   **What is the most common form of systemic vasculitis in children?**

Anaphylactoid (Henoch-Schönlein purpura).

O   **A 4-year-old presents with irritability, weakness, lethargy, dehydration, edema, petechiae, and a hepatosplenomegaly ten days after an episode of gastroenteritis. Laboratory results reveal a low platelet count and hemoglobulin level, what is the most likely diagnosis?**

Hemolytic-uremic syndrome.

O   **What are the complications of hemolytic uremic syndrome?**

Fluid overload, anemia, acidosis, hyperkalemia, congestive heart failure, hypertension, and uremia.

O   **What is the treatment for hemolytic uremic syndrome?**

Control of fluid and electrolyte balance, control of hypertension, careful use of red cell transfusions, and early initiation of dialysis for the correction of hyperkalemia, metabolic acidosis, severe uremia, or volume overload.

O   **A child presents with dysplastic nails, hypoplastic patellae, and findings consistent with nephrotic syndrome, what is the most likely diagnosis?**

Nail-patella syndrome (hereditary onycho-osteodysplasia).

O   **What disorders in the newborn and infant may lead to renal vein thrombosis?**

Shock, sepsis, dehydration, asphyxia, and umbilical vein catheterization.

O   **A patient presents with a flat nose, recessed chin, epicanthal folds, low-set abnormal ears, club feet and bilateral renal agenesis. What is the likely diagnosis?**

Potter's syndrome.

O   **What is the differential diagnosis for a flank mass in an infant?**

Nephrosis, renal vein thrombosis, tumor, or cystic disease.

O   **What is the best screening test for a bleeding diathesis?**

A good history.

O   **What is the normal protein excretion in a healthy child?**

150 mg/24 hr.

O   **What is postural (orthostatic) proteinuria?**

Significant proteinuria in the upright position with normal or slightly increased serum protein.

O   **A patient presents with proteinuria on routine urinalysis, which is absent, after obtaining a voiding specimen from the same patient upon awakening in the morning, what is the most likely diagnosis?**

Postural (orthostatic) proteinuria.

O   **What are the characteristics of the nephrotic syndrome?**

Edema, hyperlipidemia, hypoproteinemia, and proteinuria.

O   **What is the treatment for children with nephrotic syndrome due to minimal change disease?**

Corticosteroid therapy.

O   **What is a major complication of nephrotic syndrome?**

Infection.

O   **What is the most common type of infection in a patient with nephrotic syndrome?**

Peritonitis with strep pneumoniae being the most common organism.

O   **What is renal tubular acidosis?**

A clinical state of systemic hyperchloremic acidosis due to impaired urinary acidification.

O   **What syndrome is associated with phosphaturia, glucosuria, aminoaciduria, carnitinuria, and proximal renal tubular acidosis?**

Fanconi syndrome.

O   **What is proximal renal tubular acidosis (RTA)?**

A renal disorder resulting in reduced proximal tubular reabsorption of bicarbonate due to deficient carbonic anhydrase production.

O   **What are the causes of acquired Fanconi syndrome?**

Heavy metals (lead, mercury, uranium), outdated tetracycline, nephrotic syndrome, and interstitial nephritis.

O   **What is Bartter syndrome?**

A condition of generalized hyperplasia of the juxtaglomerular apparatus of the kidney resulting in hypokalemia, normal blood pressure, vascular insensitivity to pressor agents, and elevated plasma concentrations of renin and aldosterone.

O   **What is most common cause of interstitial nephritis in a hospitalized child?**

Medications.

O   **What are the predisposing causes of cortical necrosis in the newborn?**

Asphyxia, shock, dehydration, disseminated intravascular coagulation, and renal vein thrombosis.

O   **What are the causes of acute renal failure in the newborn?**

Sepsis, shock, hemorrhage, renal vein thrombosis, dehydration, congenital heart disease, obstructive uropathy, renal dysgenesis, and renovascular accidents.

O   **What are the most common causes of chronic renal failure in a child under 5 years of age?**

Anatomic abnormalities of the kidneys.

❍   **What are the most common causes of chronic renal failure in children greater than 5 years of age?**

Glomerulonephritis, hemolytic uremic syndrome, or hereditary disorders (Alport syndrome, cystic disease).

❍   **What are the mechanisms behind anemia of chronic renal failure?**

Decreased erythropoietin production, low grade hemolysis, bleeding, decreased erythrocyte survival, inadequate iron intake, inadequate folic acid intake, and inhibition of erythropoiesis.

❍   **What are the causes of hypertension in a patient with chronic renal failure?**

Sodium and water overload and excessive renin production.

❍   **What are the two most common surgically remediable causes of hypertension in children?**

Coarctation and renovascular hypertension.

❍   **A 7-year-old child presents with severe refractory hypertension, what is the most likely cause?**

Renovascular hypertension.

❍   **What are the clinical clues that suggest renovascular hypertension?**

Retinopathy, hypokalemia, epigastric or flank bruit, abrupt onset of severe hypertension, normal or elevated plasma bicarbonate level, hypertension refractory to intensive antihypertensive therapy, hypertension with a unilateral small kidney, and excellent response to angiotensin-converting enzyme inhibitors.

❍   **What are the indications for admission for nephrotic syndrome?**

Peritonitis, refractory edema, unexplained fever, renal insufficiency, severe dehydration, and first time diagnosis.

❍   **Which initial study should be used to differentiate obstructive from intrinsic renal causes of acute renal failure?**

Renal ultrasound.

❍   **What is the treatment for acute renal failure resulting from a pre-renal cause?**

Fluid resuscitation is the treatment of choice with an initial bolus of 20 ml/kg of crystalloid solution until vital signs become stable and urine flow is established.

❍   **What are the indications for dialysis in a patient with acute renal failure?**

BUN greater than 100 mg/dl, persistent hyperkalemia, persistent metabolic acidosis, uremic syndrome, persistent congestive heart failure, and acute renal failure with oliguria due to rhabdomyolysis.

❍   **A 6-year-old child presents with the following urine indices. Urine plasma urea nitrogen ratio greater than 8; urine: plasma creatinine ratio greater than 40; urine: plasma osmolality ratio greater than 500 mOsm/kg or greater than 1.5; and fractional excretion of sodium less than 1. What is the most likely cause of the renal failure?**

Prerenal cause such as decreased cardiac output or decreased intravascular volume due to hemorrhagic shock, dehydration, or third spacing of fluid.

❍ **A normally functioning glomerulus is able to filter out proteins of what molecular weight?**

60,000 daltons or greater.

❍ **At what age does the GFR approximate adult values (correcting for body surface area)?**

3 years old.

❍ **What is the formula for calculating the clearance of a substance?**

Cs (ml/min)=(Us(mg/ml)x V(ml/min))/Ps (mg/ml) (where Cs is clearance of the substance; Us is concentration of substance in urine; V is urine flow rate; and Ps is concentration of substance in plasma).

❍ **What medications can be used to prevent nephrolithiasis in a patient with idiopathic hypercalciuria?**

Thiazide diuretics, which can increase calcium reabsorption in the distal tubule.

❍ **A child complains of "red urine". What foods can cause this?**

Beets, blackberries and red food coloring.

❍ **On physical exam of a newborn infant, you notice a palpable abdominal mass. What is the most likely cause?**

A hydronephrotic kidney.

❍ **What is the recommended course of action for a child with gross hematuria?**

Hospitalize and run the following tests: CBC, BUN/Cr, 24 hr creatine/protein/calcium, urine culture, serum C3, and anti-DNAse B titer. If these do not lead to a diagnosis then get an ultrasound or IVP to look for structural abnormalities.

❍ **You still have not reached a diagnosis for the child with hematuria. Should you get a biopsy?**

Yes, if the child has unexplained gross hematuria, that is an indication in itself. A biopsy is also indicated for patients with persistent microscopic hematuria with associated hypertension, proteinuria, or decreased renal function.

❍ **A dipstick test of the urine of a child reveals 2+ proteins. How much protein is this?**

Close to 100 mg/dl.

❍ **The labs from a child with hematuria shows depressed levels of C3. What etiologies should you suspect?**

Chronic infection, lupus, PSG, or membranoproliferative disease.

❍ **What are the four most common causes of recurrent gross hematuria in the absence of trauma?**

Acute PSG, IgA nephropathy, familial nephritis (Alport syndrome), and idiopathic.

❍ **What is the prognosis of a child with Berger nephropathy?**

Most patients do not have significant renal damage and only supportive therapy is recommended. However, about 1/3 of the patients will develop progressive disease (note: this disorder is also known as IgA nephropathy).

❍   **A 13-year-old boy presents with gross hematuria and some hearing loss. What is your diagnosis?**

Alport's syndrome.

❍   **What is the most common cause of gross hematuria in children?**

IgA nephropathy.

❍   **What is the classic presentation of post-streptococcal glomerulonephritis(PSG)?**

Sudden development of gross hematuria, hypertension, edema and renal insufficiency following a throat or skin infection with group A B-hemolytic streptococcus. Patients frequently also have generalized complaints of fever, malaise, lethargy, abdominal pain, etc.

❍   **How early in the development of "strep throat" will antibiotic therapy decrease the risk for PSG?**

Antibiotics have not been found to decrease the risk for PSG.

❍   **What lab test best confirms PSG as the diagnosis?**

Anti-DNAse B antibody titer.

❍   **What is the most common form of lupus nephritis?**

Diffuse proliferative nephritis (WHO class IV). Unfortunately, this is also the most severe form.

❍   **The biopsy of the kidney from a 14-year-old boy with nephrotic syndrome shows increased mesangial cells and, on immunofluorescence, C3 deposits in the mesangium. What is the boy's diagnosis and prognosis?**

This child has membranoproliferative glomerulonephritis (a type of chronic glomerulonephritis). Prognosis is poor, with many patients progressing to end-stage renal failure.

❍   **What is the most common manifestation of Goodpasture disease?**

Hemoptysis. These patients usually develop pulmonary hemorrhage before any signs of renal failure develop.

❍   **HUS most commonly follows infection with what organism?**

E. coli (O157:H7). The disease is usually a sequelae to a bout of gastroenteritis caused by this organism. Pneumococcal pneumonia has also been associated with HUS, though this is much less common.

❍   **What is the diagnostic triad for HUS?**

Microangiopathic anemia, acute renal failure, and thrombocytopenia ($20k$-$100k/mm^3$).

❍   **What is the prognosis for patients with acute renal failure secondary to HUS?**

Over 90% survival with many patients eventually recovering normal renal function.

❍   **What is the role of corticosteroids in the treatment of HUS?**

None.

❍   **The mother of a 2 month old male infant is concerned that she cannot retract the foreskin. Should you circumcise at this point?**

No. More than 85% of uncircumcised males can retract the foreskin by the 3rd year. Before this time it is not a concern.

❍   **What is Drash syndrome?**

Nephropathy, genital abnormalities and Wilms tumor.

❍   **What is the diagnostic triad of the nephrotic syndrome?**

Edema, hyperlipidemia, and proteinuria with hypoproteinemia.

❍   **What is the most common cause of the nephrotic syndrome in children?**

Idiopathic nephrotic syndrome, of which the most common type is minimal change disease.

❍   **Below what level of serum albumin will edema appear?**

< 2.5g/dl.

❍   **A child with mental retardation and eye abnormalities is found to have Fanconi syndrome. What disease should you suspect?**

Oculocerebrorenal Dystrophy.

❍   **Is idiopathic nephrotic syndrome more common in boys or girls?**

Boys are twice as commonly afflicted.

❍   **What is the most common complication of idiopathic nephrotic syndrome?**

Infection, especially spontaneous peritonitis.

❍   **What medication can be used to ameliorate minimal change disease in the patient with corticosteroid toxicity?**

Cyclophosphamide (3 mg/kg/day).

❍   **What is the most common cause of acute scrotal pain in patients less than 6 years old?**

Testicular torsion.

❍   **How is renal tubular acidosis (RTA) classified?**

Into one of three types: Type 1-distal RTA, Type II-proximal RTA, or Type IV- mineralocorticoid deficiency. There is no type III.

❍   **What are the mechanisms for the different types of RTA?**

In Type I, there is a deficiency in the secretion of the hydrogen ion by the distal tubule and collecting duct. In mechanism for Type II is a decrease in the bicarbonate reabsorption in the proximal tubule.

O   **Which isolated form of RTA will be most likely to lead to renal failure?**

Distal (Type I), though most cases of Type I RTA have an excellent prognosis.

O   **What is Fanconi syndrome?**

Phosphaturia (with hypophosphatemia), renal glycosuria, and generalized aminoaciduria.

O   **Why do patients with Fanconi syndrome commonly present with rickets?**

This is due to both hypophosphatemia and metabolic acidosis which, among other things, is believed to decrease the conversion of vitamin D to its active metabolite.

O   **How do you treat the rickets associated with the Fanconi syndrome?**

How else but by high dose Vitamin D therapy (starting at 5,000 units/day and progressing up to 3,000 units/kg/day).

O   **What is the most common presentation of idiopathic nephrotic syndrome?**

Edema, frequently in conjunction with anorexia, diarrhea and abdominal pain.

O   **What are the roentgenographic findings in a child with renal osteodystrophy?**

Osteitis fibrosa (especially in the distal phalanges) from the increased osteoclastic bone resorption, and endosteal fibrosis from the increased bone turnover and disorganized replacement.

O   **What two common medications can induce nephrogenic diabetes insipidus?**

Lithium and amphotericin B.

O   **A child with nephrogenic diabetes insipidus has a serum sodium level of 117 mEq/l. How do you determine how much NaCl to administer to keep the risk of cerebral edema at a minimum?**

Amount of NaCl to add (in mEq/l)=0.6 x wt. (in kg) x (140 - serum sodium). The sodium should not be elevated by more than 10-12 mEq/dl/day.

O   **At what level of creatinine should you consider putting the patient on dialysis?**

9-10 mg/dl.

O   **What is the most frequent technique of dialysis employed in children?**

Continuous ambulatory peritoneal dialysis (CAPD).

O   **What is the most common cause of arterial hypertension in children?**

Chronic pyelonephritis (aka reflux nephropathy).

O   **What percentage of kidney transplants donated from a relative (usually a parent) are still functional after three years?**

75-80%.

❍   **What immunosuppressive agent, commonly used in renal transplants, have nephrotoxicity as a side effect?**

Cyclosporine.

❍   **Are circumcised males more, less, or equally likely to develop urinary tract infection when compared to their uncut counterparts?**

Less.

❍   **A urinary tract infection due to what organism may lead to hyperammonemia?**

Proteus.

❍   **What is the definitive diagnostic test for suspected acute pyelonephritis?**

CT. However, this is hardly used as a good H&P and less expensive tests are usually sufficient to make the diagnosis.

❍   **Aside from the cost factor, why should you be hesitant to order a CT scan on a child with suspected pyelonephritis?**

To protect the gonads from radiation, especially in the females. There is an increased risk of ovarian cancer from a relatively small amount of radiation.

❍   **What is the most common cause of acute hemorrhagic cystitis in males?**

Adenovirus. In females, *E. coli* is more common, followed by adenovirus.

❍   **Why should you order an ultrasound for a child with acute febrile urinary tract infection?**

To rule out an obstruction.

❍   **A concerned mother asks you whether it is common for her 5-year-old son to still be wetting his bed at night. What should you tell her?**

Not to be concerned, as about one-fifth of children his age have this problem. 15-20% of children stop having this problem each year.

❍   **The above mentioned mother is not relieved to find she and her son have to "wait it out". "Isn't there something you can do to make it better now?", she asks. What is your response?**

You can prescribe desmopressin nasal spray, which will temporarily ease the condition, but time is still the main factor in treatment.

❍   **What is the cause of primary vesicoureteral reflux?**

This is due to a congenital defect in which the valve at the vesicoureteral junction is patent or incompetent.

❍   **How do you grade a vesicoureteral reflux?**

There are 5 grades: I-no dilatation, II-no dilatation, but reflux reaches upper collecting system, III-ureter dilated and there may be blunting of the calyceal fornices, IV-ureter is grossly dilated, V-all details of calyces are lost and the entire ureter is grossly dilated and tortuous.

❍   **What is the surgery used for the correction of ureteral reflux?**

The Cohen reimplantation, which is successful in > 95% of the time.

O   **A newborn child has his urethral opening on the ventral side of the glands. What are some common abnormalities frequently seen concomitantly with this condition?**

Inguinal hernias and undescended testes.

O   **What is a circumcaval ureter?**

As the name suggests, this is due to aberrant development of the vena cava. The vena cava can thus obstruct the ureter, almost always on the right side.

O   **What is the most common cause of urethral strictures in males?**

Trauma.

O   **What are the two most severe sequelae for congenital neurogenic bladder?**

Urinary incontinence and renal damage, from high intravesical pressures caused by lack of coordination of the sphincters and detrusor muscles.

O   **What is the treatment of choice for low grade reflux in a child with neurogenic bladder?**

Intermittent catheterization, antibiotics (prophylactic), and anticholinergics.

O   **What is the treatment for paraphimosis?**

As the glans edema and venous engorgement can lead to arterial compromise, this is a true emergency. First, try to manually compress the edema, after which the foreskin may be successfully reduced. If this does not work, a superficial vertical incision of the constricting band (after local anesthetic) will decompress the gland. Obviously, this procedure should be performed by a urologist or emergency medicine physician.

O   **You are at home barbecuing a fine steak on a sunny day when a neighbor comes running to you with his little boy, who is grabbing his groin area and crying in agony. You examine the boy and it looks as if it could be testicular torsion. What do you do?**

Flip your steak, then try manual detorsion. The right testis commonly torses clockwise, and the left counterclockwise. Thus, you need to reverse the directions (as if opening a book). Obviously, this is a surgical emergency and this should be done while preparations for hospital transport is arranged.

O   **What is the treatment for minimal change disease?**

Steroids

O   **What is the most common anatomic cause of UTIs?**

Persistent vesicoureteral reflux.

HEMATOLOGY AND ONCOLOGY

❍ **Which types of blood loss are indicative of a bleeding disorder?**

1. Spontaneous bleeding from many sites.
2. Bleeding from non-traumatic sites.
3. Delayed bleeding several hours after trauma.
4. Bleeding into deep tissues or joints.

❍ **What common drugs have been implicated in predisposing to acquired bleeding disorders?**

Ethanol, ASA, NSAIDs, warfarin, and antibiotics.

❍ **Mucocutaneous bleeding, including petechiae, ecchymoses, epistaxis, GI, GU, or menorrhagia are indicative of what coagulation abnormality?**

Qualitative or quantitative platelet disorders.

❍ **Bleeding into joints or potential spaces (i.e., retroperitoneum), as well as delayed bleeding, suggests what type of bleeding disorder?**

Coagulation Factor Deficiency.

❍ **What is primary hemostasis?**

It is the platelet interaction with the vascular subendothelium that results in the formation of a platelet plug at the site of injury.

❍ **What 4 components are required for primary hemostasis?**

1. Normal vascular subendothelium (collagen).
2. Functional platelets.
3. Normal von Willebrand factor (connects the platelet to the endothelium via glycoprotein Ib).
4. Normal Fibrinogen (connects platelets to each other via glycoprotein IIB-IIIA).

❍ **What is the final end-product of secondary hemostasis (coagulation cascade)?**

Cross-linked fibrin.

❍ **What mechanism limits the size of the fibrin clots that are formed?**

The fibrinolytic system.

❍ **What is the principle physiologic activator of the fibrinolytic system?**

Tissue plasminogen activator (tPA). tPA is released from endothelial cells and converts plasminogen, adsorbed in the fibrin clot, to plasmin. Plasmin degrades fibrinogen and fibrin monomer into fibrin degradation products (FDPs [once called fibrin split products]) and cross-linked fibrin into D-dimers.

❍ **Below what platelet count is spontaneous hemorrhage likely to occur?**

$< 10,000/mm^3$.

O   **It is generally agreed that most patients with active bleeding and platelet counts $< 50,000/mm^3$ should receive platelet transfusion. How much will the platelet count be raised for each unit of platelets infused?**

$10,000/mm^3$.

O   **What groups of patients with thrombocytopenia would be unlikely to respond to platelet infusions?**

Those with platelet antibodies (ITP or hypersplenism). Also HUS may make hemolysis worse.

O   **How can an overdose of warfarin be treated? What are the advantages and disadvantages of each treatment?**

Treatment depends on the severity of symptoms, not the degree of prolongation of the prothrombin time (PT). If there are no signs of bleeding, temporary discontinuation may be all that is necessary; if bleeding is present, treatment can be initiated with fresh frozen plasma (FFP) or Vitamin K.

Advantages of FFP: rapid repletion of coagulation factors and control of hemorrhage.

Disadvantages: volume overload, possible viral transmission

Advantages of Vitamin K: ease of administration.

Disadvantages: possible anaphylaxis when given IV; delayed onset of 12-24 hours; effects may last up to 2 weeks, making anticoagulation of the patient difficult or impossible.

O   **What is the only coagulation factor not synthesized by hepatocytes?**

Factor VIII.

O   **What 4 hemostatic alterations are seen in patients with liver disease?**

1.   Decreased protein synthesis leading to coagulation factor deficiency.
2.   Thrombocytopenia.
3.   Increased fibrinolysis.
4.   Vitamin K deficiency.

O   **What 5 treatment options are available for patients who are bleeding and have liver disease?**

1.   Transfusion with PRBCS (maintains hemodynamic stability).
2.   Vitamin K.
3.   Fresh frozen plasma.
4.   Platelet transfusion.
5.   DDAVP (Desmopressin).

O   **Which test of hemostasis is most often prolonged in uremic patients?**

Bleeding time.

O   **What options are available for treatment of patients with renal failure and coagulopathy?**

1.   Dialysis.
2.   Optimize hematocrit (by recombinant human erythropoietin or transfusion with PRBCs).

3. Desmopressin.
4. Conjugated estrogens.
5. Cryoprecipitate and platelet transfusions if hemorrhage is life-threatening.

○ **What are the clinical complications of DIC?**

Bleeding, thrombosis, and purpura fulminans.

○ **What three laboratory studies would be most helpful in establishing the diagnosis of DIC?**

1. Prothrombin time—prolonged.
2. Platelet count—usually low.
3. Fibrinogen level—low.

○ **What are the most common hemostatic abnormalities in patients infected with HIV?**

Thrombocytopenia and acquired circulating anticoagulants (causes prolongation of aPTT).

○ **How much will one unit of Factor VIII concentrate raise the circulating Factor VIII level?**

2%.

○ **How much will one unit of Factor IX concentrate raise the circulating Factor IX level?**

1%.

○ **What is the most common inherited bleeding disorder?**

von Willebrand Disease.

○ **70-80% of patients with von Willebrand disease have Type I. What is currently the approved mode of therapy for bleeding in these patients? What is the dose?**

DDAVP (0.3 μg/kg IV or sc q 12h for 3–4 doses).

○ **What is the most common hemoglobin variant?**

Hemoglobin S (Valine substituted for glutamic acid in the sixth position on the ß-chain).

○ **What types of clinical crises are seen in patients with sickle-cell disease?**

1. Vasoocclusive (thrombotic).
2. Hematologic (sequestration and aplastic).
3. Infectious.

○ **What is the most common type of sickle-cell crisis?**

Vasoocclusive.

○ **What percentage of patients with sickle-cell disease have gallstones?**

75% (only 10% are symptomatic).

○ **What is the only type of vasoocclusive crisis that is painless?**

CNS crisis (most commonly cerebral infarction in children and cerebral hemorrhage in adults).

❍   **What are the mainstays of therapy for a patient in sickle-cell crisis?**

1. Hydration.
2. Analgesia.
3. Oxygen (only beneficial if patient is hypoxic).
4. Cardiac monitoring (if patient has history of cardiac disease or is having chest pain).

❍   **What is the most commonly encountered sickle hemoglobin variant?**

Sickle-cell trait.

❍   **What is the most common human enzyme defect?**

Glucose-6-phosphate Dehydrogenase Deficiency (G-6-PD).

❍   **What drugs should be avoided in patients with G-6-PD Deficiency?**

1. Drugs that induce oxidation.
2. Sulfa.
3. Antimalarials.
4. Pyridium.
5. Nitrofurantoin.

❍   **What is the single most useful test in ascertaining the presence of hemolysis and a normal marrow response?**

The reticulocyte count.

❍   **What is the most common morphologic abnormality of red cells in hemolytic states?**

Spherocytes.

❍   **In a child 6 months to 4 year of age with an antecedent URI, the findings of fever, acute renal failure, microangiopathic hemolytic anemia (MAHA), and thrombocytopenia are suggestive of what disorder?**

Hemolytic Uremic Syndrome.

❍   **What malignancy is most frequently associated with MAHA?**

Gastric Adenocarcinoma.

❍   **What is the most common worldwide cause of hemolytic anemia?**

Malaria.

❍   **What are the components of whole blood that are used for transfusion?**

1. RBCs.
2. Platelets.
3. Plasma.
4. Cryoprecipitate.

❍   **By how much will the infusion of one unit of PRBcs raise the hemoglobin and hematocrit in a 30 kg patient?**

Hemoglobin: 1 g/dL.

Hematocrit: 3%.

O   **What are the 5 contents of cryoprecipitate?**

1   Factor VIII C.
2. von Willebrand Factor.
3. Fibrinogen.
4. Factor XIII.
5. Fibronectin.

O   **What is the first step in treating all immediate transfusion reactions?**

Stop the transfusion.

O   **What type of immediate transfusion reaction is not dose-related and can often be completed following patient evaluation and treatment with diphenhydramine?**

Allergic transfusion reaction.

O   **What infection carries the highest risk of transmission by blood transfusion?**

Hepatitis C (1:3,300 units).

O   **In current practice, which blood components are routinely infused along with PRBcs in a patient receiving a massive transfusion?**

None. The practice of routinely using platelet transfusion and FFP is costly, dangerous, and unwarranted.

O   **What is the only crystalloid fluid compatible with PRBcs?**

Normal saline.

O   **What diagnosis should be considered in a patient who presents to the ED with coma, anemia and rouleau formation in the peripheral blood smear?**

Hyperviscosity Syndrome.

O   **What is the most common cause of hyperviscosity syndrome?**

Waldenstrom macroglobulinemia.

O   **Vitamin K dependent factors of the clotting cascade include:**

X, IX, VII and II.   Remember 1972.

O   **A patient receives a major head injury. He also suffers from classic hemophilia, what treatment should be given?**

Give Factor VIII 50 U/kg.

O   **What is von Willebrand's disease?**

It is an autosomal dominant disorder of platelet function. It causes bleeding from mucous membranes, menorrhagia, and increased bleeding from wounds. Patients with von Willebrand's disease have less (or dysfunctional) von Willebrand's factor.

O   **What lab abnormalities does DIC cause?**

Increased PT, elevated fibrin split products, decreased fibrinogen and thrombocytopenia.

O   **What factors are deficient in Classic hemophilia, Christmas disease, and von Willebrand's disease, respectively?**

Classic hemophilia: Factor VIII.
Christmas disease: Factor IX.
Willebrand's disease: Factor VIIIc + von Willebrand's cofactor.

O   **Which pathway involves factors VIII and IX?**

Intrinsic pathway.

O   **What effect does deficiency of factors VIII and IX have on PT and on PTT?**

Deficiency leads to increase in PTT.

O   **What pathway does the PT measure, and what factor is unique to this pathway?**

Extrinsic and factor VII, respectively.

O   **How may hemophilia A be clinically distinguished from hemophilia B?**

Hemophilia A is not clinically distinguishable from Christmas disease (Hemophilia B).

O   **Which blood product is given when the coagulation abnormality is unknown?**

FFP.

O   **The most frequently encountered platelet disorder of childhood is:**

Idiopathic thrombocytopenic purpura

O   **The characteristic bone marrow finding in ITP is:**

Increased or normal megakaryocytes

O   **Potential treatment modalities for ITP include:**

Gamma globulin, steroids, and winrho if platelets are Rh positive.

O   **How do gamma globulin and steroids work in the treatment of ITP?**

They block the uptake of antibody-coated platelets by splenic macrophages.

O   **Under what circumstances is a bone marrow aspirate crucial in the diagnosis and treatment of ITP?**

If treatment with steroids is planned, a bone marrow aspirate must be performed to rule out leukemia. Steroid treatment can delay the diagnosis of an occult leukemia.

O   **Which patients with ITP and mild head trauma without neurological findings should be treated with gamma globulin?**

Patients whose platelet count < 20,000/mm3, with signs of easy or spontaneous bleeding within one week of diagnosis, and whose follow-up is uncertain.

O   **The most common cause of neutropenia found in the evaluation of a febrile child is:**

Viral illness

O   **Ethnic groups with a high incidence of (thalassemia gene include those from which geographic areas?**

1.   Countries bordering the Mediterranean
2.   Southeast Asia

O   **The most likely diagnosis in a child with poor growth, hepatosplenomegaly, pallor, hemoglobin of 4.0 gm/dL, and an MCV of 60 is:**

Thalassemia major

O   **Long term treatment of thalassemia major includes repeated blood transfusions. An important complication of the treatment is:**

Iron overload.

O   **Cyanosis without demonstrable cardiac or pulmonary disease should prompt consideration of what condition?**

Methemoglobinemia.

O   **Why is the pulse oximetry reading normal in a patient with cyanosis and methemoglobinemia?**

Because pulse oximetry devices measure oxygen saturation of that hemoglobin available for saturation. Blood oximetry levels will be low in this condition. pO2 is normal.

O   **List drugs and other substances implicated in causing methemoglobinemia in children:**

Sulfa antibiotics, quinones, phenacetin, benzocaine, nitrites, aniline dyes, and naphthalene (moth balls).

O   **Oxygen binding of hemoglobin is severely impaired in methemoglobinemia because of what change in heme iron?**

More heme iron is present in the ferric rather than ferrous state.

O   **The definitive test for diagnosing sickling disorders is:**

Hemoglobin electrophoresis

O   **Alternatives for treating bleeding in a patient with Factor VIII deficiency and an inhibitor are:**

1.   Children with low inhibitor titers and minor hemorrhage may respond to Factor VIII
2.   Factor IX concentrates
3.   Plasmapheresis and factor replacement
4.   High dose Factor VIII (>100 units/kg)

O   **In von Willebrand's Disease there is a decrease in or a defect of what protein?**

von Willebrand's factor (vWF) which, when combined with factor VIII procoagulant protein (factor VIII:C), forms factor VIII.

O   **Typical lab findings in von Willebrand's Disease include:**

1) Normal platelet count
2) Normal pro-time
3) Normal or increase partial thromboplastin time
4) Increased bleeding time

❍ **There is simultaneous activation of coagulation and fibrinolysis in what pathologic condition?**

Disseminated Intravascular Coagulation.

❍ **The predominant symptom in DIC is:**

Bleeding.

❍ **Common ischemic complications of DIC include:**

1) Renal failure
2) Seizures/coma
3) Pulmonary infarcts
4) Hemorrhagic necrosis of the skin

❍ **The most common familial and congenital abnormality of the red blood cell membrane is:**

Hereditary spherocytosis.

❍ **The usual pattern of inheritance for hereditary spherocytosis is:**

Autosomal dominant but it may be autosomal recessive and there is a high rate of new mutations.

❍ **The most common molecular defect in hereditary spherocytosis is an abnormality in what protein?**

Spectrin.

❍ **Complications of hereditary spherocytosis include:**

1. Hyperbilirubinemia in newborn period
2. Hemolytic anemia
3. Gallstones
4. Susceptibility to aplastic and hypoplastic crises secondary to viral infections

❍ **How is the diagnosis of hereditary spherocytosis made?**

1. Blood smear
2. Splenomegaly
3. Family history
4. Osmotic fragility test

❍ **Treatment of hereditary spherocytosis may include:**

Splenectomy.

❍ **Hemosiderosis from chronic transfusion therapy for thalassemia can be successfully treated with:**

Subcutaneous deferoxamine via pump.

❍ **A cure for thalassemia major is possible with:**

Bone marrow transplant.

❍ **More than 90% of individuals with (-thalassemia trait will have diagnostic elevation of:**

Hemoglobin A2 to 3.4-7%.

❍ **A 4 month old African American male is given trimethoprim-sulfamethoxazole for otitis media and 24 hours later develops a severe hemolytic anemia. What is the most likely cause?**

G-6-PD deficiency.

❍ **G-6-PD deficiency is prevalent in what ethnic groups?**

Greek, southern Italians, Sephardic Jews, Filipinos, south Chinese, African Americans and Thai's.

❍ **A 15-year-old female has cervical adenopathy and supraclavicular nodes. The patient has had fevers which last several days, followed by afebrile periods lasting several days. The most likely malignancy would be?**

Hodgkin's Disease. The recurrent fevers and adenopathies hint at this diagnosis. Diagnosis would be obtained by lymph node biopsy.

❍ **At what age is a sickle cell patient at greatest risk for sepsis?**

Six months to 3 years.

❍ **Why is the patient from the previous question considered at high risk during this age?**

Because there is limited protective antibody, and splenic function is decreased or completely absent.

❍ **T/F: Children with hemoglobin SC disease have the same frequency of sepsis as those with hemoglobin SS during the first three years of life.**

False. 3.5/100 patient years vs. 8/100 patient years.

❍ **How should you treat hypoxia in a sickle cell patient who has acute chest syndrome?**

Red cell transfusion (simple or exchange).

❍ **What two processes are involved in the pathophysiology of a sickle cell patient with acute chest syndrome?**

Pulmonary infarction and/or pneumonia.

❍ **How does renal papillary necrosis that is secondary to sickle cell vaso-occlusion commonly present?**

Painless hematuria that may worsen the anemia, and red blood cells without casts in urine sediment.

❍ **What procedures might be included to treat the type of renal papillary necrosis mentioned in the previous question?**

Intravenous hydration, anti-fibrinolytic drugs, red blood cell transfusion or exchange transfusion.

O   **Name some options for the treatment of priapism arising secondary to sickle cell vaso-occlusive crisis.**

Intravenous hydration, analgesics, red cell or exchange transfusion, and aspiration of the penile corpora.

O   **What are some of the signs and symptoms of central nervous system infarction secondary to sickle cell vaso-occlusion?**

Mild, fleeting TIA-like symptoms, seizures, hemiparesis, coma, death.

O   **How do you treat a central nervous system vaso-occlusive crisis?**

1.5-2 volume exchange transfusion as soon as blood is ready.

O   **What are the signs and symptoms of splenic sequestration crisis?**

Pallor, weakness, lethargy, disorientation, shock, decreased level of consciousness, and an enlarged spleen.

O   **How do you treat splenic sequestration crisis?**

Rapid infusion of saline, and transfusion of red cells or whole blood.

O   **What is the most common cause of aplastic crisis in patients with hemolytic anemia?**

Parvovirus B19 infection.

O   **What percentage of hemoglobins A and F are found in a normal term infant?**

Hemoglobin A: 30%

Hemoglobin F: 70%

O   **The amount of hemoglobin F declines to <2% by what age?**

6-12 months.

O   **Increased levels of hemoglobin A2 are found in what condition?**

Σ Thalassemia-trait megaloblastic anemias secondary to vitamin B12 and folic acid deficiencies.

O   **What syndrome is characterized by macrocytic anemia, reticulocytopenia, and an absence of red cell precursors in the bone marrow aspirate during the first 6 months of life?**

Diamond-Blackfan syndrome.

O   **What is the initial treatment of Diamond-Blackfan syndrome?**

Prednisone.

O   **Normal red blood cell life span is:**

120 days.

O   **What factors contribute to the pathophysiology of chronic disease anemia?**

Decreased red cell life span (hyperactive reticuloendothelial system), hypoactive bone marrow, erythropoietin production inadequate for degree of anemia, and an abnormality of iron metabolism.

○   **What is the most important aspect in the treatment of chronic disease anemia?**

Correction of the underlying disorder.

○   **A patient receiving a transfusion of packed red cells abruptly develops fever, chills, chest pain, dyspnea and tachycardia. What is the most likely cause?**

Acute hemolytic transfusion reaction due to ABO incompatibility.

○   **Which factors contribute to physiologic anemia during infancy?**

Abrupt cessation of erythropoiesis with onset of respiration, low erythropoietin levels (made in the liver during the neonatal period), decreased half life and increased volume of distribution of erythropoietin, shortened survival of fetal RBCs, and expansion of the infant's blood volume with rapid weight gain during the first three months.

○   **At what age does the physiologic anemia of infancy peak?**

2-3 months in full term infants; 3-6 weeks in prematures.

○   **T/F: Vitamin E deficiency has been shown to contribute to anemia of prematurity:**

False.

○   **Which deficiencies cause megaloblastic anemia in children?**

Folic acid and/or vitamin B12.

○   **Which test assesses the absorption rate of vitamin B12?**

The Schilling test.

○   **T/F: Infants absorb the iron from cow's milk more efficiently than that of breast milk.**

False. Iron is absorbed 2-3 times more efficiently from breast milk.

○   **Iron deficiency anemia in an older child should prompt an investigation for what?**

Blood loss.

○   **You have just started a course of iron therapy on a child who had a significant iron deficiency. How soon can you expect to see a subjective improvement such as decreased irritability and increased appetitive?**

Twelve to 24 hours.

○   **What are the most common sites for bleeding in patients who are hemophiliacs?**

Joints, muscles, subcutaneous tissue.

○   **A 3-year-old hemophiliac presents with a swollen, warm, painful knee. You suspect hemarthrosis. Factor infusion should be administered to raise levels to what percent?**

25-30%.

○   **What serious sequela of hip hemarthrosis is common among hemophiliacs?**

Aseptic necrosis of the femoral head.

O   **A hemophiliac presents with pain in the abdomen and groin, flexion of the thigh, and paresthesia of the lower thigh. What condition do you suspect?**

Iliopsoas hemorrhage.

O   **A hemophiliac presents with a headache after minor head trauma. What should your management include?**

CT of the brain, and factor replacement.

O   **Define the drug regimen MOPP.**

Mechlorethamine, Oncovin, Prednisone, and Procarbazine.

O   **What is the MOPP regimen of drugs used to treat?**

Hodgkin's lymphoma.

O   **A patient on chemotherapy is experiencing severe nausea and vomiting. What can you prescribe to alleviate some of his symptoms?**

Serotonin-receptor antagonists, such as Granisetron and Ondansetron, or a combinations of phenothiazine and an antihistamine.

O   **After a course of chemotherapy, your patient has had a fever, neutropenia and granulocytopenia for over a week, despite antibiotic use. What should you do now?**

Add Amphotericin-B for a presumed fungal infection while continuing your search for the source of the infection.

O   **What is the mechanism of action for methotrexate?**

It inhibits the enzyme dihydrofolate reductase.

O   **What is the drug of choice for treating a Wilms' tumor?**

Actinomycin D.

O   **A patient on chemotherapy to treat Burkitt's lymphoma is found to be hyperkalemic, hypocalcemic, hyperphosphatemic, and hyperuricemic. What is the presumptive diagnosis?**

Tumor lysis syndrome.

O   **Childhood cancer is a leading cause of death. How does it rank?**

Childhood cancer is only exceeded by trauma as a leading cause of death in the 1-15-year-old population.

O   **Which chemotherapeutic agents are associated with pulmonary fibrosis?**

Bleomycin, BCNU, and Busulfan are commonly associated with pulmonary fibrosis. Cyclophosphamide and Methotrexate are rarely implicated.

O   **How may an oncologic patient with a serum calcium concentration of 13 mgs/dl may be treated?**

Furosemide and forced saline diuresis. Extreme hypercalcemia may require mithramycin.

❍ **An oncologic patient experiences a reaction to a platelet transfusion. He has a fever and chills. What medications would you prescribe?**

Acetaminophen or hydrocortisone. Reactions more severe than this may require diphenhydramine or epinephrine.

❍ **What is the most frequent soft tissue tumor in the pediatric patient?**

Rhabdomyosarcoma. This malignancy accounts for 5% of all pediatric cancers.

❍ **Which congenital anomalies can be associated with hepatoblastoma?**

Beckwith-Wiedemann syndrome, hemihypertrophy, Meckel's diverticulum, diaphragmatic hernias, umbilical hernias and renal anomalies.

❍ **What is the most common extracranial solid tumor in the pediatric patient?**

Neuroblastoma. It accounts for about 10% of all pediatric malignancies.

❍ **Most cases of neuroblastoma are diagnosed by what age?**

Eighty-five percent of cases are diagnosed before the age of five years, the median age of diagnosis is two years.

❍ **The most common form of childhood malignancy is?**

Leukemia – of which the majority are all. Approximately 2,500 children a year are affected annually in the United States.

❍ **Which chemotherapeutic agent is a known carcinogen?**

Cyclophosphamide.

❍ **Which genetic disorders increase the incidence of leukemia?**

Down's syndrome, Fanconi anemia and ataxia-telangiectasis.

❍ **What are the most frequent sites of osteosarcoma involvement?**

The femur, tibia, and humerus. Usually this tumor is found in the metaphysis of long bones.

❍ **After osteosarcoma, what is the most frequent bone tumor in children and adolescents?**

Ewing's sarcoma. This tumor accounts for about 30% of all primary bone tumors.

❍ **A 2-year-old male has a seborrheic rash, chronically draining ears, and loose teeth. What is your diagnosis?**

Histiocytosis X.

❍ **What is the most common pediatric liver tumor of childhood?**

The hepatoblastoma. The second most common is hepatocellular carcinoma.

❍ **A 7-year-old female in Tanner stage 3 has lower abdominal pain of unknown etiology, and a 4 cm abdominal mass. What is the most likely diagnosis?**

An ovarian tumor.

O   **What is the origin of most testicular childhood tumors?**

Germ cell. Germ cell tumors account for 35% to 45% of childhood testicular tumors.

O   **Urinary catecholamine metabolite levels are useful in diagnosing which common pediatric malignancy?**

Neuroblastoma. The most useful metabolites are vanillylmandelic acid and homovanillic acid.

O   **A three-year-old girl is brought in for a mass protruding from her vaginal area. There are no signs of abuse. What is the most likely diagnosis?**

Sarcoma botryoides. Adenocarcinoma is more common in adolescents.

O   **A three-year-old male presents with proptosis and periorbital ecchymosis. What is the most likely malignancy?**

Neuroblastoma. Occasionally, these patients are mistake for battered children.

O   **A 14-year-old male presents with a history of headache, morning vomiting and ataxia. What is your diagnosis?**

A posterior fossa tumor. The most likely tumor to occur at this age is a medulloblastoma.

O   **A 6-year-old male is diagnosed and treated for intussusception. What tumor is associated with this?**

After the age of 5, it would be unusual to have an intussusception without a lead point. The most likely malignancy would be a non-Hodgkin's lymphoma.

O   **How does cryptorchism effect the risk of testicular malignancy?**

The risk is 30-50 times greater than in a normal testicle. About one-eighth of testicular tumors develop in cryptorchid testes.

O   **How common is Hodgkin's disease during childhood?**

Children less than 10 years of age constitute 4% of all cases of Hodgkin's disease. Patients between the ages of 11 to 16 years of age constitute another 11%.

O   **An 8-year-old female is being treated with cyclophosphamide for a malignancy. She develops hemorrhagic cystitis. What would her treatment consist of ?**

Hydration. Correction of coagulopathies and anemia should be done as indicated. Clots in the bladder may need to be removed.

O   **A 4-year-old child with a brain tumor develops seizures. He has a history or SIADH. Serum sodium is 116 mEq/dl. What would his treatment consist of ?**

3% saline and Furosemide, if still seizing. The mainstay of therapy for a chronic or asymptomatic patient is fluid restriction. Sodium levels should never be raised more than 10 mEq/dl /day.

O   **What are the second most common neoplasms during childhood?**

Primary central nervous system tumors. These account for 20% of all cancers of childhood.

○ **Which pediatric brain tumor has the worst prognosis?**

A brain stem Glioma. Children typically die within two years of presentation.

○ **EBV has been associated with which malignancies?**

Nasopharyngeal carcinoma, Burkitt lymphoma and Hodgkin's lymphoma. Hepatocellular carcinoma is associated with Hepatitis B.

○ **A leukemia patient is exposed to Varicella, which he has never had. What is the best course of action?**

Immunize the patient with Varicella immune globulin. This is best done within three days of exposure.

○ **A leukemia patient develops a sudden onset of right lower quadrant pain. The patient is febrile, neutropenic, and has an abdominal mass. What is the most likely etiology of this child's pain?**

Typhlitis, which has a high mortality and is treated with antibiotics.

○ **What is the best treatment for superior vena cava syndrome?**

Secure the airway, supply oxygen. The next goal is to shrink the tumor with either radiation and/or surgery.

○ **The treatment for a neutropenic febrile leukemic patient includes what?**

A semisynthetic antipseudomonal penicillin, an aminoglycoside, plus a first generation cephalosporin for gram positive coverage. Ceftazidime may be used by itself, as can cefepime.

○ **What percentage of neuroblastoma patients have metastatic disease at the time of their diagnosis?**

75%. The usual sites are lymph nodes, bone marrow, liver, skin, orbit and bone.

○ **What are the typical findings in a familial erythro (hemo) phagocytic lymphohistiocytosis patient?**

Fever, organomegaly, failure to thrive, pancytopenia, hepatic dysfunction and coagulopathy. This disorder presents in early infancy, and is fatal.

○ **Name some conditions that predispose a child to adenocarcinoma of the colon.**

Inflammatory bowel disease, polyposis syndromes, nodular lymphoid hyperplasia, retinitis pigmentosa, and ureterosigmoidostomy.

○ **What is the most common thyroid tumor in childhood?**

Papillary adenocarcinoma. This accounts for about three-quarters of malignant thyroid tumors.

○ **A 2-year-old male is brought in by his mother because he has a flank mass. He is hypertensive and polycythemic. Urinalysis reveals hematuria. What is your diagnosis?**

Wilms tumor. Typically, the mass is noted by the patient's primary caregiver. Hypertension, hematuria, and (less commonly) polycythemia may be seen.

O **A 15-year-old male complains of tibial pain after playing football. X-ray shows an "onion skin" appearance of the tibia. What condition is the patient likely to have?**

Ewing Sarcoma. The onion skin appearance is characteristic of this tumor.

O **What is the most common sites of involvement of a rhabdomyosarcoma?**

The head and neck regions. Other areas that can be involved are the genitourinary tract, the extremities, and the trunk.

O **What is the leading cause of death from leukemia?**

Infection. The second leading cause is hemorrhage.

O **A 6-year-old known leukemic appears pale. Hemoglobin is 4 gm/dl. Evidence of congestive heart failure exists. What would be the most appropriate treatment?**

Slow transfusion of irradiated PRBCs. Transfuse three to five cc/kg over four hours and give furosemide, 1 mg/kg, to avoid volume overload.

O **What are the most common malignancies to cause tumor lysis syndrome?**

Advanced leukemia and non-Hodgkin's lymphoma. Large tumor burdens with aggressive chemotherapy are risk factors.

O **What are the major toxicities of Vincristine?**

Peripheral neuropathy, SIADH, and cardiomyopathy (long-term).

O **What are the major toxicities of cyclophosphamide?**

Myelosuppression, hemorrhagic cystitis and infertility.

O **What do the major toxicities of I-asparaginase include?**

Coagulopathy, pancreatitis, and hepatitis.

O **Which conditions increase the risk for development of non-Hodgkin's lymphoma?**

Ataxia-telangiectasia, Wiskott-Aldrich, SCID, transplant recipients. Immunodeficient states are associated with non-Hodgkin's lymphoma.

O **What is the proposed etiology of idiopathic thrombocytopenic purpura (ITP)?**

Viral infections (esp rubella, rubeola, and URIs) leading to an immune mechanism. There is increased IgG bound to platelets.

O **In what percentage of patients with ITP was there an antecedent viral illness?**

Roughly 70% of the time. Interval between infection and onset of purpura is usually about 2 weeks.

O **What is the test of choice for the serological diagnosis of ITP?**

No specific test exists. Platelet count is usually very low (<20K k) with megathrombocytes. The WBC and RBC counts are usually normal.

O **What is the prognosis for ITP?**

Usually excellent, with >90% of children regaining normal platelet count; though it may take up to a year for them to do so. Most children recover completely within 8 weeks.

❍   **What is the treatment of ITP?**

Infusions of IV gamma globulin (IVIG) at the rate of 1 g/kg/24hr reduces the severity and frequency of thrombocytopenia. Severe cases may benefit from corticosteroids. Unless there is evidence of life threatening hemorrhage, platelet concentrates have minimal effect as they are quickly destroyed.

❍   **What is the therapy for chronic ITP?**

Splenectomy.

❍   **On average, how many acute vasoocclusive crises do patients with sickle-cell disease experience?**

4 attacks/year.

DERMATOLOGY

○ **A 16-year-old slender female with no history of diabetes or other endocrine problem is found to have acanthosis nigricans on routine examination. What might you want to work her up for?**

Underlying malignancy. Acanthosis nigricans is often a marker for malignancy, especially of the GI tract. It is the velvety brown hyperpigmentation and thickening of the flexures common in the axilla and the groin. It is also associated with obesity, diabetes, and endocrine disorders.

○ **What is a Bartholin's cyst?**

An obstructed Bartholin's duct resulting in an abscess.

○ **What are Beau lines?**

Transverse grooves in the nailbed caused by the disruption of the nailbed matrix secondary to systemic illness. Illness can actually be dated by these lines as nails grow 1 mm/month.

○ **Candida albicans infections of the skin are <u>most</u> <u>commonly</u> located where?**

In the intertriginous areas (i.e., in the folds of the skin, axilla, groin, under the breasts, etc.) Candida albicans appears as a beefy red rash with satellite lesions.

○ **What is a carbuncle?**

A deep abscess that interconnects and extends into the subcutaneous tissue. Commonly seen in patients with diabetes, folliculitis, steroid use, obesity, heavy perspiration, and in areas of friction.

○ **Patients with untreated orbital or central facial abscesses are at risk for developing what serious complication?**

Cavernous sinus thrombosis.

○ **A mother is worried that her 5-year-old will get chicken pox because she was playing with her neighbor who was diagnosed with chicken pox and had crusty lesions all over his body. If this was the only day she played with the neighbor will she develop chicken pox too?**

No. Chicken pox is only contagious 48 hours before the rash breaks out and until the vesicles have crusted over.

○ **What are the <u>most</u> <u>common</u> causes of allergic contact dermatitis?**

Poison ivy, poison sumac, poison oak, ragweed, topical medications, nickel, chromium, rubber, glue, cosmetics, and hair dyes.

○ **A mother brings her 14-year-old boy to you a week after you prescribed ampicillin for his pharyngitis. Mom says he developed a rash over his torso, arms, legs, and even the palms of his hands. On examination the patient has a erythematous, maculopapular rash in the places described. What might the child have other than pharyngitis?**

Infectious mononucleosis. In almost 95% of patients with Epstein Barr viruses that are treated with ampicillin, a rash will develop. The rash and subsequent desquamation will last about a week.

❍   **Ecthyma <u>most</u> <u>commonly</u> presents on what body parts?**

The lower legs. Ecthyma is similar to impetigo but can also be associated with a fever and lymphadenopathy. The most common infecting agent is *Staphylococcus aureus*. This infection is most prevalent in moist warm climates.

❍   **What is the <u>most</u> <u>common</u> bullous disease?**

Erythema multiforme. The typical erythema multiforme lesion is the iris lesion (a gray center with a red rim). These lesions are symmetrical and most frequently found on the distal extremities spreading proximally. Patients may also have plaques, papules, and bullous lesions. The disease is most common in children and young adults.

❍   **What is the <u>most</u> <u>common</u> cause of erythema multiforme?**

Repetitive minor herpes simplex infections (90%). Drug reactions are the second most common cause for erythema multiforme. The rash generally erupts 7–10 days after a bout of herpes.

❍   **What is the <u>most</u> <u>common</u> location of erythema nodosum?**

The shins. They can also be found on the extensor surfaces of the forearms. Erythema nodosum are erythematous subcutaneous nodules which result from inflammation of subcutaneous fat and small vessels.

❍   **A patient presents with a raised, red, small, and painful plaque on the face. On exam, a distinct, sharp, advancing edge is noted. What is the cause?**

Erysipelas is caused by group A streptococci. When the face is involved, the patient should be admitted.

❍   **What type of reaction is erythema multiforme?**

Hypersensitivity. Bullae are subepidermal, the dermis is edematous, and a lymphatic infiltrate may be present around the capillaries and venules. In children, infections are the most important cause; in adults, drugs and malignancies are more common causes. EM is often seen during epidemics of adenovirus, atypical pneumonia, and histoplasmosis.

❍   **What is the <u>most</u> <u>common</u> cause of erythema nodosum in the Western world?**

Drug reactions - most commonly due to sulfonamides. Erythema nodosum is also associated with the following systemic diseases: fungal infection, inflammatory bowel disease, sarcoidosis, streptococcal infection, and tuberculosis.

❍   **What are the causes of exfoliative dermatitis?**

Chemicals, drugs, and cutaneous or systemic diseases. Usually scaly erythematous dermatitis involves most or all of the surface skin. It can be recognized by erythroderma with epidermal flaking or scaling. Acute signs and symptoms may include low-grade fever, pruritus, chills, and skin tightness. The chronic condition may produce dystrophic nails, thinning of body hair, and patchy hyperpigmentation or hypopigmentation. Cutaneous vasodilation may result in increased cardiac output and high-output cardiac failure. Splenomegaly suggests leukemia or lymphoma.

❍   **What is a furuncle?**

A deep-inflammatory nodule which grows out of superficial folliculitis.

❍   **What is hidradenitis suppurativa?**

Chronic suppurative abscesses found in the apocrine sweat glands of the groin and/or axilla. Proteus *mirabilis* overgrowth is common.

❍   **Your neighbor brings her 4-year-old little girl to you because she has a "disgusting" rash. The child's face is patched with vesiculopustular lesions covered in a thick, honey-colored crust. Just two days ago, these lesions were small red papules. Diagnosis?**

Impetigo contagiosa. This is most common in children and usually occurs on exposed areas of skin. Treat by removing the crusts and cleansing the bases and prescribing systemic antibiotics (erythromycin, cephalosporin, or dicloxacillin).

❍   **What is the <u>most</u> <u>common</u> organism responsible for the above child's infection?**

50–90% of impetigo contagiosa cases are caused by *Staphylococcus aureus* alone. *β-Hemolytic streptococcus* is the second most common infecting agent, being the sole affecting agent in 10% of cases or coinfecting with *staphylococcus aureus*.

❍   **What is the Koebner phenomenon?**

The development of plaques in areas where trauma has occurred. Just a scratch can trigger the development of a plaque. This is most common in patients with psoriasis and lichen planus.

❍   **What are the ABCDEs of melanomas?**

<u>A</u>symmetry.
<u>B</u>order irregularity.
<u>C</u>olor variation.
<u>D</u>iameter > 6 millimeters.
<u>E</u>levation above skin.

❍   **A patient of yours has dysplastic nevus syndrome. She comes to you depressed because her aunt has just been diagnosed with melanoma. What is her risk of developing melanoma too?**

100%. People with familial dysplastic nevus syndrome have a genetic disposition for melanoma. If diagnosis is made in the family, then the remaining members who also have the above syndrome will inevitably develop melanoma too.

❍   **What are the <u>most</u> <u>common</u> locations for melanomas for African-American and Caucasian-Americans respectively?**

<u>African-Americans</u>: hands, feet, and nails.

<u>Caucasian-Americans</u>: back and lower legs.

❍   **Differentiate between pigmented and dysplastic nevi.**

Pigmented nevi are benign moles that are uniform in appearance. They are most common in sun exposed areas. Pigmented nevi are suspicious and warrant biopsy if they grow suddenly, change color, bleed, or begin to hurt. Dysplastic nevi are not uniform in appearance and they are frequently larger than 5–12 mm in diameter. 50% of malignant melanomas originate from the melanocytes in moles.

❍   **What is the <u>most</u> <u>common</u> cause of onychomycosis?**

Trichophyton rubrum and *Trichophyton mentagrophytes*.

❍   **What is a pilonidal abscess?**

An abscess which occurs in the gluteal fold as a result of disruption of the epithelial surface.

❍   **Where does a perirectal abscess originate?**

Anal crypts and burrows through the ischiorectal space. They may be perianal, perirectal, supralevator, or ischiorectal. Perianal abscesses which involve the supralevator muscle, ischiorectal space, or rectum require operative drainage.

❍   **How may the *Toxicodendron* species be recognized?**

Poison oak and ivy have leaves with 3 leaflets per leaf. They also have U- or V-shaped leaf scars. The milky sap becomes black when exposed to air.

❍   **How quickly will people react to the *Toxicodendron* antigen?**

Contact dermatitis typically develops within 2 days of exposure; cases have been reported as quickly as 8 hours to as long as 10d. Lesions appear in a linear arrangement of papulovesicles or erythema. Fluid from vesicles does not contain antigen and does not transmit the dermatitis.

❍   **What is the <u>most</u> <u>common</u> cause of secondary pyodermia?**

Like impetigo and ecthyma, this superinfection of the skin is caused predominantly by *Staphylococcus aureus* (80–85%). Other responsible organisms are *Streptococcus, Proteus, Pseudomonas,* and *E. coli.*

❍   **A 17-year-old female comes to your office complaining of a rash over her elbows and her knees. On examination you find that she has several clearly demarcated erythematous plaques that are covered with silvery scales that can be removed with scraping. These lesions are on her extensor surfaces only in the areas previously mentioned. Examination of her nails reveals pitting in the nailbed. What is her prognosis?**

Psoriasis is an intermittent disease that may spontaneously disappear or may be life long. There may be associated arthritis in the distal interphalangeal joints; otherwise, the disease is limited to the skin and nails. Treatment is with hydration of the skin and topical mid-potency steroids.

❍   **A 12-year-old female comes to your office complaining of intense itching in the webs between her fingers that worsens at night. On close examination you see a few small squiggly lines 1 cm x 1 mm where the patient has been scratching herself. Diagnosis?**

Scabies. Scabies are due to the mite *Sarcoptes scabiei* var. *hominis.* Scabies are spread by close contact; therefore, all household contacts should also be treated.

❍   **A 16-year-old patient presents to your office complaining of greasy, red, scaly, plaques in her eyebrows, eyelids and nose that are spreading to the naso-labial folds. What patient population is this disease more likely to occur in?**

The above patient has seborrheic dermatitis. This can occur in anyone but is also a common problem in patients with HIV and Parkinson's disease. The infant form of the disease is "cradle cap."

❍   **A 14-year-old female comes to your office complaining of a painful red rash with crops of blisters on erythematous bases in a band-like distribution on the right side of her lower back spreading down and out towards her hip. Diagnosis?**

Shingles or herpes zoster disease. This is due to a reactivation of the dormant varicella virus in the sensory root ganglia of a patient with a history of chicken pox. The rash is in the distribution of the dermatome, in this case L5. It is most common in the elderly population or in patients who are immunocompromised. Treatment is with acyclovir and oral analgesics. This will help decrease the post herpetic neuralgia that is frequently associated with the disease.

❍   **Where is the <u>most</u> <u>common</u> site of eruption of herpes zoster?**

The thorax. Unlike chicken pox, shingles can recur.

❍   **A patient with shingles extending to the tip of his nose is at risk for what?**

Corneal ulceration and scarring. Lesions on the tip of the nose indicate that the nasociliary branch of the ophthalmic nerve is affected and the cornea is at risk. This is a medical emergency and needs immediate referral.

❍   **What are the 2 distinct causes of toxic epidermal necrolysis (scalded skin syndrome)?**

(1) Staphylococcal and (2) drugs or chemicals. Both begin with appearance of patches of tender erythema followed by loosening of the skin and denuding to glistening bases.

Staphylococcal scalded skin syndrome is commonly found in children younger than 5 and is due to toxin that cleaves within the epidermis under the stratum granulosum.

❍   **What areas does Staphylococcal scalded skin syndrome (SSSS) usually affect?**

The face around nose and mouth, neck, axillae, and groin. Disease commonly occurs after upper respiratory tract infections or purulent conjunctivitis. Nikolsky's sign is present when lateral pressure on the skin results in epidermal separation from the dermis.

❍   **How can SSSS be distinguished from scalded skin syndrome caused by drugs or chemicals?**

In drug or chemical etiologies, the skin separates at the dermoepidermal junction. This drug-induced TEN carries up to 50% mortality as a result of fluid loss and secondary infection. On microscopic exam of SSSS, intraepidermal cleavage occurs, and a few acantholytic keratinocytes can be seen. In non-staphylococcal type, cellular debris, inflammatory cells, and basal cell keratinocytes are present.

❍   **What is the treatment of SSSS?**

Oral or IV penicillinase-resistant penicillin, baths of potassium permanganate or dressings soaked in 0.5% silver nitrate, and fluids. Corticosteroids and silver sulfadine are contraindicated.

❍   **A patient presents with fever, myalgias, malaise, and arthralgias. On exam, findings include bullous lesions of the lips, eyes, and nose. The patient indicates eating is very painful. What should the family be told about the patient's prognosis?**

Stevens-Johnson syndrome has a mortality of 5–10% and may have significant complications including corneal ulceration, panophthalmitis, corneal opacities, anterior uveitis, blindness, hematuria, renal tubular necrosis, and progressive renal failure. Scarring of the foreskin and stenosis of the vagina can occur. Treatment in a burn unit is supportive; steroids may provide symptomatic relief; however, they are not of proven value and may be contraindicated.

❍   **What is the <u>most</u> <u>common</u> cause of Stevens-Johnson syndrome?**

Drugs, most commonly sulfa drugs. Other causes are responses to infections with *Mycoplasma pneumonia* and herpes simplex virus. The disease is self-limiting but severely uncomfortable.

❍   **What is the treatment of a tetanus prone wound?**

Surgical debridement, 3,000–10,000 units of human tetanus immune globulin [TIG (hours), (Hyper-tet)], IM (do not inject into wound), penicillin G, or metronidazole.

❍   **What is the danger of giving tetanus toxoid boosters in a pleonastic fashion (e.g. with only a 9 months interval)?**

Arthus-type hypersensitivity reaction, with onset about 4–6 hours after injection. History of a severe hypersensitivity reaction or of a severe neurologic reaction are the only contraindications to tetanus toxoid.

❍   **A patient who was born with a diffuse capillary hemangioma in the distribution of the ophthalmic division of the trigeminal nerve will have what neurological findings?**

Epilepsy (usually generalized seizures), mental retardation, and/or hemiparesis. This is Sturge-Weber syndrome. The patient is born with a hemangioma of the ophthalmic nerve and ipsilateral angiomas of the pia matter and cortex (most commonly in the parieto-occipital area).

❍   **Tinea capitis is <u>most</u> <u>commonly</u> seen in what age group?**

Children aged 4–14. This is a fungal infection of the scalp that begins as a papule around one hair shaft and then spreads to other follicles. The infection can cause the hairs to break off, leaving little black dot stumps and patches of alopecia. Trichophyton tonsurans is responsible for 90% of the cases. Wood's lamp examination will fluoresce only Microsporum infections, which are responsible for the remaining 10%. This is also called "ringworm of the scalp".

❍   **What organisms are <u>most</u> <u>commonly</u> implicated in causing tinea pedis or tinea manuum?**

Trichophyton rubrum and trichophyton mentagrophytes.

❍   **What are the 3 <u>most</u> <u>common</u> causes of acute urticaria?**

1.   Medications.
2.   Arthropod bites.
3.   Infection.

Urticaria, also known as hives or wheels, is a localized swelling due to a cytokine mediated increase in vascular permeability.

❍   **What is the <u>most</u> <u>common</u> cause of physical urticaria?**

Dermatographism. In this case, urticaria develops after firm, rapid stroking of the skin with a blunt surface. Such urticaria generally resolves within the hour.

❍   **What is the <u>most</u> <u>common</u> location of verrucae vulgaris?**

This is the common wart. It is usually located on the back of the hands or fingers and is caused by HPV.

❍   **What can be done to prevent the development of decubitus ulcers?**

Frequently change the patients position (q 2 hours), keep the skin dry and clean, use protective padding at potential sites of ulceration (i.e., heel pads or ankle pads), and keep patients on "egg-crate" mattresses or the like.

❍   **What foods cause acne?**

There is no evidence that any particular foods cause acne.

❍   **Does stress exacerbate acne?**

Yes, though the mechanism is unclear.

❍   **What is the causative agent of acne?**

Propionibacterium acnes, and the resulting obstruction and inflammatory response.

❍   **How effective are alcohol cleaning pads at preventing acne?**

There is no evidence to suggest they are effective at all.

❍   **Can prolonged treatment with systemic antibiotics be used to treat acne?**

Yes.

❍   **A 16-year-old male complains of persistent acne on the forehead. What should you tell him?**

That this is most likely due to greasy hair preparations (Pomade acne). Changing or stopping those products should improve symptoms.

❍   **What is the most effective medication for acne?**

Tretinoin (Retin-A).

❍   **What is the treatment of choice for an adolescent with severe nodulocystic acne unresponsive to conventional therapy?**

Accutane (isotretinoin), 0.5-1.0 mg/kg/day for 4 months.

❍   **Why should you never prescribe tetracycline for a patient on Accutane?**

Either drug can cause benign intracranial hypertension, but the two drugs together are especially predisposing for this disorder.

❍   **Does cleansing of the face with soap and water decrease the incidence of comedones on an adolescent face?**

No. It may decrease surface lipids so the skin looks cleaner, but surface lipids are not involved in comedone generation.

❍   **What organism is the most common cause of bullous impetigo?**

Coagulase positive *Staph. aureus.*

❍   **What is the best treatment for impetigo?**

Oral erythromycin mupirocin (Bactroban) topical lotion.

❍   **What is the treatment for atopic dermatitis?**

Oral antihistamines, topical steroids, emollients, and avoidance of irritants.

❍   **Elevations of which immunoglobulin is common in atopic dermatitis?**

IgE.

❍   **Of gels, creams, lotions, and ointments, which has the highest fat content?**

Ointment >cream > gel > lotion. The more fat, the greater the lubricating effect.

○   **What are the two main organisms responsible for Tinea Capitus?**

Microsporum canis and Trichophyton tonsurans. Of these two, T. tonsurans is the most contagious.

○   **How do you make the diagnosis of Tinea Versicolor?**

Examination under a Wood's lamp would show yellow fluorescence. Also, a KOH prep is useful in confirming diagnosis.

○   **What is the recommended therapy for Tinea Capitis?**

Oral Griseofulvin (15-20 mg/kg/day) and shampooing twice a week with 2.5% Selenium Sulfide.

○   **If you want to sound more sophisticated while writing your H&P on a child with Tinea Capitis and a tender, fluctuant mass, what would you call it?**

A kerion.

○   **What is the causative agent of Tinea Versicolor?**

Pityrosporum orbiculare (Malassezia furfur), a fungus.

○   **Patients with what conditions are more likely to develop vitiligo?**

Diabetes, Addison's disease, thyroid disorders and pernicious anemia.

○   **Which areas of the body are normally most affected by vitiligo?**

Areas that are normally hyperpigmented (i.e. face, areolae) and areas subject to friction (i.e. hands, elbows).

○   **What is telogen effluvium?**

Significant hair loss seen after significant stress (severe illness, surgery, tumor therapy, etc.).

○   **Who is more likely to present with pediculosis capitis, Caucasians or African Americans?**

Caucasians are 30% more likely to acquire this organism.

○   **What is the drug of choice for head lice?**

Permethrin (Nix).

○   **How fast does human hair grow?**

1 cm per month.

○   **Where is the best place to get a scraping to rule out scabies?**

The web spaces between the fingers and toes.

○   **What is the treatment of choice for scabies?**

5% Permethrin cream.

○   **Generally speaking, a collodion baby develops what skin condition?**

Ichthyosis.

❍   **What is the hair loss pattern of seborrheic dermatitis?**

Localized.

❍   **Viewing a Giemsa stain of a scraping of a newborn infant with irregular blotchy yellow papules, you notice eosinophils. What is the diagnosis?**

Erythema toxicum.

❍   **What is the life expectancy of the newborn that develops erythema toxicum three days after his birth?**

Normal. This is a benign and self-limited disease that is extremely common in the neonate.

❍   **A child is brought to your office for the first time. You notice that the child is clearly ataxic. You suspect ataxia-telangiectasia. Where would you expect the dermatological lesions to first present?**

Bulbar conjunctiva, bridge of nose, ears, and the anterior chest.

❍   **What is the Auspitz sign?**

When, after removal of a psoriatic scale, you notice multiple distinct bleeding points.

❍   **Is childhood psoriasis usually bilaterally symmetrical?**

Yes.

❍   **Psoriatic arthritis classically attacks which joints?**

The DIPs of hands and feet.

❍   **Are freckles inherited?**

Yes, they are inherited in an autosomal dominant pattern.

❍   **Are freckles a risk factor for the development of melanoma?**

Yes.

❍   **An 11-year-old female presents with a maculopapular rash on trunk and upper legs. The rash is in lines along the long axis of the ovoid lesions. The patient states that 1 week ago, she had only 1 lesion which was round and "about as wide as a golf ball". What is your diagnosis?**

Pityriasis rosea.

❍   **What is the distribution of the rash in pityriasis rosea?**

"Christmas tree" pattern with parallel rows of lesions on the trunk.

❍   **A 1 week old infant is brought to the ED with multiple purpuric, firm lesions on her back, buttocks, and thighs. The child was born post-term and the delivery was complicated by a shoulder dystocia. What is the most likely diagnosis?**

Subcutaneous fat necrosis.

❍   **What potentially life-threatening complication of subcutaneous fat necrosis should you be vigilant for?**

Hypercalcemia. This is due to rupture of calcium deposits in the area and usually presents at 1 to 6 months of age.

❍   **Which races most commonly develop Mongolian spots?**

African-Americans > Native Americans > Haitians > Latin Americans > Caucasian.

❍   **What maneuver can you perform to diagnose urticaria pigmentosa?**

The Darier sign - stroking the lesion, which releases histamine from mast cells which leads to urticaria.

❍   **What percentage of hemangiomas resolve spontaneously?**

90-95%. However, they may take up to 10 years to disappear.

❍   **What is the therapy for port wine stains in children?**

Flash lamp pulsed-dye laser.

❍   **Is there a role for topical steroids in acute severe sunburn?**

Yes. It may relieve pain and inflammation.

❍   **Patients on which antibiotic are most likely to have photoallergic drug reaction?**

Tetracycline and sulfonamides.

❍   **A 17-year-old girl complains that she can't wear gold earring without developing a localized rash. This is true not only in her earlobes, but also in all the pierced body parts (nose, navel, and eyebrows). What is her allergy to?**

Nickel, which is commonly found in some jewelry. She would have to wear either stainless steel or pure gold to avoid the allergy.

❍   **In a child with scalded skin syndrome (SSS), you notice that pressing on the blister enlarges it laterally. What is the name of this phenomenon?**

Nikolsky sign-A sign of epidermal fragility.

❍   **Can you develop Rhus dermatitis from physical contact with someone who already has the condition?**

Not unless they have not yet washed off the allergen.

❍   **What is the treatment for scalp lesions of seborrheic dermatitis?**

Antiseborrheic shampoo (i.e. tar, selenium sulfide).

❍   **Which responds more rapidly to topical steroids - seborrheic dermatitis or atopic dermatitis?**

Seborrheic dermatitis. This is used when the lesions are inflamed.

GENETICS

○ **What does a "dominate" mutation mean?**

A single mutant gene of a pair is dominant if it causes a evident abnormality. The chance of inheriting this mutant gene is 50%.

○ **What does a "heterozygous recessive" mutation mean?**

A single mutant gene which causes no evident abnormality. The individual with this gene is called a heterozygous carrier.

○ **What does "homozygous recessive" mean?**

When both genes of a pair are mutant the abnormal effect is expressed. The parents are usually carriers and have a 25% chance of having an affected offspring.

○ **What are the defects seen in the DiGeorge syndrome?**

Hypoplasia to plasia of thymus (immunity problems), hypoplasia to plasia of the parathyroids (hypocalcemia and seizures), and cardiac anomalies.

○ **Prenatal exposure to cocaine has been associated with what anomalies?**

Genitourinary abnormalities, microcephaly, IUGR, and an increased incidence of SIDS and developmental delays.

○ **What is VATER Syndrome/Sequence?**

Stands for Vertebral defects, Anal atresia, Tracheo-Esophozeal fistula with esophageal atresia, Radial limb hypoplasia, and Renal defects. Cardiac defects, prenatal growth deficiency and a single umbilical artery may also be seen. The majority have a normal brain.

○ **What is CHARGE association?**

This association includes Cholaboma (80%), Heart defect, Atresia Choanae (58%), Mental deficiency (Retardation, 94%), Growth deficiency (87%), Genital hypoplasia (75%), and Ear anomalies (88%).

○ **What are some effects of alcohol on the fetus?**

Effects may include: prenatal and postnatal growth deficiency, mental retardation (average IQ 63), microcephaly, short palpebral fissures, maxillary hypoplasia, short nose, smooth philtrum with thin and smooth upper lip, altered palmar creases, and VSD.

○ **What are some effects of Dilantin on the fetus?**

Mild to moderate prenatal growth deficiency, borderline to mild mental retardation, wide anterior fontanelle, broad depressed nasal bridge, short nose, bowed upper lip, low set hairline, small nails, and strabismus.

○ **What is Kartanger Syndrome?**

Situs inversus, sinusitis, bronchiectasis and immotile sperm. Etiology is autosomal recessive.

O   **What is the mode of inheritance for Albinism?**

Autosomal recessive.

O   **What is the mode of inheritance for Cystic Fibrosis?**

Autosomal recessive (4% of US whites).

O   **What is the mode of inheritance for Galactosemia?**

Autosomal recessive.

O   **What is the mode of inheritance for Hemoglobin SS (sickle cell anemia)?**

Autosomal recessive (1 in 400 are affected).

O   **What is the mode of inheritance for Hemoglobin S-C?**

Autosomal recessive.

O   **What is the mode of inheritance for S-B thalassemia?**

Autosomal recessive.

O   **What is the mode of inheritance for B thalassemia?**

Autosomal recessive.

O   **What is the mode of inheritance for Phenylketonuria?**

Autosomal recessive.

O   **What is the mode of inheritance for Tay-Sachs disease?**

Autosomal recessive (3% US Askkenazi Jews).

O   **What is the mode of inheritance for Achondroplasia?**

Autosomal dominant.

O   **What is the mode of inheritance for Aniridia?**

Autosomal dominant.

O   **What is the mode of inheritance for Neurofibromatosis?**

Autosomal dominant.

O   **What is the mode of inheritance for all types of polycystic kidneys?**

Autosomal dominant.

O   **What is the mode of inheritance for Retinoblastoma?**

Autosomal dominant.

○ **What is the mode of inheritance for Tuberous Sclerosis?**

Autosomal dominant.

○ **What is the mode of inheritance for Bruton agammaglobulinemia?**

X-linked recessive.

○ **What is the mode of inheritance for Ocular Albinism?**

X-linked recessive.

○ **What is the mode of inheritance for Red-Green Color blindness?**

X-linked recessive.

○ **What is the mode of inheritance for nephrogenic Diabetes insipidus?**

X-linked recessive.

○ **What is the mode of inheritance for Glucose-5-phosphate dehydrogenase deficiency?**

X-linked recessive (affects 10-14% of black Americans).

○ **What is the mode of inheritance for Duchenne muscular dystrophy?**

X-linked recessive.

○ **What is the mode of inheritance for Factor VIII Deficiency (Hemophilia A)?**

X-linked recessive.

○ **What is the mode of inheritance for Factor IX deficiency?**

X-linked recessive.

○ **What is the mode of inheritance for Hunter Syndrome?**

X-linked recessive.

○ **What is the mode of inheritance for Vitamin D resistant rickets?**

X-linked dominant.

○ **Name some clinical features of Trisomy-21 (Down's Syndrome).**

Mental retardation, hypotonia, flat occiput, epicanthal folds, Sieman crease, gap between 1st and 2nd toes, endocardial cushion defects, and Brunsfield spots (speckled iris).

○ **Name some clinical features of Trisomy-18.**

Mental retardation, hypertonia, low birth weight, prominent occiput, micrognathia, malformed ears, VSD and PDA, cleft lip, TEF, flexion deformities of fingers and rocker bottom feet.

○ **Name some clinical features of Trisomy-13.**

Mental retardation, seizures, microcephaly, cleft lip and/or palate, microphthalmia, polydactyly, and Sieman crease.

○   **What is the incidence of Down's Syndrome?**

1:800 (correlated with maternal age).

○   **What is the incidence of Trisomy 13?**

1:20,000.

○   **What is the incidence of Trisomy 18?**

1:2000.

○   **What type of cancer is more common in individuals with Down's Syndrome?**

Acute leukemia (mostly lymphoblastic type).

○   **Deletion of 5p chromosome results in what syndrome?**

Cri du Chat Syndrome (the cry of these infants sounds like a cat). The characteristic cry disappears in late infancy. Infants have mental retardation, microcephaly, low set ears, low birth weight, and partial syndactyly.

○   **What is significant about deletion of chromosome 11?**

The result is aniridia and sometimes Wilms Tumor (ambiguous genitalia in male patients, and gonadoblastoma in females is sometimes associated).

○   **What is the Karyotype of Turner Syndrome?**

45, X (45XO). Incidence is 1:10,000 for female births. Analysis of the products of spontaneous abortion reveal 45X karyotype to be the most common chromosomal alteration.

○   **What are some common clinical features of Turner Syndrome?**

Short stature, streak gonads, and primary amenorrhea.

○   **What is the genotype of Klinefelter Syndrome?**

Two or more X chromosomes and one or more Y chromosomes (usually 47 XXY).

○   **What are some common clinical features of Klinefelter Syndrome with 47XXY?**

Mental retardation is only 10%. 100% of affected males are infertile (impaired spermiogenesis), with 99% having small testes.

○   **What is "Fragile X" syndrome?**

Syndrome of mental retardation with macroorchidism in males.

○   **What are some effects seen in Fetal Rubella Syndrome?**

Growth deficiency, microcephaly (with M.R.), deafness, cataracts, P.D.A., thrombocytopenia, jaundice, and pneumonia. (Cultures of the rubella virus may be present up to 3 years.)

❍   **What are some "Fetal Varicella effects"?**

Mental deficiency and/or seizures, cutaneous scars, limb hypoplasia, and paralysis with atrophy of limb. (Most cases occur between 8-19 weeks gestation).

❍   **What are the four types of major mutant gene inheritance?**

Autosomal dominant, autosomal recessive, X-linked dominant, and X-linked recessive.

❍   **What is the mode of inheritance for Huntington Chorea?**

Autosomal dominant.

SURGERY, TRAUMA AND ORTHOPEDIC

○ **How many days should sutures remain in the following areas: face, scalp, trunk, hands and back, and the extremities?**

Face: 3-5; scalp: 5-7; trunk: 7-10; hands and back: 10-14; extremities: 10-21.

○ **Which is more painful to the patient, plain lidocaine or lidocaine with epinephrine?**

Lidocaine with epinephrine, because it has a very low pH. To avoid pain, buffer the solution with sodium bicarbonate. The injection should be given very slowly and subdermally.

○ **Why is epinephrine added to local anesthesia?**

To increase the duration of the anesthesia. However, epinephrine also causes vasoconstriction and decreased bleeding, which weakens tissue defenses and increases the incidence of wound infection.

○ **How should hair be removed prior to wound repair?**

Clip the hair around the wound. Do not use a razor during the preparation, as it will increase the infection rate.

○ **Lidocaine with epinephrine is a useful combination for anesthesia and the cessation of bleeding. On which parts of the body is this mixture contraindicated?**

The nose, ears, digits, and penis. Epinephrine causes local constriction of the blood vessels, which can also increase infection.

○ **What is the rate of wound infection in the average surgical service?**

4–7%. Clean wound infection rate is 2%, clean-contaminated wounds 3–4%, contaminated wounds 10–15%, and dirty wounds 25–40%. Wound infection is dependent on the degree of contamination, viability of tissue, blood supply to the tissue, dead space, amount of foreign material, age, concomitant infections, nutrition, and immunocompromised status.

○ **How long can wound care be delayed before proliferation of bacteria (that may result in an infection) occurs?**

3 hours.

○ **What mechanisms of injury create wounds that are most susceptible to infection?**

Compression or tension injuries. They are 100 times more susceptible to infection.

○ **A 15-year-old stepped on a nail that went right through her shoe and into her foot. Aside from normal skin flora, what organism might infect her puncture wound?**

Pseudomonas aeruginosa.

O   **Which has a greater resistance to infection, sutures or staples?**

Staples.

O   **What is the amount of bacteria necessary to cause wound infection, with and without a foreign body?**

With foreign body: 100 bacteria.
Without foreign body: > 1 million bacteria.

O   **Which two factors determine the ultimate appearance of a scar?**

Static and dynamic skin tension on surrounding skin.

O   **Can tetanus occur after surgical procedures?**

Yes. While most cases of tetanus in the US occur after minor trauma, there have been numerous reports of tetanus following general surgical procedures, especially those involving the GI tract.

O   **What are the characteristics of tetanus prone wounds?**

Age of wound:	> 6 hours
Configuration:	Stellate wound
Depth:	> 1 cm
Mechanism of injury:	Missile, crush, burn, frostbites
Signs of infection:	Present
Devitalized tissue:	Present
Contaminants:	Present
Denervated and/or ischemic tissue:	Present

O   **How long should one wait before delayed primary closure?**

4 days. This will decrease the infection rate; it is used for severely contaminated wounds.

O   **How long should an area of abraded skin or a laceration be kept out of the sun?**

For at least 6 months. Abraded skin will develop permanent hyperpigmentation after exposure to the sun.

O   **What is the most common organism in wound infections?**

Staphylococcus.

O   **A patient who develops a reddish-brown exudate within 6 hours of an appendectomy most likely has a wound with what type of infection?**

Clostridium. Necrotizing fasciitis, dehiscence, and sepsis may result if not treated promptly.

O   **What is the appropriate bolus for a dehydrated child who weighs 15 Kg?**

300 ml (20 ml/kg).

O   **Normal saline and Ringer's lactate have how many mEq/L of sodium, respectively?**

154 mEq/L, 130 mEq/L.

O   **What are the laboratory criteria for putting a patient on mechanical ventilation?**

$PO_2 < 70$ on 50% O_2
$PO_2 < 55$ on room air
$PCO_2 > 50$
$pH < 7.25$

○ **What negative pressure must be generated by an intubated patient for weaning to be successful?**

At least -20 cm of H_2O. Other factors are important as well: PaO_2, arterial saturation, pH, respiratory rate, minute volume, tidal volume, A-a oxygen tension, and dead space to tidal volume ratio.

○ **Matching transplants:**

1.	Autograft	a.	Donor and recipient are genetically the same.
2.	Heterotrophic	b.	Donor and recipient are the same person.
3.	Isograft	c.	Donor and recipient are of the same species.
4.	Orthotopic	d.	Donor and recipient belong to different species.
5.	Allograft	e.	Transplantation to a normal anatomical position.
6.	Xenograft	f	Transplantation to a different anatomical position.

Answers: (1) b, (2) f, (3) a, (4) e, (5) c, and (6) d.

○ **What transplant organ can be preserved the longest?**

The kidney. Kidneys can be preserved in cold storage for up to 48 hours, the pancreas and liver for 8 hours, and the heart for 4 hours. Viability can be extended by using cold storage solutions, such as Collins solution and UW-Belzer solution.

○ **What is the most common cause of bleeding in a postoperative patient?**

Poor local control.

○ **A 15-year-old fire victim is burned over both legs, his entire back, and his right arm. What percentage of his body is burned?**

63%. Follow the adult rule of 9s. Face = 9%. Arms = 9% each. Front = 18%. Back = 18%. Legs = 18% each.

○ **A 14-year-old patient who has been burned over the entire top of his body (arms and torso, front and back) develops severe difficulty breathing and appears to be going into respiratory arrest. What should you do?**

Perform an escharotomy. The patient is most likely suffering ventilatory restriction due to the circumferential eschar about his chest that is constricting the chest cavity. Escharotomies need not be performed with anesthesia, not even local anesthesia, because third degree burns involve the nervous tissue and are thus insensitive to pain.

○ **What does an increase in pulmonary arterial wedge pressure indicate?**

Fluid overload. Normal pulmonary wedge pressure is 4–12 mm Hg. Higher levels can indicate left ventricular failure, constrictive pericarditis, or mitral regurgitation with stenosis.

○ **At what point of airway obstruction will inspiratory stridor become evident?**

70% occlusion.

○ **What is the initial treatment of tension pneumothorax?**
Large bore IV catheter placed in the second intercostal space (not a chest tube).

O   **How much fluid needs to collect in the chest if it is to be seen on a decubitus or upright chest x-ray?**

200–300 ml; if supine, greater than 1 L may be necessary to be seen on AP CXR.

O   **What should be checked prior to inserting a chest tube in an intubated patient with respiratory distress and decreased breath sounds on one side?**

Position of the ET tube.

O   **What is Kehr's sign?**

A pain in the left shoulder made worse in Trendelenburg. This is a sign of splenic injury or inflammation.

O   **What postoperative complication does a patient most likely have if he has a fever and shoulder pain occurring four days after a splenectomy?**

Subphrenic abscess. This can cause fever and irritation to the diaphragm and the branch of the phrenic nerve that innervates it.

O   **Which organisms are <u>most</u> <u>commonly</u> responsible for overwhelming postsplenectomy sepsis?**

Encapsulated organisms: pneumococcus (50%); meningococcus (12%); *E. Coli* (11%); *H. Influenza* (8%); staphylococcus (8%); and streptococcus (7%).

O   **What is a sentinel loop?**

A distended loop of bowel seen on x-ray that lies near a localized inflammatory process. This is a clue to an underlying inflammatory process adjacent to the distended bowel. It can often be seen in pancreatitis or appendicitis.

O   **Which types of nodules, when viewed on thyroid scan, are more likely to be malignant: hot or cold?**

Cold. This is not, however, diagnostic. Cysts and benign adenomas can also read as cold on thyroid scan, and some thyroid cancers will read as warm.

O   **Which test should be done to differentiate a benign cystic nodule from a malignant one?**

Fine needle aspiration biopsy and cytology.

O   **When does a subdural hematoma become isodense?**

Between 1–3 weeks after the bleed. At that time, it may not show up on a CT unless you use contrast.

O   **What percentage of C-spine fractures will be identified on a lateral x-ray?**

90%.

O   **A 16-year-old female comes to your office complaining of a mass in the center of her neck, near the hyoid bone. It is tender and rises if she sticks her tongue out. What is the diagnosis?**

Infected thyroglossal duct cyst. This is a remnant of the embryological descent of the thyroid in the neck. Thyroid tissue is actually found in 10–45% of these cysts. Treat with antibiotics, drainage, and then excision, once inflammation has decreased. If the cyst is found in a noninfected state, elective surgery would also be the treatment of choice, since most of these cysts eventually become infected.

❍   **What is the most common acute surgical condition of the abdomen?**

Acute appendicitis.

❍   **Why would you order a chest x-ray in a case of acute abdomen (no one said anything about an "acute chest")?**

An upright chest x-ray can more easily show air under the diaphragm, an indication of a ruptured viscous. In addition, subdiaphragmatic abscesses or pancreatitis can cause pleural effusions that are evident on chest x-ray. Lastly, lower lobe pneumococcal pneumonia can present as abdominal pain.

❍   **What might the abdominal films reveal on a patient with appendicitis?**

Sentinel loops with air fluid levels in the RLQ, a gas filled appendix or a fecalith (pathognomonic). A barium enema may show a partially filled appendix, a mass effect on the medial/inferior boarder of the cecum, and mucosal changes on the terminal ileum.

❍   **What is the most common cause of appendicitis?**

Fecaliths. Fecaliths are found in 40% of uncomplicated appendicitis cases, 65% of cases involving gangrenous appendices that have not ruptured, and in 90% of cases involving ruptured appendices. Other causes of appendicitis include lymphoid tissue hypertrophy, inspissated barium, foreign bodies, and strictures.

❍   **How does retrocecal appendicitis most commonly present?**

Dysuria and hematuria (due to the proximity of the appendix to the right ureter). Poorly localized abdominal pain, anorexia, nausea, vomiting, diarrhea, mild fever, and peritoneal signs are also frequently common.

❍   **What is the characteristic temporal sequence of the following signs and symptoms of appendicitis?**

Anorexia, abdominal pain, and vomiting are the order of occurrence in 95% of patients with acute appendicitis.

❍   **Differentiate between McBurney's point, Rovsing's sign, the obturator sign, and the psoas sign.**

McBurney's point —   Point of maximal tenderness in a patient with appendicitis. Location is 2/3 of the way between the umbilicus and the iliac crest on the right side of the abdomen.
Rovsing's sign   —   Palpation of LLQ causes pain in the RLQ.
Obturator sign   —   Internal rotation of a flexed hip causes pain.
Psoas sign   —   Extension of the right thigh causes pain. This is also indicative of an inflamed appendix.

❍   **What is the higher rupture rate in appendicitis?**

The pediatric population has a rupture rate of 15–50%, and an associated mortality rate of 3%.

❍   **What kind of wound closure should be used in a patient with a perforated appendix?**

Delayed primary closure with direct drainage of the infection. Wound infection occurs in 20% of patients with perforated appendices.

❍   **What is the most common site of intracranial aneurysms?**

The circle of Willis (most common in the anterior communicating artery). A ruptured aneurysm presents as a headache followed by altered consciousness. .

○   **What is the most common brain tumor in the pediatric population?**

Medulloblastoma.

○   **What are the most common organisms found in brain abscesses?**

Enteric Gram-negative bacilli and anaerobes, *nocardia, staphylococci, streptococci*, and *toxoplasma*.

○   **How many minutes of cerebral anoxia will result in irreversible brain injury?**

Over 8 minutes. Six to eight minutes of anoxia will produce injury that is reversible.

○   **Matching:**

1. Neuropraxia   a.   Damage to the axon, no damage to the sheath
2. Axonotmesis   b.   Temporary loss of function, no damage to axon
3. Neurotmesis   c.   Damage to axon and sheath

Answers: (1) b, (2) a, and (3) c.

○   **You detect a hard mass in the upper outer quadrant of the right breast of a 15-year-old patient. What is your next step?**

Excision biopsy. A negative needle aspiration cannot rule out malignancy. False negative rates for fine-needle biopsy are 3–30%.

○   **A 16-year-old female fears she has cancer in both breasts. Her breasts are lumpy with mild swelling. She has a greenish-yellow discharge from her nipples and is sore in the upper outer quadrants of her breasts, and she says the pain usually begins one week before menstruation, and disappears when her menses is over. Does she have breast cancer?**

Probably not. These symptoms indicate fibrocystic breast changes, which is not a premalignant syndrome.

○   **What is the most common non-cystic breast tumor?**

Fibroadenomas. These small, painless, mobile round tumors are most common in women under the age of twenty-five.

○   **What does a high cathepsin D level indicate in a female with breast cancer?**

A high risk of metastasis.

○   **Tachycardia, hypotension, and distended neck veins are the classic signs of what?**

Pericardial tamponade.

○   **What is the most common tumor of the first year of life?**

Wilms tumor. Hepatoma is second.

○   **What is the average age of diagnosis of Wilms tumors?**

3 years old. Cure rates are as high as 90% in patients with no metastasis.

○   **What are the most common sites of secondary malignancies in patients who have had Wilms tumors?**

Hepatocellular carcinoma, leukemia, lymphoma, and soft tissue sarcoma. 1–2% of patients with Wilms tumors will develop secondary malignancies.

○   **What are Grey-Turner's and Cullen's signs?**

Grey-Turner's sign–flank ecchymosis indicative of pancreatic disease.

Cullen's sign- periumbilical ecchymosis indicative of pancreatic disease. Both are caused by dissection of blood retroperitoneally.

○   **What common electrolyte disturbances occur in patients with acute pancreatitis?**

Hypocalcemia and hypomagnesemia.

○   **Serum amylase is frequently elevated in acute pancreatitis. What other conditions can cause a similar rise in amylase?**

Bowel infarct, cholecystitis, mumps, perforated ulcer, and renal failure. A lipase level is more specific for pancreatitis.

○   **What is the most common cause of pancreatic pseudocysts in children ?**

Trauma. Pseudocysts are generally filled with pancreatic enzymes and are sterile. They appear as upper abdominal pain with anorexia and weight loss, about one week after a bout of acute pancreatitis. 40% of them regress on their own.

○   **What is the treatment for pancreatic pseudocysts?**

Initial therapy is to wait 4-6 weeks for regression. If there is no improvement, or if superinfection occurs, surgical drainage or excision is required.

○   **What is the most common location of pancreatic cancer?**

80% of cases are located in the head of the pancreas; 20% are in the tail. Pancreatic cancer is generally adenocarcinoma and located in the ducts.

○   **What is the most common endocrine tumor of the pancreas?**

An insulinoma. Only 10% are malignant. Gastrinomas are second most common, and are malignant 50% of the time.

○   **Which type of operation is associated with a higher incidence of common bile duct injury, laparoscopic cholecystectomy or conventional cholecystectomy?**

Laparoscopic.

○   **What is the average size of an adrenal carcinoma on diagnosis?**

90% are larger than 6 cm in diameter.

○   **Vanillylmandelic acid, normetanephrine, and metanephrine found in the urine are indicative of what illness?**
Pheochromocytoma.

O   **Pheochromocytomas produce what?**

Catecholamines. Symptoms include increased blood pressure, perspiration, heart palpitations, anxiety, and weight loss.

O   **Where are the majority of pheochromocytomas located?**

90% are found in the adrenal medulla. The remaining 10% are found in other tissues originating from neural crest cells.

O   **What is the pheochromocytoma rule of 10's?**

10% are malignant, 10% are multiple or bilateral, 10% are extra-adrenal, 10% occur in children, 10% recur after surgical removal, and 10% are familial.

O   **What is the most common benign tumor of the liver?**

Cavernous hemangiomas.

O   **Hepatic cancer most commonly metastasizes to what organ?**

The lung (bronchiogenic carcinoma).

O   **Surgery is curative for liver cancer in what percentage of resectable asymptomatic tumors?**

> 70% of children without cirrhosis. If the patient has cirrhosis and a tumor < 2 cm, then surgery is curative 70% of the time. If the patient has cirrhosis and a tumor > 3 cm, then cure rates are only 10%.

O   **What is the two year survival rate for patients who have had liver transplants to cure liver cancer?**

25–30%.

O   **In what types of tumors will Σ-fetoprotein (AFP) be elevated?**

Primary hepatic neoplasms and endodermal sinus or yolk sac tumors of the ovaries and testes. AFP is present in 30% of patients with primary liver cancer.

O   **What is the most common cause of portal hypertension?**

Intrahepatic obstruction (90%). Cirrhosis is the most common cause of intrahepatic obstruction.

O   **What is the most commonly isolated organism in pyogenic hepatic abscesses?**

E. coli or other Gram-negative bacteria. The source of such bacteria is most likely infection in the biliary system.

O   **Which has a higher mortality rate, amebic or pyogenic liver abscesses?**

Pyogenic. The mortality rate for a singular pyogenic abscess is 25%, whereas multiple abscesses can have a mortality rate of up to 70%. Treatment of amebic abscesses is with amebicidal drugs and surgical drainage only if secondary infection develops or the abscess persists. Mortality rates for these abscesses are only 7% if uncomplicated with superinfections. Amebic abscesses are more likely to be singular in nature while pyogenic abscesses can be solitary or multiple.

O   **What clinical sign can help in the diagnosis of cholecystitis?**

Pain on inspiration with palpation in RUQ. This is called Murphy's sign. As the patient breaths in, the gallbladder is lowered in the abdomen and comes in contact with peritoneum just below the examiner's hand. An inflamed gallbladder will be greatly aggravated by this event, and the patient will discontinue her deep breath.

○   **What is the difference between cholelithiasis, cholecystitis, choledocholithiasis, and cholangitis?**

Cholelithiasis: The existence of gallstones in the gallbladder.
Cholecystitis: The inflammation of the gallbladder secondary to gallstones.
Choledocholithiasis: The existence of gallstones in the common bile duct that have migrated from the gallbladder.
Cholangitis: The inflammation of the common bile duct often secondary to bacterial infection or choledocholithiasis.

○   **Which ethnic group has a proportionately larger number of people with symptomatic gallstones?**

Native Americans. By the age of 60, Eighty percent of Native-Americans with previously asymptomatic gallstones will develop symptoms, as compared to only 30% of Caucasian-Americans, and 20% of African-Americans.

○   **What percentage of patients with cholangitis are also septic?**

50%. Chills, fever, and shock can occur.

○   **After a cholecystectomy, can gallstones reform?**

Yes. They can recur in the bile ducts.

○   **Where do most hernias occur?**

In the groin (75%). Incisional and ventral hernias account for 10%, and umbilical hernias account for 3%.

○   **The majority of inguinal hernias in infants and children are what kind of hernias?**

Indirect inguinal hernias.

○   **Differentiate between reducible, incarcerated, strangulated, Richter, and complete hernias.**

Reducible: The contents of the hernia sac return to the abdomen spontaneously, or with slight pressure, when the patient is in a recumbent position.

Incarcerated: The contents of the hernia sac are irreducible and cannot be returned to the abdomen.

Strangulated: The sac has compromised blood flow.

Richter: Only part of the hernia sac and its contents becomes strangulated. This hernia may spontaneously reduce and be overlooked.

Complete: An inguinal hernia that passes all the way into the scrotum.

○   **What are the boundaries of Hesselbach's triangle?**

The triangle is medial to the inferior epigastric artery, superior to the inguinal ligament, and lateral to the rectus sheath. Hesselbach's triangle is the site through which direct hernias pass.

O   **A direct hernia is due to a weakness in what tissue?**

The transversalis fascia, which composes the floor of the Hesselbach triangle.

O   **Indirect inguinal hernias occur secondary to what defect?**

A failure of the processus vaginalis to close. The resulting hernia can then pass through the inguinal ring.

O   **What is the most common hernia in females?**

Direct hernias. Indirect hernias are the most common hernias overall (i.e. in both sexes combined).

While *femoral* hernias are more common in females than in males, they are still not as common as direct hernias.

O   **Of all the hernias in the groin area, which type will most likely strangulate?**

A femoral hernia. Femoral hernias occur in the femoral canal, an unyielding space between the lacunar ligament and the femoral vein.

O   **Which is more common, sliding or paraesophageal hiatal hernias?**

Sliding hiatal hernias, which account for 95% of hiatal hernias.

O   **In paraesophageal hiatal hernias, does the stomach most commonly herniate to the left or the right of the esophagus?**

The left. Paraesophageal hiatal hernias have a higher rate of strangulation that can quickly lead to death. These hernias should be surgically repaired. Treat sliding hernias with antacids, H2 blockers, and changes in eating and sleeping habits, with surgery as a last resort.

O   **What is the most common site for duodenal ulcers?**

The duodenal bulb (95%). Surgery is indicated only if perforation, gastric outlet obstruction, intractable disease or uncontrollable hemorrhage occur.

O   **What is the most common site for gastric ulcers?**

The lesser curvature of the stomach. Surgery is considered earlier in gastric ulcers because of the higher recurrence rate after medical treatment and because of the higher malignant potential.

O   **What are the signs and symptoms of intestinal obstruction in a newborn?**

Maternal polyhydramnios, abdominal distention, failure to pass meconium, and vomiting.

O   **A newborn's vomit will be stained with bile if the obstruction is distal to what anatomical structure?**

The ampulla of Vater.

O   **What are the common causes of neonatal obstruction?**

Annular pancreas, Hirschsprung's disease, intestinal atresia, malrotation and volvulus or peritoneal bands, meconium plug, small left colon syndrome, and stenosis.

O   **Where does atresia of bowel most commonly occur?**

The duodenum (40%), jejunum (20%), ileum (20%), and colon (10%).

O   **What is the double bubble sign?**

The appearance of the distended stomach and duodenum on x-ray in a patient with duodenal obstruction. This is classically seen in duodenal atresia of the newborn.

O   **What is the most common cause of obstruction in children?**

Hernia.

O   **Volvulus of the colon most frequently involves which segment?**

The sigmoid (65%), cecum (30%), transverse colon (3%) and splenic flexure (2%). Volvulus is the cause of 5–10% of all large bowel obstructions.

O   **What is the most common site of intestinal obstruction secondary to gall stones?**

The terminal ileum. 55–60% will have associated air in the biliary tree.

O   **What is Rendu-Osler-Weber syndrome?**

Hereditary hemorrhagic telangiectasias found in the small intestine.

O   **Rebleeding is most common in patients with upper GI bleeds due to what?**

PUD and esophageal varices.

O   **Which type of ulcer is more likely to rebleed?**

Gastric ulcers, which are three times as likely to rebleed as are duodenal ulcers.

O   **If blood is recovered from the stomach after an NG tube is inserted, where is GI bleeding likely?**

Above the ligament of Treitz.

O   **Where are the majority of Mallory-Weiss tears found?**

In the stomach (75%), esophagogastric junction (20%), and distal esophagus (5%).

O   **What is the major cause of death in patients with Hirschsprung's disease?**

Enterocolitis.

O   **Is Hirschsprung's disease more common in males or females?**

Males. The ratio is 5:1.

O   **Are tumors found in the jejunum and ileum more likely to be malignant or benign?**

Benign. Tumors of the jejunum and ileum only compromise 5% of all GI tumors. The majority of these tumors are asymptomatic.

❍   **What is the Meckel's diverticulum rule of 2's?**

2% of the population has it, it is 2 inches long, it is 2 feet from the ileocecal valve, it most commonly occurs in children under 2, and is symptomatic in 2%.

❍   **Rectal bleeding in a patient with Meckel's diverticulum most likely due to what condition?**

Ulceration of ectopic gastric mucosa.

❍   **Cellulitis of the umbilicus in a pediatric patient with an acute abdomen is most likely due to what condition?**

A perforated Meckel's diverticulum.

❍   **What is the difference in prognosis between familial polyposis and Gardner's disease?**

Although both are inheritable conditions of colonic polyps, Gardner's disease rarely results in malignancy, while familial polyposa virtually always results in malignancy.

❍   **Which is more likely to become malignant: villous adenomas, tubulovillous adenomas or tubular adenomas?**

40% of villous adenomas will become malignant as compared to 22% of tubulovillous and 5% of tubular adenomas.

❍   **Which are more likely to turn malignant: pedunculated or sessile lesions?**

Sessile.

❍   **What is the treatment of choice for plantaris warts?**

Cryosurgery with liquid nitrogen. First, the callus should be shaved off with a razor. If possible, the keratin plug should be dug out. Lastly, liquid nitrogen should be applied. The wart will fall off in 3–4 weeks.

❍   **Soft tissue sarcomas are most often found where?**

In the lower extremities. They are fairly rare. The most common sarcomas are liposarcomas, leiomyosarcomas, fibrosarcomas, rhabdomyosarcomas, and malignant fibrous histiocytomas.

❍   **What percentage of patients with familial polyposis will go on to develop carcinoma of the colorectum?**

100%. Due to the imminent development of cancer, these patients are advised to have total colectomies and ileostomies.

❍   **A 17-year-old patient complains of severe spasms of rectal pain, but no blood. He has been stressed and over-taxed at school. What is the diagnosis?**

Proctalgia Frugux. These short rectal spasms last less than 1 minute and occur infrequently. They are associated with anxious and overworked people or people with irritable bowel syndrome. No cause is known; therefore, treatment is with analgesic suppositories, heating pad, and relaxation techniques.

❍   **A patient complains of severe pain with defecation, constipation, and blood streaked stools, which contain bloody discharge, following bowel movements. What is the diagnosis, and what is the most common place this will be found?**

Anal fissure. 90% of anal fissures are found in the posterior midline. If fissures are found elsewhere in the anal canal, anal intercourse, TB, carcinoma, Crohn's disease, or syphilis should be considered.

○   **Which are more painful, internal or external hemorrhoids?**

External. The nerve supply above the pectinate or dentate line is supplied by the autonomic nervous system and has no sensory fibers. The nerve supply below the pectinate line is supplied by the inferior rectal nerve and does have sensory fibers.

○   **Differentiate between mucosal rectal prolapse, complete rectal prolapse, and occult rectal prolapse.**

Mucosal rectal prolapse: Involves only a small portion of rectum protruding through the anus. This will look like radial folds.

Complete rectal prolapse: Involves all the layers of the rectum protruding through the anus. Clinically this appears as concentric folds.

Occult rectal prolapse: Does not involve protrusion through the anus but rather intussusception.

○   **What are some extraintestinal manifestations of ulcerative colitis?**

Ankylosing spondylitis, sclerosing cholangitis, arthralgias, ocular complications, erythema nodosum, aphthous ulcers in the mouth, thromboembolic disease, pyoderma gangrenous, nephrolithiasis, and cirrhosis of the liver.

○   **What is the most frequent site of carcinoid tumors?**

The appendix accounts for 50% of carcinoid tumors. The second most common site is the small bowel (the ileum).

○   **What carcinoid tumors have the highest rate of metastasis?**

Ileal carcinoids. Malignancy is highly dependent on the size of the tumor: only 2% of tumors under 1 cm in diameter are malignant, while 80–90% of tumors over 2 cm are malignant.

○   **A 16-year-old male presents with jaundice, upper GI bleeding, anemia, a palpable non-tender gallbladder, a palpable liver, and rapid weight loss. What is the diagnosis?**

This is the clinical picture of tumor of the ampulla of Vater.

○   **Magnesium-ammonium phosphate stones most commonly are formed secondary to what?**

UTIs due to *proteus,* a bacteria that produces urease. These are infected stones and need to be removed. Antibiotics will help end the UTI and will generally cease stone formation and urinary acidification. A urease inhibitor like acetohydroxamic acid will also prevent stone growth.

○   **What is the most common germinal tumor of the testes?**

Seminoma (40%). The overall survival rate for seminomas is 85%, as hematogenous spread does not occur until late in the disease. Other germinal tumors are embryonic cell carcinoma (25%), teratocarcinoma (25%), and choriocarcinoma. Germinal cell tumors of the testes are the most common malignant tumors of the testes.

○   **In what age group is torsion of the testicles most common?**

Adolescents.

O   **What is the maximum amount of time a testes can remain torsed without irreversible damage being done?**

4–6 hours.

O   **What lab value is indicative of bony metastasis?**

Increased alkaline phosphatase.

O   **What are mycotic aneurysms?**

Mycotic aneurysms are true aneurysms that have become infected or false aneurysms that have occurred because of an arterial infection. The femoral artery is the most common site for such aneurysms.

O   **Is mesenteric ischemia more serious in the small or large bowel?**

The small bowel. Embolization in the superior mesenteric artery effects the entire small bowel. Mortality from small bowel ischemia is 60%. Embolization to the large bowel is not as serious due to collateral circulation to the large bowel. Rarely does ischemia of the large bowel result in full thickness injury or perforation.

O   **Is venous thrombosis more common in the upper or lower extremities?**

The lower. There is decreased fibrocytic activity in the lower extremities compared to the upper.

O   **What is the treatment for paronychia?**

Wedge resection in which the ingrown part of the nail is cut at a 30° angle. This treatment is recommended only after a conservative approach of soaking in warm water and hydrogen peroxide, wide shoes, good hygiene, and a course of antibiotics has been tried.

O   **Describe the key features of spinal shock.**

Sudden areflexia which is transient and distal and lasts hours to weeks. BP is usually 80–100 mmHg with paradoxical bradycardia.

O   **The corneal reflex tests:**

Ophthalmic branch (V_1) of the trigeminal (fifth) nerve afferent and the facial (seventh) nerve efferent.

O   **Define increased intracranial pressure.**

ICP > 15 mmHg.

O   **What drug is used to reverse heparin after open heart surgery?**

Protamine.

O   **What is the most sensitive indicator of shock in children?**

Tachycardia.

O   **What is the initial fluid bolus that should be given to children in shock?**

20 ml/kg.

❍   **A radial pulse on exam indicates a BP of at least:**

80 mmHg.

❍   **A femoral pulse on exam indicates a BP of at least:**

70 mm Hg.

❍   **A carotid pulse indicates a BP of at least:**

60 mm Hg.

❍   **Do post-traumatic seizures occur more frequently in children or young adults?**

Children.

❍   **What is the most common long bone fractured?**

The tibia.

❍   **What is the most common site of osteomyelitis of the vertebral column?**

The lumbar spine.

❍   **What is the most common cause of pyogenic osteomyelitis of the vertebral column?**

Staphylococcus aureus, secondary to hematogenous spread.

❍   **A felon is a subcutaneous infection of the pulp space of the fingertip, usually *Staphylococcus aureus*. What is the treatment for this disorder?**

Treat by incising the pulp space.

❍   **Describe a common patient with a slipped capital femoral epiphysis.**

Obese boy, 10–16 years old. Groin or knee discomfort increases with activity; her may have a limp. Often bilateral. The slip is best seen on a lateral view.

❍   **What is the most common ankle injury?**

75% of ankle injuries are sprains with 90% of these involving the lateral complex. 90% of lateral ligament injuries are anterior talofibular.

❍   **What is the most helpful physical exam test for anterior talofibular ligament injury?**

Anterior drawer test. > 3 mm of excursion might be significant (compare sides); > 1 cm is always significant.

❍   **How are sprains classified?**

1°—stretching of ligament, normal x-ray.
2°—severe stretching with partial tear, marked tenderness, swelling, pain, normal x-ray (now stressed).
3°—complete ligament rupture, marked tenderness, swollen and/or obviously deformed joint. x-ray may show an abnormal joint.

❍   **A 17-year-old female complains of pain and a "clicking" sound located at the posterior lateral malleolus. You sense fullness beneath the lateral malleolus. What is the diagnosis?**

Peroneal tendon subluxation, with associated tenosynovitis.

O   **Which bone is most commonly fractured at birth?**

The clavicle.

O   **A patient cannot actively abduct her shoulder. What injury does this suggest?**

Rotator cuff tear. The cuff is comprised of the supraspinatus, infraspinatus, subscapularis, and the teres minor muscles and tendons.

O   **Why is a displaced supracondylar fracture (of distal humerus) in a child considered a true emergency?**

The injury often results in injury to brachial artery or median nerve. It can also cause compartment syndrome.

O   **What is the significance of the fat pad sign with an elbow injury?**

Fat pad sign or radiolucency just anterior to the distal humerus is indicative of effusion or hemarthrosis of the elbow joint; this suggests an occult fracture of the radial head.

O   **What type of Salter-Harris fracture has the worst prognosis?**

Type V—compression injury of the epiphyseal plate.

O   **Which is the more sensitive test used to determine an anterior cruciate ligament tear in the knee: the anterior drawer test or the Lachman test?**

Lachman test. While the knee is held at 20° flexion and the distal femur is stabilized, the lower leg is pulled forward. Greater than 5 mm anterior laxity compared to the other knee is evidence of an anterior cruciate ligament tear.

O   **What is a stress fracture?**

A stress or "fatigue" fracture is caused by small, repetitive forces usually involving the metatarsal shafts, the distal tibia, and the femoral neck. These fractures may not be visible on initial radiographs.

O   **What is "nursemaid's elbow"?**

Subluxation of the radial head. During forceful retraction, some fibers of the annular ligament that encircle the radial neck become trapped between the radial head and the capitellum. On presentation, the arm is held in slight flexion and pronation.

O   **Why "tap" a knee with an acute hemarthrosis?**

To relieve pressure and pain and see if fat globules are present, indicating a fracture. This should only be done if absolutely necessary as the hemarthrosis commonly recur, and the joint may become infected.

O   **Where is the most common site of compartment syndrome?**

Anterior compartment of the leg. Contains tibialis anterioris, extensor digitorum longus, extensor hallucis longus, and peroneus muscles, as well as anterior tibial artery and deep peroneal nerve.

O   **What are the most common lower extremity injuries to bone in children?**

Tibial and fibular shaft fractures, usually secondary to twist forces.

○   **What radiograph would one order with suspected patellar fracture in a child?**

Standard radiographs including patellar or "sunrise" views, plus comparison radiographs of uninvolved knee.

○   **What are the differences between avulsion of tibial tubercle and Osgood-Schlatter disease?**

Both occur at tibial tubercle. Avulsion presents with acute inability to walk, lateral view of the knee is most diagnostic; treatment is surgical. Osgood-Schlatter's has vague history of intermittent pain, is bilateral in 25% of cases, has pain with range of motion but not with rest; treatment is symptomatic and not surgical.

○   **What is a toddler fracture?**

Common cause of limp or refusal to walk in this age group is a spiral fracture of the tibia, without fibular involvement.

○   **What is the <u>most</u> <u>common</u> Salter-Harris class fracture?**

Type II. A triangular fracture involving the metaphysis and an epiphyseal separation.

○   **A pneumatic tourniquet can be inflated on an extremity to more than a patient's systolic blood pressure for how long without damaging underlying vessels or neurons?**

2 hours.

○   **What is the basic disorder contributing to the pathophysiology of compartment syndrome?**

Increased pressure within closed tissue spaces compromising blood flow to muscle and nerve tissue. There are three prerequisites to the development of compartment syndrome:

1.   Limiting space
2.   Increased tissue pressure
3.   Decreased tissue perfusion

○   **What are the two basic mechanisms for elevated compartment pressure?**

1.   External compression—by burn eschar, circumferential casts, dressings, or pneumatic pressure garments.
2.   Volume increase within the compartment—hemorrhage into the compartment, IV infiltration, or edema due to post-ischemic (postischial) swelling or secondary to injury.

○   **Which two fractures are most commonly associated with compartment syndrome?**

Tibia (resulting most often in anterior compartment involvement), and supracondylar humerus fractures.

○   **What are the early signs and symptoms of compartment syndrome?**

1.   Tenderness and pain out of proportion to the injury.
2.   Pain with active and passive motion.
3.   Hypesthesia (paresthesia)—abnormal two point discrimination.

○   **What are the late signs and symptoms of compartment syndrome?**

1.   Compartment is tense, indurated, and erythematous
2.   Slow capillary refill

3.   Pallor and pulselessness

○   **What signs and symptoms would be noted for a compartment syndrome involving the deep posterior compartment of the leg?**

Pain on foot eversion or toe dorsiflexion. Hypesthesia of plantar surface of foot.

○   **What is the most common ligamentous injury to the knee?**

Anterior cruciate ligament, usually from non-contact injury.

○   **How long does it take to prepare fully crossmatched blood?**

30–60 minutes.

○   **When is a scar considered mature so that scar revision can be performed?**

6–12 months.

○   **What is the risk associated with not treating a septal hematoma of the nose?**

Aseptic necrosis followed by absorption of the septal cartilage, resulting in septal perforation.

○   **What are the important structures to be considered when repairing lacerations of the cheek?**

Facial nerve, parotid duct, and gland.

○   **What is the formula for calculating the internal diameter of a pediatric ET tube?**

ID mm = (age in years +16) / 4.

○   **What procedure should be considered as an alternative to cricothyroidotomy in children?**

Needle cricothyroidotomy with jet insufflation.

○   **Why is maintenance of core body temperature more difficult in a small child?**

A child has a larger surface area to volume ratio, and is therefore more susceptible to heat loss.

○   **At what age is an intraosseous line considered an alternative for IV access?**

Although an IO line can be used on a patient of any age, it is generally reserved for patients less than 8 years old.

○   **Where does one place an Intraosseous Line?**

Unless there is an injury to the extremity, the anterior tibial plateau and the distal femur should be the first sites considered.

○   **What are the features of central cord syndrome?**

There is a loss of motor function, worse in the upper extremities than the lower extremities. There is often sparing of perianal sensation. It is usually caused by hyperextension of the neck.

○   **What are the features of the Brown-Sequard syndrome?**

Caused by penetrating injury to one side of the spinal cord, it presents with ipsilateral motor deficit and contralateral loss of pain and temperature sensation. Light touch is usually absent on the side of the lesion.

❍   **Which pattern of partial cord injury has the worst rate of functional recovery?**

Anterior cord syndrome.

❍   **At what level of the cervical vertebrae is *pseudosubluxation* most commonly seen in children?**

C2 on C3, and C3 on C4.

❍   **What is the upper limit for the normal Atlas-dens interval on a pediatric C-spine x-ray?**

4 mm. In an adult the space should be no wider than 2-3 mm.

❍   **How is Cerebral Perfusion Pressure calculated?**

CPP=MAP-ICP. Ideal CPP is 50-60 mm Hg.

❍   **Are epidural hematomas more common in children or adults?**

Children. This is thought to be the case because the dura mater is not as tightly adhered to the skull.

❍   **What is the most likely cause of a subdural hematoma with retinal hemorrhages in a child?**

Child abuse.

❍   **A child is intubated following a closed head injury. Hyperventilation should be instituted with what target arterial PCO_2?**

22-30 mm Hg. Unlike adults who are susceptible to reductions in cerebral blood flow with PCO_2's below 30 mm Hg, children show beneficial reductions in their ICP with lower PCO_2's.

❍   **What is SCIWORA?**

Spinal Cord Injury Without Radiographic Abnormality. This can be seen at any age, but more commonly in children under 8. Thought to be related to the deformability and elasticity of the pediatric spine.

❍   **What is the weakest portion of a child's bone?**

The physis.

❍   **What is the major concern with injury to the physis?**

The potential for subsequent growth arrest.

❍   **What is the most common physeal injury?**

The distal radius.

❍   **What is a Type I Salter-Harris fracture?**

A separation of the epiphysis from the metaphysis. Usually caused by avulsion or shearing forces. Prognosis is good.

❍   **What is a Type II Salter-Harris fracture?**

A fracture through the physis which exits the metaphysis. Prognosis is good.

○ **What is a Type III Salter-Harris fracture?**

A fracture through the physis which exits the epiphysis into the articular surface. Much worse prognosis than Types I & II. ORIF is often required.

○ **What is a Type IV Salter-Harris fracture?**

A fracture extending through the metaphysis, physis and epiphysis. Carries a high rate of premature physeal arrest.

○ **What is a Type V Salter-Harris fracture?**

A crushing injury of the physis. Often difficult to pick up radiographically. Usually diagnosed retrospectively after growth arrest occurs.

○ **What is the most common cause of painful hip in older children?**

Transient synovitis. It can be difficult to distinguish from septic arthritis.

○ **What is the resultant deformity if an auricular hematoma is not properly treated?**

Cauliflower ear.

○ **What is a "green stick" fracture?**

A long bone fracture in which there is 'bending' of the bone with cortical disruption on the convex side of the bone. The cortex and periosteum is intact on the concave side of the bone.

○ **What percent of pediatric burns are inflicted?**

16-20%.

○ **A child sustains an electrical burn to the corner of his mouth from chewing an electrical cord. What complication should be anticipated?**

Delayed hemorrhage from the labial artery in 10-15 days.

○ **What clinical features differentiate partial thickness from full thickness burns?**

Partial thickness: Pink to mottled red, blisters, bullae or moist weeping surface, painful.
Full thickness: Waxy white, charred or dark red, dry leathery, insensate.

○ **In estimating the size of a burn, which body part varies most as a percent body surface area with age?**

The head. At birth the head accounts for 19% BSA. At age 1 it is 17%, age 5=13%, age 10=11%, age 15=9%, adult =7%.

○ **What are some of the proposed etiologies of acute osteomyelitis in children?**

Possible mechanisms include transient bacteremia, trauma, malnutrition, and recent illness.

○ **What are some possible findings in a child with a septic hip joint?**

The hip may be held in external rotation and flexed. Any motion of the joint will be very painful.

❍   **What bacterial pathogens are associated with osteomyelitis in children?**

Staph aureus is the most common (40-80% of cases), H. influenza type b (especially in unimmunized children less than 3 years old). Less common: S. pneumoniae, S. pyogenes, Salmonella, Brucella, Kingella, Serratia, coagulase negative Staph and Neisseriae (the latter two occasionally associated with sepsis and osteomyelitis in neonates). Pseudomonas must be considered, especially with puncture wounds to the foot (especially through a gym shoe); N. gonorrhea must be considered in sexually active patients.

❍   **Are x-rays helpful in diagnosing osteomyelitis?**

X-rays done within the first week may be negative; periosteal reaction and bony destruction take about 10-14 days to become radiographically evident.

❍   **What is the treatment of osteomyelitis in children? Of a septic joint?**

Pending culture results, treatment with broad-spectrum antibiotics including coverage for S. aureus is recommended; neonates should also be covered for group B strep, and gram negative coliforms; treatment for osteomyelitis associated with puncture wounds should provide coverage for Pseudomonas. Treatment for a septic joint should also provide coverage for H. flu type b (incidence of this has decreased as immunization for H. flu increases). Primary treatment for a septic joint is irrigation and drainage of the joint in the operating room, obtaining cultures prior to starting antibiotics. Sexually active patients should be covered for N. gonorrhea.

❍   **What is toxic synovitis?**

It is a noninfectious inflammatory condition that is seen in children approximately 3-7 years old, often involves the hip, and may follow a viral upper respiratory infection. It may be confused with a septic hip (which must be ruled out first) or Legg-Calve-Perthes. There may be decreased medial rotation of the hip in flexion, and some decreased abduction and extension. The child may have low grade fever, but unlike a septic hip, the CBC and ESR are usually normal, the child does not appear toxic, and has better range of motion of the hip. Ultrasonography can help to visualize a distended capsule as distinguished from synovial thickening which may be seen in Perthes' disease. Aspiration of the hip may be required to distinguish synovitis from a septic joint. It is treated with bed rest, anti-inflammatories, and the patient should be re-evaluated to assure resolution of symptoms has occurred.

❍   **What is lordosis?**

It is the anterior convex curvature of the lumbar spine; lordosis may also be used to describe pathologic excess anterior curvature.

❍   **What is a physis?**

A cartilaginous growth plate which appears lucent on x-ray; also called the epiphyseal growth plate.

❍   **What is an epiphysis?**

A secondary ossification center at the ends of long bones, which is separated by the physis from the remainder of the bone.

❍   **What is an apophysis?**

A secondary bone growth center at the insertion of tendons onto bones; it does not participate in a joint. Traction on immature apophyses may cause a variety of painful conditions.

❍   **What is a metaphysis?**

The flared portion at the ends of a bone next to the physis, where the calcified cartilage from the physis is replaced by endochondral bone.

O   **What is a diaphysis?**

The shaft of a long bone.

O   **What is equinus?**

Plantar flexed position or deformity of the foot so that the person walks on their toes.

O   **What is osteochondrosis?**

It refers to pathological changes in a secondary growth center (either epiphysis or apophysis) involving infarction, revascularization, reabsorption, and replacement of affected bone. It may also be seen after traction on bone.

O   **What is Sever disease?**

It refers to calcaneal apophysitis, a common cause of heel pain.

O   **What is Freiberg disease?**

It is idiopathic avascular necrosis of the head or epiphysis of the second or, less commonly, third metatarsal head. Radiographic findings include sclerosis, partial collapse, and eventual flattening of the affected area. It is relatively uncommon.

O   **What is Kohler disease?**

It is an idiopathic avascular necrosis (osteochondrosis) of the tarsal navicular bone. It is unique among the osteochondroses in that it occurs more commonly in school-aged rather than adolescent children.

O   **What is a valgus deformity? Varus deformity?**

Valgus deformity is angulation of an extremity at a joint with the more distal part angled away from the midline. Varus deformity is angulation of an extremity at a joint with the more distal part angled toward the midline.

O   **What are some common terms used in describing orthopedic findings?**

Pes: refers to the foot
Genu: refers to the knee
Coxa: refers to the hip
Cubitus: refers to the elbow
Talipes: a general term for foot deformities
Cavus: abnormally arched foot
Dislocation: complete loss of contact between two joint surfaces
Planus: flat two joint surfaces
Subluxation: incomplete loss of contact between two joint surfaces

O   **Are dislocations and sprains more common in children or adults?**

Dislocations and ligamentous injuries are uncommon in prepubertal children as the ligaments and joints are quite strong as compared to the adjoining growth plates. Excessive force applied to a child's joint is more likely to cause a fracture through the growth plate than a dislocation or sprain.

O   **Can fractures result in overgrowth or undergrowth of the involved bone?**

Both. Fractures involving the growth plate may result in arrest of growth and severe shortening or uneven arrest of growth leading to angular deformities. Fractures can also result in overgrowth as some fractures stimulate growth at the physis of the fractured bone.

○   **Which type of fracture deformity can be particularly difficult to correct?**

Rotational deformities do not correct spontaneously and require meticulous realignment.

○   **What factors help in determining whether angular deformities will correct?**

Angular deformities are more likely to correct through bony remodeling the younger the child is and the closer the fracture is to the physis.

○   **What is a torus fracture?**

A torus, or buckle, fracture is a metaphyseal fracture unique to children secondary to compressive forces causing buckling of the bone, leaving the cortices intact.

○   **The Salter-Harris classification refers to what type of fractures unique to children?**

It refers to physeal fractures.

○   **Can other signs be helpful in diagnosing occult fractures?**

Fracture should be suspected when there is significant swelling and if there is hemarthrosis in or around the joint. This may be seen at the elbow joint as elevation of the fat pad in the coronoid fossa (the anterior fat pad sign, which can be normal in children), or in the olecranon fossa (the posterior fat pad sign, which is abnormal).

○   **What possibilities should not be overlooked when evaluating fractures in children?**

Intrinsic bone disease (e.g. osteogenesis imperfecta), metabolic diseases (especially calcium related) and child abuse.

○   **What are some possible clues to the diagnosis of child abuse?**

Fractures in children less than 3 years of age, especially those less than 1-year-old should raise suspicion (roughly 50% of fractures in children less than one-year-old and 30% of fractures in children less than 3 years old are related to child abuse). Delay in seeking treatment, evidence of other bruising, inconsistent history of the injury, social risk factors, and behavioral problems in the child may be clues to the presence of non-accidental injury.

○   **Which fractures are thought to be specific for child abuse?**

Metaphyseal fractures (chip fractures in a corner), posterior rib fractures, acromioclavicular fractures, and multiple fractures of different ages.

○   **Which bony lesions suggest possible child abuse?**

Spinal fractures, digital fractures, complex skull fractures, spiral long bone fractures, scapular fractures, sternal fractures, and periosteal separation.

○   **What findings comprise the shaken baby syndrome?**

Retinal hemorrhage, subdural hematoma, and rib fractures.

O   **What is Volkmann's ischemia?**

It is pain worsened by passive motion of a muscle and associated neurologic deficits secondary to ischemia of the muscles and nerves; it is usually associated with a compartment syndrome.

O   **What is Volkmann's contracture?**

It is the result of untreated Volkmann's ischemia, a contracture deformity secondary to muscle necrosis.

O   **What is an antalgic limp?**

It is a painful limp characterized by a shortened stance phase to decrease time on the affected extremity.

O   **What is a Trendelenburg gait?**

It is a non-painful limp, indicative of underling hip instability or muscle weakness, characterized by an equal stance phase between the involved and uninvolved side. The child will attempt to shift the center of gravity over the involved side for improved balance.

O   **What are some causes (according to age) of painful limping?**

Antalgic gait may be caused by: (1-3-year-old): infection, occult trauma, or neoplasm; (4-10-year-old): infection, transient synovitis of the hip, Legg-Calve-Perthes disease, rheumatologic disorder, trauma, or neoplasm; (11+-year-old): slipped capital femoral epiphysis, rheumatologic disorder, trauma. It may also be seen in sickle cell disease.

O   **What are some causes of Trendelenburg gait?**

(1-3-year-old): hip dislocation, neuromuscular disease
(4-10-year-old): hip dislocation, neuromuscular disorder

O   **What is developmental dysplasia of the hip (DDH)?**

It is the current term to describe a spectrum of hip deformities, usually manifest in the neonatal period, where the hip joint is dislocatable.

O   **What are the two major groups into which DDH is classified?**

Typical and teratologic. They are differentiated as listed below.
Typical: in a neurologically intact child
Teratologic: an underlying neurologic disorder is present (e.g. myelodysplasia, arthrogryposis)

O   **What is arthrogryposis?**

Arthrogryposis (curved joints) refers to a group of diseases characterized by immobile joints at birth. Arthrogryposis multiplex congenita is a descriptive term that signifies multiple congenital contractures. Etiologies include primary myopathic disease and neurogenic disorders.

O   **What is amyoplasia?**

The major form of arthrogryposis multiplex congenita, AMC, is called amyoplasia, a syndrome involving both the upper and lower extremities.

O   **What are some intrauterine factors that may predispose to DDH?**

Breech position, first born (smaller, more constraining uterus), or anything else that restricts fetal movement.

O   **What is the Ortolani maneuver?**

Gentle abduction with the hip in flexion while lifting up on the greater trochanter which results in reduction of a dislocated hip with an palpable "clunk" as the femoral head slips over the posterior rim of the acetabulum.

O   **What is the Barlow maneuver?**

Adduction of the hip in flexion while pushing down gently on the on the femoral head, in a dislocatable hip, will cause dislocation as the femoral head slips out of the acetabulum.

O   **What is the most sensitive indicator of hip disease?**

Decreased internal rotation of the hip.

O   **What is a Pavlik harness?**

It is a harness that is the major mode of treatment in 1-6 month old infants to attempt reduction of the femoral head into the acetabulum. It attempts to flex the hips at greater than 90 degrees and maintain abduction.

O   **What makes the blood supply to the capital femoral epiphysis vulnerable?**

The retinacular vessels lie on the surface of the femoral neck and are intracapsular; they enter the epiphysis from the periphery and are subject to damage from trauma, joint infection, and other vascular insults.

O   **What is Legg-Calve-Perthes disease (LCPD)?**

It is an idiopathic avascular necrosis of the capital femoral epiphysis in a child (usually male) aged 2-12 years (mean: 7 years). Male to female ratio: 4-5:1.

O   **What is the treatment of LCPD?**

The treatment is directed at maintaining the femoral head within the acetabulum which acts as a mold for the re-ossifying femoral head. The treatment goal is to prevent femoral head deformity and osteoarthritis. Treatments may be surgical or non-surgical.

O   **What are some clinical manifestations of LCPD?**

Antalgic gait, muscle spasm (with restricted abduction and internal rotation), proximal thigh atrophy, thigh pain, and mild shortness of stature.

O   **What is the most common adolescent hip disorder?**

Slipped capital femoral epiphysis (SCFE).

O   **What is SCFE?**

It is an inferior and posterior slippage of the head of the femur off the femoral neck. Slips can be either chronic or acute. It most typically presents in summer months, and is coincident with increased physical activity.

O   **SCFE typically occurs in which individuals?**

Obese adolescents with delayed skeletal maturation or in tall, thin children after a recent growth spurt. If a slip occurs before the age of ten, endocrine disorder or systemic disorder should be suspected. It is seen in males much more commonly than females.

O   **Is SCFE bilateral or unilateral?**

The disease usually presents unilaterally with thigh, knee, or groin pain and a limp. Up to 30-40% of children with one slip will develop bilateral disease eventually and must be followed for this possibility.

O   **What radiographic views may be helpful in diagnosing SCFE or LCPD?**

Anteroposterior and Lauenstein (frog-leg) radiographs.

O   **What is the treatment of SCFE?**

SCFE is one of the few pediatric orthopedic emergencies. Weight bearing must cease to prevent a partial slip from becoming complete (complete slips carry an increased risk of vascular compromise and aseptic necrosis). The treatment is surgical by performing an epiphysiodesis of the capital femoral epiphysis with in situ pinning with cannulated screws.

O   **What are the two major complications of SCFE?**

Osteonecrosis (secondary to damage to the retinacular vessels) and chondrolysis (degeneration of the articular cartilage) of the hip.

O   **What are growing pains?**

They are nighttime thigh and calf pains most commonly seen in 4-10 year olds with symmetric limb pains unaccompanied by systemic symptoms such as fever or weight loss. Although termed growing pains, they are usually not seen in adolescents who undergo a faster rate of growth than younger children.

O   **What is scoliosis?**

Scoliosis is an alteration in normal spinal alignment occurring in the AP or frontal plane, i.e., it is a lateral spine curvature.

O   **What is postural scoliosis?**

It is due to leg length discrepancy, also termed transient, functional, or compensatory scoliosis.

O   **What is structural scoliosis?**

All other types of scoliosis.

O   **What are the general categories of scoliosis?**

Idiopathic, congenital, neuromuscular (e.g. cerebral palsy, Duchenne muscular dystrophy), "other" including spina-bifida, Marfan syndrome, neurofibromatosis, osteogenesis imperfecta, cord tumor, spondyloepiphyseal dysplasia, osteoid osteoma (painful), and Ehler-Danlos syndrome.

O   **What is the most common form of scoliosis?**

Idiopathic (by definition, idiopathic curves are those in which all specific causes have been ruled out). It occurs in healthy, neurologically normal children.

O   **To which side does the thoracic convexity usually curve?**

To the right (radiographs of the spine are viewed as the physician would view the back).

O   **What are some concerning findings with scoliosis suggesting underlying disease?**

Left thoracic curve, pain, stiffness, and overlying skin lesion.

O   **What is the most common form of idiopathic scoliosis?**

Adolescent onset scoliosis accounts for approximately 80% of idiopathic scoliosis, occurring at ages 11 and older. Infantile onset, birth-3 years, is very rare in the U S. and juvenile onset occurs at ages 4-10 years.

O   **What radiographic evaluations are obtained to evaluate scoliosis?**

PA and lateral standing radiographs of the entire spine are obtained. Increased use of MRI has identified children with otherwise inapparent abnormalities of their spinal cords.

O   **In which patients should MRI be seriously considered?**

Patients with neurologic findings, left thoracic curve, age less than 10 years, rapidly progressive curve, or vertebral abnormalities.

O   **What is the treatment of scoliosis?**

Treatment is based on etiology of the scoliosis, degree of deformity, degree of skeletal maturity, and curve progression. Observation is indicated for mild, idiopathic curve (less than 20 degrees) with clinical exam and x-rays every six months. Orthosis is indicated for those in whom the curve is considered acceptable at diagnosis, but whose curve is likely to progress. Surgical correction is usually indicated for curves greater than approximately 40 degrees or those with significant cosmetic deformity.

O   **What are risk factors for progression of idiopathic curves?**

Female sex, pre-menarche, curve location, curve magnitude, and absence of bony maturity.

O   **What are the classifications of congenital scoliosis?**

1)   Partial or complete failure of vertebral bodies (wedge vertebrae or hemivertebrae)
2)   Partial or complete failure of segmentation (unsegmented bars which "tether" one side of the vertebral column)
3)   Mixed processes

O   **What other abnormalities may be found in patients with congenital scoliosis?**

There may be malformations in other organ systems that are differentiating at the same time as the spine. Congenital genitourinary malformations-20%, congenital heart disease-10-15%, spinal dysraphism-20% (The numbers represent the percentage of children with congenital scoliosis having these associated organ findings).

O   **What is the most common GU abnormality in children with congenital scoliosis?**

Unilateral renal agenesis.

O   **What is spinal dysraphism?**

It is a general term for coexistent vertebral and spinal cord defects including spina bifida occulta, myelomeningocele, and other intradural and extradural lesions.

O   **What is Klippel-Feil syndrome?**

It is failure of segmentation of two or more cervical vertebrae. A short, webbed neck with a low hair line may be seen. Renal, cardiac, scapular, and hearing abnormalities should be sought.

O   **What is Sprengel deformity?**

It is a congenital undescended scapula manifested by elevation and medial rotation of the inferior pole of the scapula. It is often associated with other congenital abnormalities especially those of the spine, ribs, heart, and kidney.

O   **What is the VATER association?**

Vertebral anomalies
Imperforate Anus
Tracheoesophageal fistula
Radial dysplasia (clubhand)
Renal abnormalities

O   **What classifications of kyphosis are there?**

Postural (flexible, round-back deformity without vertebral deformity), idiopathic, and congenital.

O   **What is Scheuermann disease?**

It is an idiopathic rigid kyphosis of the dorsal spine; it is second only to idiopathic scoliosis as a cause of spinal deformity. Treatment is similar to that for scoliosis; surgical treatment is rarely needed.

O   **What radiographic findings are seen with Scheuermann disease?**

1) Narrowing of the disc space
2) Anterior wedging of at least three adjacent vertebrae
3) Irregularities of the endplate
4) Schmorl nodes

O   **Is back pain in children common?**

No, it is unusual and frequently due to organic causes. Etiologies include inflammatory diseases, rheumatologic diseases, developmental diseases, mechanical trauma, and neoplastic diseases.

O   **What is Panner disease?**

It is an osteochondrosis of the ossific nucleus of the capitellum (the lateral aspect of the distal humeral epiphysis).

O   **What types of tumors may be found in children who have back pain?**

Tumors may involve the vertebral column or the spinal cord. Benign tumors include osteoid osteomas, osteoblastoma (giant osteoid osteoma-greater than 20 mm), solitary bone cysts, and eosinophilic granuloma. Malignant tumors may be osseous (osteogenic or Ewing's sarcoma), neurogenic (neuroblastoma), or metastatic.

O   **What is torticollis?**

It refers to twisted or wry, neck, where the head is tipped to one side, with the occiput rotated toward the shoulder. Etiologies include soft tissue trauma, rotary subluxation of the cervical spine, dystonic reactions, muscular causes (e.g. viral myositis), osseous causes, neurogenic causes, and Sandifer syndrome (Gastroesophageal reflux, iron deficiency anemia, vomiting, and a head-tilting trait).

○ **What is "Little League elbow"?**

It is medial epicondylitis or osteochondritis desiccans of the capitellum and/or radial head laterally. Children usually present with pain after throwing or after gymnastics.

○ **What is osteochondritis desiccans?**

Osteochondritis desiccans is a degenerative process in a localized area of bone and its articular surface that may be due to ischemia or repeated trauma; the exact cause is unknown. The bone becomes avascular and ultimately separates from the underlying proximal bone. The lateral aspect of the medial condyle is the most common site.

○ **What is the most common site of osteochondritis desiccans?**

The lateral aspect of the medial femoral condyle is the most common site; it may also be seen in the ankle and the elbow.

○ **What is a ganglion?**

It is a fluid-filled cyst at the wrist where a defect in the joint capsule allows herniation of the synovium. If the synovium ruptures, fluid collects in the soft tissue where it gets walled off by fibrous tissue. They are benign and tend to disappear over time.

○ **What is radial clubhand?**

It is total or partial absence of the radius resulting in radial deviation of the hand and abnormal function.

○ **Which carpal bones form the articular surface of the hand?**

The scaphoid and lunate bones.

○ **What is polydactyly?**

Extra digits which may be simple skin tags and digit remnants which do not have palpable bone within or complex varieties which require formal amputation.

○ **What is syndactyly?**

It is fusion of one digit to its neighbor. It may be bony or cutaneous.

○ **Where is syndactyly most often seen?**

It is most often seen between the third (long) and fourth (ring) fingers and the second and third toes.

○ **What is clinodactyly?**

It is curving of a digit, most often the fifth digit and may be directed either radially or in an ulnar direction. It often results from hypoplasia of the middle phalanx and is usually a minor anomaly.

○ **What causes trigger finger?**

Thickening of the tendon of the flexor hallucis longus (in the thumb) or the flexor digitorum longus (of the fingers) in the flexor sheath causing a flexion deformity (triggering). This may be a fixed deformity.

○ **What are the three regions of the foot?**

The hindfoot (the calcaneus and the talus), the midfoot (the navicular, the cuboid, and the three cuneiform bones), and the forefoot (the metatarsals and toes).

O   **What is the joint between the calcaneus and the talus?**

The talocalcaneal or subtalar joint.

O   **What is metatarsus adductus?**

It is incurving (adduction) of the forefoot with the lateral border of the foot appearing convex. Forefoot mobility can be either flexible or rigid.

O   **What is the treatment for metatarsus adductus?**

Treatment varies with the degree of rigidity of the foot and ranges from stimulating the peroneal musculature, corrective shoes and orthotics, serial casting, and, rarely, surgery for older children who have not achieved satisfactory correction.

O   **What other disorder should be ruled out in children with metatarsus adductus?**

Hip dysplasia (acetabular dysplasia) which is found in approximately 10% of children with metatarsus adductus.

O   **What is calcaneovalgus foot?**

It is a relatively common finding in the newborn secondary to inutero positioning. The foot is hyperdorsiflexed with forefoot abduction and increased heel valgus and is usually associated with external tibial torsion.

O   **What is the treatment for calcaneovalgus foot?**

This condition usually corrects without specific treatment by the age of two.

O   **What is talipes equinovarus?**

Clubfoot. It consists of forefoot adduction, heel inversion or varus with the sole of the foot pointed medially, and ankle equinus with the foot in a plantarflexed position. Mild calf atrophy, and mild hypoplasia of the tibia, fibula, and bones of the feet may also be seen.

O   **What are the classifications of clubfoot?**

Congenital, teratologic, and positional. The congenital form is usually an isolated abnormality whereas the teratologic form is associated with a neuromuscular or syndrome complex.

O   **What is the treatment?**

Taping, malleable splints, and serial plaster casts. Failure to achieve correction by three months of age is an indication for surgical correction.

O   **What is Kite's angle?**

It is the angle formed by the long axes of the calcaneus and talus. It is normal (approximately 25 degrees) in all but the most severe forms of metatarsus adductus. It is always much smaller in clubfoot.

O   **What congenital deformity causes "rocker-bottom" foot?**

Congenital vertical talus (congenital convex pes valgus); it may be idiopathic, but is often associated with an underlying neurologic or orthopedic disorder or syndrome.

○   **What is hypermobile pes planus?**

It is hypermobile flat feet or pronated feet. Children usually show improvement by six years of age, as there is decreased laxity in the bony-ligamentous complexes of the feet in the area of the medial longitudinal arch.

○   **What is tarsal coalition?**

It is also called peroneal spastic flatfoot characterized by a painful, rigid flatfoot deformity and lateral calf (peroneal) muscle spasm. A congenital fusion or failure of segmentation between two or more tarsal bones causes it.

○   **What are the most common tarsal coalitions?**

Coalitions occur at the medial talocalcaneal (subtalar) facet and between the calcaneus and navicular tarsal bones. Coalitions can be osseous, cartilaginous, or fibrous.

○   **What is the treatment for tarsal coalition?**

Treatment varies dependent on degree of disability, age, type of coalition, presence of arthritis and extent of coalition. It may be operative or non-operative (casts or orthotics).

○   **What is cavus foot?**

It is an increase in the medial longitudinal arch of the foot commonly associated with varus deformity at the hindfoot. Etiologies such as peripheral neuropathies (e.g. Charcot-Marie-Tooth) and spinal cord disease must be ruled out.

○   **What is the treatment of cavus foot?**

Treatment is often surgical if there is persistent pain or to prevent worsening deformity with asymmetrical weight-bearing.

○   **What is curly toe deformity?**

It refers to flexion deformity at the proximal interphalangeal joint with lateral rotation and varus alignment of the affected toe. It is secondary to tightness in the flexor tendons. The fourth and fifth toes are most commonly involved.

○   **What is the treatment of curly toes?**

Initially the child is observed as up to 50% will resolve spontaneously. If it persists beyond age 3 or 4 years, surgery (flexor tenotomy or PIP fusion) may be required.

○   **What is hammer toe?**

It is a flexion deformity at the PIP of the toe with extension at the metatarsophalangeal joint.

○   **What is mallet toe?**

It is a flexion deformity at the distal interphalangeal joint, which usually requires release of the flexor digitorum longus tendon.

○   **When does physiological bowing of the lower extremities usually resolve?**

It usually resolves with 6-12 months of ambulation.

O   **When is physiologic genu valgum (knock knees) usually seen?**

Between the ages of three and four years; it typically resolves with growth between the ages of five and eight years.

O   **What is the most common cause of in-toeing in children two years of age and older?**

Internal femoral torsion, usually due to generalized ligamentous laxity; the entire lower extremity is inwardly rotated during gait.

O   **What is the treatment for internal femoral torsion?**

It is initially observed and takes one to three years to resolve depending on sitting habits of the child. Older children may require surgical correction.

O   **What is the most common cause of in-toeing in children younger than two years old?**

Internal tibial torsion, which is secondary to normal in utero positioning. Other causes of in-toeing include metatarsus adductus and internal femoral rotation (femoral anteversion).

O   **What is the treatment for internal tibial torsion?**

It is a physiological condition and usually resolves with normal childhood growth within approximately 6-12 months of the child walking independently.

O   **What are two common causes for out-toeing gait?**

External femoral torsion (also known as femoral retroversion) and external tibial torsion.

O   **What disorder must be ruled out in femoral retroversion?**

External femoral torsion (femoral retroversion) is uncommon unless it occurs in association with SCFE (slipped capital femoral epiphysis) which must be ruled out, especially if the torsion is unilateral and diagnosed in obese young adolescents. The idiopathic form of external femoral torsion is usually bilateral.

O   **External tibial torsion is associated with which other orthopedic finding?**

Calcaneovalgus foot.

O   **What is genu varum?**

Bow-legs. It may be physiologic (secondary to intrauterine positioning) or due to asymmetric growth, dysplasia, or metabolic disorders.

O   **What is Blount disease?**

Tibia vara (Blount disease) is a localized growth disturbance of the medial aspect of the proximal tibial epiphysis. This results in progressive deformity with varus angulation below the knee. It may be due to increased loading and compressive forces over the medial aspect of the tibia.

O   **What are the various classifications of Blount disease?**

Infantile (1-3 year), juvenile (4-10 year), or adolescent (11 year or older) dependent on the age at which it occurs; the infantile form is the most common.

❍ **What is the treatment of Blount disease?**

Non-surgical treatment with braces to resist varus angulation can be considered for onset of disease before age three. In those who are older than three years, those with severe deformity, or those failing to respond to bracing, surgical correction (usually with osteotomy) is indicated.

❍ **What is congenital fibular hemimelia?**

It is congenital absence of the fibula and is usually also associated with congenital absence of the lateral portion of the foot.

❍ **What is a Baker cyst?**

A popliteal or Baker cyst is a benign, fluid-filled cyst of the popliteal space caused by outpouchings of the knee joint capsule or bursae between the gastrocnemius and semimembranosus tendons. Most are idiopathic and resolve spontaneously.

❍ **An adolescent boy presents with pain over the tibial tubercle after athletic activity and presents with a tender prominent tibial tubercle. What is the diagnosis?**

Osgood-Schlatter disease; complete resolution of symptoms over 1-2 years is expected as physeal closure of the tubercle occurs. Symptomatic care with rest, anti-inflammatories, and non-steroidal medication is the usual treatment.

❍ **What is patella alta?**

High riding patella.

❍ **What is the apprehension test?**

Attempts to displace the patella laterally gives a subjective feeling of imminent patellar subluxation in patients with maltracking patellas who are predisposed to dislocation. The apprehension test refers to the patient's anxiety over this imminent subluxation during the above described maneuver.

❍ **What is bony dysplasia?**

Dysplasias of bone (and cartilage) refers to a variety of conditions involving metaphyses, diaphyses, epiphyses, and cartilage usually associated with short stature. As a group, they are common and associated with a high rate of stillbirths and early postnatal deaths. Most are genetically based, but some drugs (e.g. warfarin) or Vitamin K deficiency may also cause dysplasia. Some examples include epiphyseal dysplasias, metaphyseal dysplasias, metaphyseal dysostosis, hypochondroplasia, achondroplasia, osteogenesis imperfecta, and diaphyseal dysplasia.

❍ **What is genu recurvatum?**

It refers to hyperextension at the knee joint usually associated with benign hyperlaxity.

❍ **What is rhizomelia?**

It refers to shortening of the proximal segment of the limb (e.g. humerus or femur) relative to more distal limb segments.

❍ **What is mesomelia?**

It refers to segmental shortening of the middle portion of the limb (e.g. radius/ulna or tibia/fibula).

❍   **What is acromelia?**

It is shortening of the distal portion of the limb (e.g. hands or feet).

❍   **What are some additional features that may be seen with skeletal disproportion?**

Club feet, increased skin creases, prominent forehead, macrocephaly, joint prominence, craniotabes, restricted or excess joint motion, skin dimpling at the pretibial area, dislocations, fractures, camptodactyly, and clinodactyly. Cystic ears, cleft palate, polydactyly, encephalocele, and hemivertebrae should prompt a search for possible underlying skeletal dysplasia.

❍   **What is SD/MCA?**

It refers to skeletal dysplasia combined with multiple congenital anomaly syndrome.

❍   **What is platyspondylia?**

Flat vertebral bodies.

❍   **What is pseudoachondroplasia?**

It refers to spondylometal-epiphyseal dysplasias.

❍   **What is schneckenbecken dysplasia?**

It refers to a snail-like pelvis.

❍   **In which dysplasia is a wrench-like proximal femur found?**

Desbuquois syndrome, a lethal autosomal recessive disorder.

❍   **What are some of the general categories into which late onset dwarfing conditions are classified?**

They are classified as those affecting predominantly the spine, metaphysis, epiphysis, or single geographic area, those associated with increased bony density disorders, and storage disorders (e.g. mucopolysaccharidoses).

❍   **What are some of the usually fatal causes of neonatal dwarfism?**

Thanatophoric dwarfism, achondrogenesis, short rib polydactyly, homozygous achondroplasia, congenital osteopetrosis, camptomelic dysplasia, Silverman-Handmaker dys-segmental dysplasia, osteogenesis imperfecta-type II, hypophosphatasia-congenital, and rhizomelic chondrodysplasia punctata.

❍   **What is achondroplasia?**

It is a pure autosomal dominant skeletal spondylometaphyseal dysplasia.

❍   **What are some of the features of achondroplasia?**

Short trunk and limbs, large cranium with frontal bossing, flattened nasal bridge, hypoplasia of the maxilla, relative mandibular prognathism moderate brachydactyly, wide hands, with hypotonia noted in infancy.

❍   **What are some of the non-skeletal features that may be associated with achondroplasia?**

Dental malocclusion, recurrent otitis media, chronic serous otitis media, sleep apnea, and early child death may be seen secondary to cervical cord compression due to a small foramen magnum, and hydrocephalus secondary to obstruction of the foramen magnum.

○   **What is the prognosis for children with achondroplasia?**

They usually have a normal life span except for the uncommon patient with hydrocephalus or spinal cord compressions.

○   **What is thanatophoric dysplasia?**

It is a lethal neonatal dwarfing condition associated with a large head, short bowed limbs, very small thorax, brachydactyly, platyspondylia, metaphyseal flaring and, rarely, congenital suture fusions.

○   **What is diastrophic dysplasia?**

It is an autosomal recessive disorder characterized by short bowed limbs, club feet, knee contractures, low-set thumbs, clino-camptodactyly, ear cysts, broad arched palate; laryngomalacia, frontal hemangiomas, cleft palate, micrognathia prominent forehead, pre-tibial dimples and joint dislocations may be seen. Diastrophic refers to twisting, such as with scoliosis.

○   **What is Ellis-van Creveld dysplasia?**

It is a syndrome of skeletal dysplasia/multiple congenital anomalies that is autosomal recessive and characterized by polydactyly, nail dysplasia, oligodontia with cone shaped teeth, multiple gingival frenula, tube shaped trunk, and a high incidence of congenital heart abnormalities.

○   **Among which population is there a high frequency of Ellis-van Creveld dysplasia?**

It has a high frequency among the Amish of Pennsylvania, Ohio, and West Virginia.

○   **What is camptomelia?**

It refers to a bent or bowed limb.

○   **What is camptomelic dysplasia?**

It is a usually lethal dysplasia characterized by sharp angulations of the tibiae, pre-tibial skin dimpling, brachydactyly, frequent cleft palate, micrognathia, and prominent forehead. Patients usually experience severe respiratory distress, mental retardation, and often anatomic brain anomalies.

○   **When does limb bud development usually begin?**

It begins at four to five weeks of gestation. A thin ridge of ectoderm caps the limb buds and is the prerequisite for normal limb and finger development.

○   **What are osteochondrodysplasias?**

This group of disorders leads to skeletal hyperplasia or hypo-plasia due to development of abnormally placed cartilage or fibrous elements.

○   **What are some of the osteochondrodysplasias due to anarchic proliferation of cartilage?**

These include dysplasia epiphysealis hemimelica, multiple cartilaginous exostoses, Langiedion syndrome (multiple cartilaginous exostoses-peripheral dysplasia), multiple enchondromatosis (Ollier), enchondromatosis with hemangioma (Maffucci), and metachondromatosis.

○   **Name some osteochondrodysplasias associated with anarchic development of fibrous tissue?**

Fibrous dysplasia (Jaffe-Lichtenstein), fibrous dysplasia associated with precocious puberty and skin pigmentation (McCune-Albright) cherubism, and neurofibromatosis.

○ **What is enchondroma?**

It refers to development of cartilage within bone.

○ **What is Trevor disease?**

It is dysplasia epiphysealis hemimelica with asymmetric excess growth of the epiphyses, tarsal centers, and occasionally carpal centers. It is usually noted in the first years of life as foot or knee deformity, limp, painful gait and medial or lateral firm swelling at the knee or tibiotarsal joint.

○ **What is MCE?**

It refers to multiple cartilaginous exostoses--bony prominences found near the ends of the tubular bones and ribs, vertebral bodies, the scapulae, and the iliac crests.

○ **What is Langer-Giedion syndrome?**

It is a multiple cartilaginous exostosis-peripheral dysplasia syndrome also known as trichorhinophalangeal syndrome type II. It is characterized by acromelia or acromesomelia with short stature, abnormal facies, mild microcephaly and multiple cartilaginous exostoses.

○ **What is Ollier disease?**

It is a syndrome of multiple enchondromata with widespread involvement of the skeleton, including the hands, usually associated with bony pain or deformity.

○ **What is Maffucci syndrome?**

It is a syndrome of enchondromatosis with hemangiomatosis in which multiple enchondromata and hemangiomata of bone and overlying skin develop during childhood years. The lesions initially appear during infancy. Hemangiomas may also develop on mucous membranes and viscera. Maffucci syndrome leads to severe deformation of the skeleton with short stature and lesions may undergo malignant transformation.

○ **What is osteopenia?**

It refers to generalized decrease in bone mass. It may be due to decreased production of bone or increased resorption and is a feature of several inherited and acquired disorders of childhood.

○ **What is osteoporosis?**

It is the clinical syndrome secondary to osteopenia, with increased susceptibility to fractures.

○ **What is osteogenesis imperfecta?**

It is the most prevalent of the osteoporotic syndromes in children. It is the result of a variety of defects in the production of type I collagen, with mutations in one of the two genes for type I procollagen. It is divided into four types. Type II is usually lethal in the perinatal period and characterized by "crumpled bone" syndrome and beaded ribs. Approximately 50% are stillborn and most die of respiratory insufficiency. Type III and IV are rare.

○ **What are some of the characteristics of Osteogenesis Imperfecta Type I?**
Characteristics include bones with thin cortices, osteoporosis, multiple bone fractures usually occurring between ages 2 and 3 years and continuing through early adolescence. Patients may present with

hypermobile joints, kyphoscoliosis, joint dislocations, bowed limbs, increased capillary fragility, thin skin, and scleras which often appear blue. Most have hearing loss secondary to osteosclerosis. Type I-B patients have dentinogenesis imperfecta (dentin is rich in type I collagen). This condition is inherited as an autosomal dominant disorder.

○   **Why do the sclerae appear blue in many patients with Osteogenesis Imperfecta?**

The thin sclerae allows for choroidal pigment to show through and this appears blue.

○   **What are wormian bones (in most patients with Osteogenesis Imperfecta)?**

This refers to the wiggled markings seen on x-rays of the skull. Multiple small bony islands, separated by sutures, are seen.

○   **What is osteopetrosis?**

It refers to conditions in which generalized increased bone density is found ("marble bone disease"). There are several different forms. Osteopetrosis with precocious manifestations is present at an early age and has a progressive course associated with early death.

○   **What is Albers-Schönberg disease?**

It is osteopetrosis tarda which presents in childhood, adolescence, or young adult life associated with mild craniofacial disproportion, mild anemia, neurologic symptoms, fractures (10%), or osteitis (usually of the mandible).

○   **What is Caffey disease?**

It is a condition of unknown etiology also referred to as infantile cortical hyperostosis. It is characterized by a febrile course with swelling of soft tissues over the face and jaws, with progressive cortical thickening of flat and long bones. It must be distinguished from hyperphosphatasia with osteoectasia.

○   **What is pyknodysostosis?**

It is an autosomal recessive disorder with postnatal onset of short stature, generalized hyperostosis, large skull with frontal and occipital bossing; short, broad hands and feet and nail deformities. Blue sclerae may be seen.

○   **What is Marfan syndrome?**

It is a syndrome characterized by tall, slim stature secondary to a defect in fibrillin (a major component of extracellular microfibrils contributing to the structural integrity of connective tissue). Patients may exhibit scoliosis, joint hyperextensibility, striae, pectus, hernias, aortic valve dilatation, and mitral valve prolapse, and a high incidence of upward dislocation of the lens of the eye.

○   **What is dolichostenomelia?**

Long, thin limbs.

○   **What is arachnodactyly?**

Long thin fingers.

○   **What is rickets?**

It is a group of diseases secondary to mineral deficiency at the growth plate slowing growth with decreased bone age. It can be caused by vitamin D deficiency, renal tubular wasting of phosphate, or a miscellaneous group of conditions including: hypophosphatasia (deficiency of alkaline phosphatase), hyperphosphatasia, renal osteodystrophy (with hyperphosphatemia and secondary hypocalcemia). Rickets is characterized by generalized osteoporosis with curving of weight-bearing bones, fraying of metaphyses, and increased width of growth plates.

O   **What drugs may be associated with rickets?**

Chronic use of anticonvulsants (especially a combination of phenytoin and phenobarbital) may contribute to rickets in a small number of children.

O   **What is hypophosphatasia?**

It is an autosomal recessive inborn error of metabolism where there is deficient activity of tissue non-specific alkaline phosphatase (kidney/bone/liver). It ranges from mild (bowing of legs with shortened stature) to lethal forms with severe deficiency of ossification.

O   **What is primary chondrodystrophy?**

Also known as metaphyseal dysplasia, it is a condition of lowing of the legs, shortened stature, and waddling gait in the absence of abnormalities in calcium, vitamin D, phosphate, or alkaline phophatase.

O   **What is Pyle disease?**

It is metaphyseal dysostosis secondary to defects in endochondral bone formation and metaphyseal modeling with splaying of the ends of bones without associated short stature.

O   **What is hyperphosphatasia?**

It is excess elevation of the bone isozyme of alkaline phosphatase with significant growth failure. Periosteal elevation, bowing and thickening of the diaphyses, and osteopenia may be present.

O   **What is spondylolysis?**

It refers to a defect, lysis, or stress fracture of the pars interarticularis; the pars interarticularis is the bony connection between the superior facet of one vertebra and the posterior elements of the vertebra above it. Symptomatic children may experience low back pain worsened with activity and hamstring tightness.

O   **What is spondylolisthesis?**

It refers to anterior slippage of the superior vertebra on the lower one. Symptoms of nerve root compression (usually L-5) such as muscle weakness, sphincter problems, and sensory loss may be present.

O   **What is juvenile rheumatoid arthritis?**

It is a disease or group of diseases with chronic synovitis and extra-articular manifestations. By definition, it must be present for six weeks in children sixteen years of age or younger, after other causes have been ruled out. (Most post-infectious arthritis is gone by six weeks.) It may be monoarticular or pauciarticular (involving four or fewer joints). Knees are affected in approximately 75% of children with monoarticular JRA, with the elbow the next most common affected.

❍   **What is a synostosis?**

An osseous (bony) union between two bones.

❍   **What is a synchondrosis?**

A cartilaginous union between two bones.

❍   **What is a syndesmosis?**

A fibrous union between two bones.

HEAD AND NECK

○ **What is the range of normal intraocular pressure?**

10–23 mmHg. Patients with acute angle closure glaucoma generally have pressures elevated to 40–80 mmHg.

○ **Topical steroids for the eyes are absolutely contraindicated in what cases?**

When the patient has a herpetic lesion in the eye (often seen as dendritic lesions on slit lamp) or a herpetic infection elsewhere.

○ **What is the most common finding on funduscopic examination of the AIDS patient?**

Cotton wool spots due to disease of the microvasculature. Other findings are hemorrhage, exudate, or retinal necrosis.

○ **If you suspect rupture of the round or oval window in a patient that comes to you for acute hearing loss what test might you perform?**

Applying positive pressure to the tympanic membrane will cause the patient to have ipsilateral nystagmus if there is a rupture.

○ **What is the prognostic significance of vertigo in a patient with sudden sensorineural hearing loss?**

Vertigo is a poor prognostic sign. Young patients (under 40) regain their normal hearing in 50% of cases. Recovery correlates with degree of hearing loss and length of time hearing has been altered. Hearing loss lasting greater than 1 month is most likely permanent.

○ **What systemic sexually transmitted disease is associated with sensorineural hearing loss?**

Syphilis. 7% of patients with idiopathic hearing loss test positive for treponemal antibodies.

○ **Acute tinnitus is associated with toxicity of what medication?**

Salicylates. Other causes of tinnitus are vascular abnormalities, mechanical abnormalities, and damaged cochlear hair cells. Unilateral tinnitus is associated with chronic suppurative otitis, Ménière's disease, or trauma.

○ **Hairy leukoplakia is characteristic of what two viruses?**

HIV and Epstein-Barr virus. Hairy leukoplakia is usually found on the lateral aspect of the tongue. Oral thrush may also be associated with patients with HIV.

○ **What is the most common cause of odontogenic pain?**

Carious tooth. The offending tooth when percussed with a tongue blade will produce a sharp pain. The pain may be felt in the ear, throat, eyes, temple, or other side of the jaw.

○ **A child falls and knocks out his front tooth. How would treatment differ if the child was age 3 versus age 13?**

With primary teeth, no reimplantation should be attempted because of the risk of ankylosis or fusion to the bone. However, with permanent teeth reimplantation should occur as soon as possible. Remaining periodontal fibers are a key to success. Thus, the tooth should not be wiped dry as this may disrupt the periodontal ligament fibers still attached.

○ **A 18-year-old presents with both his upper central incisors in hand after an altercation. How can you tell which is the right tooth and which is left?**

When looking at the facial (anterior) surface of the tooth, the sharper angle faces midline. So when replacing the teeth, the two sharp angles should be midline.

○ **What is the best transport medium for an avulsed tooth?**

Hank's solution, a pH balanced cell culture medium, which can even help restore cell viability if the tooth has been avulsed for more than 30 minutes. Milk is an alternative, or the patient, if able to keep from aspiration, may place the tooth underneath his/her tongue.

○ **A patient accidentally swallowed his crown while eating. He cannot afford another crown and wants to know if this one could be used again once it passes?**

Yes. It can be sterilized and replaced.

○ **A patient complains of a tongue irritation from a slightly chipped tooth after a fall. No dentin is exposed. What treatment can be offered to this patient?**

Tooth fractures only involving the enamel are called Ellis Class I fractures. The sharp edges can be filed with an emery board for immediate relief and the patient can be referred to a dentist for cosmetic repair.

○ **How can one differentiate Ellis class II and III fractures?**

Class II: Fractures involving the dentin and enamel. The exposed dentin will be pinkish.
Class III: Fractures involving the enamel, dentin, and pulp. A drop of blood is frequently noted in the center of the pink dentin.

○ **Why should topical analgesics not be used in Ellis class III tooth fractures?**

Severe tissue irritation or sterile abscesses may occur with their use. Treatment includes application of tinfoil, analgesics, and immediate dental referral.

○ **A patient presents with gingival pain and a foul mouth odor and taste. On exam, fever and lymphadenopathy are present. The gingiva is bright red and the papillae are ulcerated and covered with a gray membrane. What is the diagnosis and treatment?**

Acute necrotizing ulcerative gingivitis. Antibiotics (tetracycline or penicillin) and topical anesthetic. A possible complication of this disease is destruction of alveolar bone.

○ **What is the most common oral manifestation of AIDS?**

Oropharyngeal thrush. Some other AIDS-related oropharyngeal diseases are Kaposi's sarcoma, hairy leukoplakia, and non-Hodgkin's lymphoma.

○ **A 17-year-old female presents complaining of excruciating waxing and waning "electric shock type" pain in the right cheek. What is the diagnosis and treatment?**

Tic douloureux. The most significant finding is that the pain follows the distribution of the trigeminal nerve. Often minor trigger zone stimulation can consistently reproduce the pain. Carbamazepine (100 mg bid starting dose and increasing to 1200 mg daily if needed). Refer to a neurologist and a dentist to rule out cerebellopontine angle tumors, MS, nasopharyngeal carcinoma, cluster headaches, polymyalgia rheumatica, temporal arteritis, and oral pathology.

❍   **A three-year-old child presents with a unilateral purulent rhinorrhea. What is the most likely diagnosis?**

Nasal foreign body.

❍   **What potential complications of nasal fractures should always be considered on physical examination?**

Septal hematoma and cribriform plate fractures. A septal hematoma appears as a bluish mass on the nasal septum and if not drained aseptic necrosis of the septal cartilage and septal abnormalities may occur. A cribriform plate fracture should be considered in a patient who has a clear rhinorrhea after trauma.

❍   **What physical exam findings would make posterior epistaxis more likely than anterior epistaxis?**

1. Inability to see the site of bleeding. Anterior nosebleeds usually originate at Kiesselbach's plexus, an area easily visualized on the nasal septum.
2. Blood from both sides of the nose. In a posterior nosebleed the blood can more easily pass to the other side because of the proximity of the choanae.
3. Blood trickling down the oropharynx.
4. Inability to control bleeding by direct pressure.

❍   **What is the most common site of bleeding in posterior nosebleeds?**

The sphenopalatine artery's lateral nasal branch.

❍   **A patient returns to the emergency department with fever, nausea, vomiting and hypotension, two days after having nasal packing placed for an anterior nosebleed. What potential complication of nasal packing should be considered?**

Toxic shock syndrome.

❍   **A child with a sinus infection presents with proptosis, a red swollen eyelid and a inferolaterally displaced globe. What is the diagnosis?**

Orbital cellulitis and abscess associated with ethmoid sinusitis.

❍   **A patient with a frontal sinusitis presents with a large forehead abscess. What is the diagnosis?**

Pott's puffy tumor. This is a complication of frontal sinusitis where the anterior table of the skull is destroyed allowing the formation of the abscess.

❍   **An ill-appearing patient presents with a fever of 103°F, bilateral chemosis, third nerve palsies, and untreated sinusitis. What is the diagnosis?**

Cavernous sinus thrombosis. This life-threatening complication occurs from direct extension through the valveless veins. Complication of sinusitis may be local (osteomyelitis), orbital (cellulitis), or within the central nervous system (meningitis or brain abscess).

❍   **Retropharyngeal abscess is most common in what age group, and why?**

Six months to three years. This is due to size regression of the retropharyngeal lymph nodes after the age of three.

O   **How do patients with retropharyngeal abscesses appear?**

Febrile, ill-appearing, stridorous, drooling, and in an opisthotonic position. These children may complain of difficulty swallowing, or may refuse to feed.

O   **What radiographic sign can be used to make the diagnosis of a retropharyngeal abscess?**

A widening of the retropharyngeal space (normal 3-4 mm or less than half the width of the vertebral bodies). False widening may occur if the x-ray is not done during inspiration with the patient's neck extended (occasionally, an air fluid level may be noted in the retropharyngeal space).

O   **What is the most common organism to cause a retropharyngeal abscess?**

β-hemolytic streptococcus.

O   **A 15-year-old male presents with a high fever, trismus, dysphagia, and swelling inferior to the mandible in the lateral neck. What is the diagnosis?**

Parapharyngeal abscess.

O   **What is the <u>most</u> <u>common</u> origin of Ludwig's angina?**

Lower second and third molar. It is a swelling in the region of the submandibular, sublingual, and submental spaces. This soft tissue swelling may cause displacement of the tongue upward and posteriorly. The most common organisms are hemolytic Streptococci, Staphylococcus, and mixed anaerobes and aerobes.

O   **Why is needle aspiration preferred over incision and drainage for a fluctuant acute cervical lymphadenitis?**

Development of a fistula tract is possible if the patient has atypical mycobacterium or cat scratch fever rather than a bacterial lymphadenitis.

O   **A 16-year-old female presents with dull right ear and jaw pain and a burning sensation in the roof of her mouth, which is worse in the evening. She also hears a "popping" sound when she opens and closes her mouth. Exam reveals tenderness of the joint capsule. What is the diagnosis and treatment?**

TMJ syndrome. Treat with physiotherapy, analgesia, soft diet, muscle relaxants and occlusive therapy. Apply warm moist compresses 4–5 times daily for 15 minutes for 7–10 days.

O   **A 14-year-old diabetic male presents with pain, itching, and discharge from the right ear. The tympanic membrane is intact. What is the diagnosis?**

Otitis externa. Treat by suctioning ear and 1 week of antibiotic steroid otic solution. An ear wick may improve delivery of the antibiotic. Suspect malignant otitis externa in the diabetic patient.

O   **A patient presents with ear pain and fluid-filled blisters on the tympanic membrane. What is the diagnosis?**

Bullous myringitis, commonly caused by Mycoplasma or viruses. Treat with erythromycin.

O   **A patient presents with a swollen, tender, red left auricle. What is the diagnosis?**

Perichondritis caused by Pseudomonas.

❍   **What is the most frequent cause of hearing loss?**

Cerumen impaction.

❍   **What would the physical finding be in unilateral sensory hearing loss?**

The patient will lateralize and have air conduction greater than bone conduction (i.e. normal Rinne test) indicating no conductive loss. The Weber test will lateralize to the normal ear. The most common cause of this is viral neuritis.

❍   **If a patient has bilateral sensory hearing loss, what causes should be suspected?**

Noise or ototoxics, such as certain antibiotics, loop diuretics, or antineoplastics.

❍   **What is the most common neuropathy associated with acoustic neuroma?**

Due to trigeminal nucleus involvement, the corneal reflex may be lost.

❍   **Name some causes of tympanic membrane perforation.**

Blast injuries (water or air), foreign bodies in the ear (particularly Q-tips), lightning strikes, otitis media, associated temporal bone fractures.

❍   **What is the most common organism which causes pediatric acute otitis media?**

Streptococcus pneumoniae, followed by *Haemophilus influenzae* and *Moraxella catarrhalis*.

❍   **What is a Bezold abscess?**

A complication of acute mastoiditis where infection spreads to the soft tissues below the ear and sternocleidomastoid muscle.

❍   **What is the most common cause of sialoadenitis?**

Mumps.

❍   **A patient presents with trismus, fever, and an erythematous, tender parotid gland. Pus is expressed from Stensen's duct. What conditions may predispose a person to bacterial parotitis?**

Any situation which decreases salivary flow. Irradiation, phenothiazine, antihistamines, parasympathetic inhibitors, dehydration or debilitation. Up to 30% of cases occur postoperatively.

❍   **In which salivary gland do stones most likely occur?**

80% are submandibular. The least likely is the sublingual gland.

❍   **What does grunting versus inspiratory stridor indicate?**

Grunting is specific for lower respiratory tract disease, such as pneumonia, asthma, or bronchiolitis. Stridor localizes respiratory obstruction to the level at or above the larynx.

❍   **What is the most common cause of epiglottitis?**

Hemophilus influenzae (as of the latest literature, though, incidence has dropped dramatically and *Streptococcus* is becoming the more common pathogen since the Hib vaccine).

❍   **A lower airway foreign body is suspected. What will plain films show?**

Plain films will show air trapping on the affected side. Inspiration and expiration views demonstrate mediastinal shift away from the affected side.

❍   **A patient presents with an itching, tearing, right eye. On exam huge cobblestone papillae are found under the upper lid. What is the diagnosis?**

Allergic conjunctivitis.

❍   **A patient is seen with herpetic lesions on the tip of the nose. Why is this a problem?**

The tip of the nose and the cornea are both supplied by the nasociliary nerve. Thus, the cornea may also be involved.

❍   **A patient presents with inflammation of the conjunctiva and lid margins. Slit lamp exam reveals a "greasy" appearance of the lid margins with scaling, especially around the base of the lashes. What is the diagnosis?**

Blepharitis. Often caused by staphylococcal infection of the oil glands and skin next to the lash follicles. Treatment consists of scrubbing with baby shampoo, and, in consultation with an ophthalmologist, sulfacetamide drops and steroids.

❍   **A patient presents with a pustular vesicle at the lid margin. What is the diagnosis and treatment?**

Hordeolum (stye). An acute inflammation of the meibomian gland most commonly of the upper lid. Treat with topical antibiotics and warm compresses. Surgical drainage may be necessary.

❍   **A patient presents with a chronic non-tender, uninflamed nodule of the upper lid. What is the diagnosis?**

Chalazion. Treat with surgical curettage.

❍   **A patient presents with the sensation of a foreign body in the eye. Slit-lamp reveals a dendritic figure which has a Christmas tree pattern. What is the appropriate treatment?**

Antiviral agents and cycloplegics are used to treat herpes simplex keratitis. Steroids spell disaster!

❍   **What are complications of a hyphema?**

The 4 S's.

Secondary rebleeds, which usually occur between the second and fifth days post injury since this is the time of clot retraction. Rebleeds tend to be worse than the initial bleed.

Significantly increased intraocular pressure which can lead to acute glaucoma, chronic late glaucoma, and optic atrophy.

Staining of the cornea due to hemosiderin deposits.

Synechiae which interfere with iris function.

❍   **Why do patients with sickle cell anemia and a hyphema require special consideration when presenting with ophthalmologic concerns?**

Increased intraocular pressure can occur if the cells sickle in the trabecular network, preventing aqueous humor from leaving the anterior chamber. Medication, such as hyperosmotics and Diamox, which increase the likelihood of sickling, must be avoided

O   **A patient presents with a history of trauma to the orbit with dull ocular pain, decreased visual acuity, and photophobia. Exam reveals a constricted pupil and ciliary flush.   What will be found on a slit-lamp exam?**

Flare and cells in the anterior chamber are present with traumatic iritis.

O   **What are causes of a subluxed or dislocated lens?**

Trauma, Marfan's syndrome, homocystinuria, Weill-Marchesani syndrome.

O   **Physiologically, what causes flare?**

Flare is caused by inflammatory proteins resulting in the "dust in the movie projector lights" or "fog in the headlights" phenomena in slit-lamp examination.

O   **When should an eye not be dilated?**

With known narrow angle glaucoma and with an iris-supported intraocular lens.

O   **Why shouldn't topical ophthalmologic anesthetics be prescribed?**

The anesthetics inhibit healing and decrease the patient's ability to protect his eye due to the lack of sensation.

O   **What is the most common organism in contact lens associated corneal ulcers?**

Pseudomonas.

O   **How can Krazy-Glue (cyanoacrylate) be removed if a patient has stuck their eyelids together?**

Copious irrigation immediately, and then mineral oil. Acetone and ethanol are unacceptable in the eyes. Surgical separation must be done with extreme care to prevent laceration of the lids or globe. Often the patient will have a corneal abrasion, which should be treated in the usual manner.

O   **An anxious 15-year-old female presents with a complaint of blurred vision made worse when looking at objects far away. On exam, the eyes converge, the pupils constrict, and accommodation is at a maximum. What is the diagnosis?**

Spasm of accommodation. Treat anxiety. A short-acting cycloplegic may stop the cycle.

O   **What test can a physician use to determine if blindness is of a hysterical origin?**

An optokinetic drum can be used. If nystagmus eye movements occur, the patient is seeing the stripes. Prisms may also be used.

O   **A patient presents with traumatic pain behind the left eye, a left pupil afferent defect, central visual loss, and a left swollen disc. What is the diagnosis and potential causes?**

Optic neuritis. This may be idiopathic or may be associated with multiple sclerosis, Lyme's disease, neurosyphilis, lupus, sarcoid, alcoholism, toxins, or drug abuse.

O   **A patient's cornea fluoresces prior to instillation of fluorescein. What should be considered?**

Pseudomonal infection. Several species fluoresce on their own.

O   **In what age group is retropharyngeal abscess most common?**

Children less than four years of age. Symptoms may include difficulty breathing, fever, enlarged cervical nodes, difficulty swallowing, and a stiff neck. Exam may reveal a mass or fullness in the posterior pharyngeal area.

O   **In what age group are peritonsillar abscesses most common?**

Adolescents and young adults. Symptoms may include ear pain, trismus, drooling, and alteration of voice.

O   **What is the most common sight-threatening ocular infection in AIDS patients?**

Cytomegalovirus (CMV) retinitis occurs in 15-40% of AIDS patients.

O   **What are the ocular manifestations of Lyme disease?**

Uveitis, keratitis, and optic neuritis.

O   **"River blindness", a major cause of blindness worldwide, characterized by uveitis, chorioretinal changes and optic atrophy, is caused by what organism?**

Microfilariae of Onchocerca volvulus causes this disease, which is also known as onchocerciasis.

O   **What are the two major risk factors for ocular candidiasis?**

Indwelling venous catheters and intravenous drug abuse.

O   **What are the ocular manifestations of congenital rubella?**

Retinitis with fine, powdery retinal pigmentation (most common), cataract, glaucoma (10%), microphthalmos (10%), corneal edema, and iris atrophy.

O   **Which is the more effective therapy for corneal epithelial herpes simplex keratitis, topical or systemic antivirals?**

Topical antivirals.

O   **Treatment with oral acyclovir has been shown to be most effective in treating which disease, recurrent herpes simplex keratitis or herpes zoster ophthalmicus?**

Herpes Zoster ophthalmicus.

O   **Extended wear contact lenses worn overnight increase the risk of infectious keratitis by how much compared to daily wear?**

Approximately 10-fold.

O   **What type of conjunctivitis is caused by adenovirus?**

Acute follicular conjunctivitis.

O   **Are topical antivirals effective in the treatment of adenoviral keratoconjunctivitis?**

No.

❍ **How long from the onset of symptoms in the second eye do patients with adenoviral epidemic keratoconjunctivitis shed infectious virus?**

2 weeks.

❍ **What are the ocular signs of cat-scratch disease?**

Follicular conjunctivitis with granulomatous nodules on the palpebral conjunctiva, swollen preauricular or submandibular lymph nodes.

❍ **How is chlamydial inclusion conjunctivitis transmitted?**

Sexual contact.

❍ **What is the most common cause of ophthalmia neonatorum in the U.S.?**

Chlamydia trachomatis.

❍ **What diagnosis is most probable in a newborn who develops "hyperacute" conjunctivitis with copious mucopurulent discharge?**

Neisseria gonorrhea.

❍ **A patient with chronic follicular conjunctivitis is found to have several smooth, centrally umbilicated papules on the eyelids. What is the most likely diagnosis?**

Molluscum contagiosum.

❍ **Is it likely for an untreated corneal ulcer caused by *Pseudomonas aeruginosa* to progress to a corneal perforation?**

Yes.

❍ **What retinal involvement can be associated with infectious mononucleosis (Epstein-Barr Virus)?**

Macular edema, retinal hemorrhages, chorioretinitis, punctate outer retinitis, multifocal chorioretinitis and panuveitis.

❍ **What is the most common cause of endogenous bacterial endophthalmitis?**

Bacillus cereus.

❍ **What two organisms are most likely to cause endogenous bacterial endophthalmitis in a host not otherwise predisposed to infection?**

Neisseria meningitidis and *Haemophilus influenzae*

❍ **Topical natamycin is the treatment of choice for what ocular infection?**

Fungal keratitis.

❍ **What is the most frequent condition associated with orbital cellulitis?**

Sinusitis.

❍ **Is orbital aspergillosis seen in immunocompetent patients?**
Yes, but it is more common in immunocompromised patients.

❍   **What is the most common viral cause of neonatal keratoconjunctivitis?**

Herpes simplex.

❍   **At what age does chronic endophthalmitis from toxocariasis usually present?**

Between the ages of 2 - 9.

❍   **How common is strabismus during the first few months of life?**

Strabismus during infancy occurs in approximately one-third of infants during the first six months of life.

❍   **What causes the appearance of pseudoesotropia?**

A wide nasal bridge and/or prominent epicanthal folds.

❍   **How can pseudoesotropia be differentiated from true esotropia?**

Using the corneal light reflex or alternate cover test when possible.

❍   **What can often be documented in parents of children with infantile esotropia?**

Reduced binocular vision. This has been suggested to be a subthreshold effect of the "gene(s)" that cause the disorder.

❍   **Describe the characteristics of intermittent exotropia.**

Intermittent exotropia is a divergent strabismus that may be latent or manifest. The tropic stage may be seen when the patient is tired, ill or if fusion is interrupted, such as when one eye is covered.

❍   **What is the natural course of intermittent exotropia?**

The long-term course of intermittent exotropia is unknown as most patients with the disorder generally undergo treatment at sometime in their lives. Most authorities believe that, left untreated, the disorder will worsen.

PSYCHOSOCIAL PEARLS

○ **Is violence more likely between family members or non-family members?**

Between family members. 20–50% of murders in the US are committed by members of the victims' families. Spouse abuse is as high as 16% in the US.

○ **In what percentage of cases of child sexual abuse is the abuser known by the child?**

90%.

○ **In what percentage of cases of child abuse is the mother also abused?**

50%.

○ **What are the most common ages for child physical abuse?**

Two-thirds of physically abused children are under the age of 3, and one-third are under the age of 6 months.

○ **In addition to an evaluation for child abuse, what laboratory studies should be done in the child with multiple bruises?**

CBC with differential, platelet count, PT, and UA.

○ **According to our best knowledge, what is the frequency of rape?**

The 1987 Uniform Crimes Report states that at least one in eight women have been raped, and it is estimated that only 25% of all rapes are reported.

○ **What are the clinical clues of domestic violence?**

Any evidence of injury during pregnancy or late entry into prenatal care. Also, look for injuries presenting after significant delay or in various stages of healing—especially to the head, neck, breasts, abdomen, or areas suggesting a defensive posture such as forearm bruises. Vague complaints or unusual injuries, such as bites, scratches, burns, or rope marks, as well as suicide attempts and/or rapes, should raise suspicion.

○ **Name a few substances that may mimic generalized anxiety when ingested.**

Nicotine, caffeine, amphetamines, cocaine, and anticholinergics. Alcohol and sedative withdrawal can also mimic this disorder.

○ **What are 8 common medical causes of anxiety or anxiety attacks?**

(1) Alcohol withdrawal, (2) thyrotoxicosis, (3) caffeine, (4) stroke, (5) cardiopulmonary emergencies, (6) hypoglycemia, (7) psychosensory/psychomotor epilepsy, and (8) pheochromocytoma.

○ **What is the most common cause of referral to child psychiatrists?**

Attention Deficit Hyperactivity Disorder. ADHD accounts for 30–50% of child psychiatric outpatients.

○ **The brother of a female patient with ADHD is at increased risk for what other disorders?**

329

Conduct, mood, anxiety, and antisocial disorders, substance abuse, and of course ADHD. Relatives of girls with ADHD are at higher risk of disorders than relatives of boys.

○   **What effect does ADHD have on sleep?**

ADHD causes restless sleep and decreases the time from the onset of sleep until actual REM sleep (REM latency).

○   **What are the side-effects of Ritalin?**

Ritalin (Methylphenidate) is a psychostimulant used to treat ADHD. Side-effects include depression, headache, hypertension, insomnia, and abdominal pain.

○   **What chromosomal abnormalities do autistic patients commonly have?**

8% have a fragile X syndrome.

○   **What percentage of autistics are mute?**

50%.

○   **Which has an earlier onset, bipolar disorder or unipolar disorder?**

Onset of bipolar disorder is usually in the patient's twenties or thirties. Unipolar onset is not until 35–50.

○   **Differentiate between Bipolar I, Bipolar II, and Hypomania.**

Bipolar I: Mania and major depression.
Bipolar II: Hypomania and major depression
Hypomania: Mania without severe impairment and psychotic features.

○   **Are the majority of affective disorder patients bipolar or unipolar?**

Unipolar (80%).

○   **Are females with an affective disorder more likely to be bipolar or unipolar?**

Unipolar (70–80%).

○   **What is the most frequent first episode of bipolar disease, mania or depression?**

Mania. Depression is rarely the first symptom. In fact, only 5–10% of patients that develop depression first go on to have manic episodes. 1/3 of manic patients never have a depressive episode.

○   **First degree relatives of bipolar patients are at a greater risk for what mental illnesses?**

Unipolar disorders and alcoholism.

○   **Other than the classic mania, what can lithium be used to treat?**

Bulimia, anorexia nervosa, alcoholism in patients with mood disorders, leucocytosis in patients on antineoplastic medication, cluster headaches, and migraine headaches.

○   **Postural tremor is a major side-effect of lithium. How is this side-effect controlled?**

Minimize the dose during the work day and give small doses of beta blockers.

○   **Should people who are physically active and taking lithium have their lithium dosage increased or decreased?**

Increased. Lithium, a salt, is excreted more than sodium during sweating.

○   **T/F: A patient starting lithium will be expected to gain weight.**

True. All psychotropic medications cause weight gain, hence lithium's usefulness in treating anorexia nervosa.

○   **What is the potential complication of a manic depressive who is also being treated for congestive heart failure?**

Lithium toxicity. Low salt diet and/or sodium-losing diuretics can cause lithium retention and toxicity.

○   **Lithium toxicity begins at what level?**

14 mg/L. Above this level nausea, diarrhea, vomiting, rigidity, tremor, ataxia, seizures, delirium, coma, and death can all occur.

○   **Why might a patient taking lithium experience polyuria?**

Long term lithium ingestion can cause nephrogenic diabetes.

○   **What is the most common clinical symptom of a patient with a borderline personality disorder?**

Chronic boredom. Other symptoms include severe mood swings, volatile relationships, continuous and uncontrollable anger, and impulsiveness.

○   **A patient presents to your office with parotid gland swelling and erosion of the enamel on her teeth. What findings might you expect to find in this patient?**

The patient described most likely has bulimia. Elevated serum amylase and hypokalemia are associated with bulimia.

○   **List some common laboratory findings associated with eating disorders?**

Hyponatremia, hypokalemia, hypocalcemia, hypophosphatemia, anemia, hypoglycemia, starvation ketoacidosis, abnormal glucose tolerance, hypothyroidism due to low T3 levels, persistently elevated cortisol due to starvation, low FSH, LH and estrogens, and elevated growth hormone.

○   **What are criteria A–D for the diagnosis of catatonic disorder?**

A: Manifestations of any of the following: echolalia, echopraxia, excessive purposeless motor activity, motor immobility, extreme negativism, resistance to external instruction or movement, or peculiar involuntary movements, such as bizarre posturing or grimacing.
B: Evidence from the history, exam, and lab findings that the catatonia is a result of a medical condition.
C: The criterion A actions are not attributed to another mental condition.
D: The criterion A actions do not occur in a bout of delirium only.

○   **What is the most common cause of catonia?**

Affective disorder.

○   **What is the prevalence of conduct disorder?**

10%. It is much more common in boys and is familial.

O   **Children with conduct disorder are most likely to develop what adult disorder?**

About 40% will have some pathology as adults. The most common disorder is antisocial personality disorder.

O   **What is conversion disorder?**

Internal psychological conflict that manifests itself as somatic symptoms. Voluntary motor or sensory function is affected. Examples include weakness, imbalance, dysphagia, and changes in vision, hearing, or sensation. These symptoms are not feigned or intentionally produced. They are also not fully explained by medical conditions.

O   **Delirium is most likely to occur in what kinds of patients?**

Those with multiple medical problems, decreased renal function, high WBC count, anticholinergic, propranolol, scopolamine, or flurazepam drug use.

O   **Describe delirium.**

"Clouding of consciousness" resulting in disorientation, decreased alertness, and impaired cognitive function. Acute onset, visual hallucinosis, and fluctuating psychomotor activity are all commonly seen. All symptoms are variable and may change over hours.

O   **Delirium versus dementia: Who is more likely to die within a month of onset, and who is more likely to fully recover after onset?**

Delirious persons are 15–30% more likely to die within a month of onset of delirium and are also more likely to fully recover from their delirium than are patients with dementia. Delirium is reversible.

O   **Name some over-the-counter and "street" drugs that may produce delirium or acute psychosis.**

Salicylates, antihistamines, anticholinergics, alcohols, phencyclidine, LSD, mescaline, cocaine, and amphetamines.

O   **What are some common medical causes of depression?**

Stroke, viral syndromes, corticosteroids, Cushing's disease, antihypertensive medication, SLE, multiple sclerosis, and subcortical dementias (Huntington's and Parkinson's diseases and HIV encephalopathy).

O   **Name some symptoms of major depression.**

IN SAD CAGES:

Interest

Sleep
Appetite
Depressed mood

Concentration
Activity
Guilt
Energy
Suicide

O   **Name some vegetative symptoms of major depression.**

Loss of appetite, lack of concentration, chronic fatigue, agitation, restlessness, inability to sleep, and weight loss.

O   **What is dysthymia?**

Dysthymia is a chronic disorder lasting more than 2 years. The severe symptoms of depression, such as delusions and hallucinations are absent. Patients with dysthymia have some good days, they react to their environment, and they have no vegetative signs. 10% of patients with dysthymia develop major depression.

O   **What is the Omega sign?**

A fixed furrowed brow associated with melancholia.

O   **Wild and abundant dreams may result from withdrawal of what drug?**

Antidepressants. Other side-effects of withdrawal are anxiety, akathisia, bradykinesia, mania, and malaise.

O   **What is a dystonic reaction?**

It is a very common side-effect of neuroleptics. Muscle spasm of tongue, face, neck, and back are seen. Severe laryngospasm and extraocular muscle spasm may occur also. Patients may bite the tongue leading to potential airway compromise because of an inability to open the mouth, tongue edema, or hemorrhage.

O   **How do you treat a dystonic reaction?**

Diphenhydramine (Benadryl), 25–50 mg IM or IV or benztropine (Cogentin), 1–2 mg IV or PO. Remember that dystonias can recur acutely.

O   **What are the 5 Kübler-Ross stages?**

1) Denial.
2) Anger.
3) Bargaining.
4) Depression.
5) Acceptance.
Patients may undergo all or only a few of these stages.

O   **Define the following dyspraxias: ideomotor, kinesthetic, and constructional.**

Ideomotor: The patient is unable to perform simple motor tasks despite adequate understanding, sensory and motor strength.
Kinesthetic: The patient is unable to position his extremities on command despite adequate understanding, sensory and motor strength.
Constructional: The patient cannot copy simple shapes despite adequate understanding, sensory and motor strength.

O   **Match the disease with the appropriate EEG pattern.**

1) Multiple sclerosis.   a) Diffuse or focal spikes and slow waves. Can be uni- or bilateral.
2) Complex partial epilepsy.   50% show diffuse, choppy wave forms.
3) Generalized epilepsy.   b) Slow progression to low voltage rhythms
4) Stroke.   c) Slow spike waves in the clonic phase, rapid rhythmic onset with a.
5) Huntington's chorea   frequency and an amplitude that increases.
                                 d) 50% have focal or generalized slowing.

e) Nonspecific local increase in slow activity and decrease in fast activity. A reduction or complete loss of background rhythms.

Answers: (1) d, (2) a, (3) c, (4) e, and (5) b.

○   **You are a consistently bright, efficient, and responsible M-4 working under the guidance of the same attending every day. One day he thinks you are the most brilliant student he has ever come across and he wants to write you a personal letter of introduction to his best friend, chief of staff at Johns Hopkins. The very next day he decides you are worthless and should consider a job in custodial engineering. What ego defense mechanism might he be exhibiting?**

Ego splitting. This is associated with borderline personality disorders. The patient sees either all good or all bad in individuals he comes in contact with.

○   **This same attending locks you in the x-ray room with no lead protection. He then goes to the controls threatening to turn the x-ray machine on and leave you there to radiate until his shift is over. Instead, he quickly flicks it off after about 2 seconds and unlocks the door. What ego defense mechanism is he now exhibiting?**

Doing and undoing. The patient enacts and counteracts unconscious wishes that are unacceptable to his conscious self. By counteracting the original action, the patient feels as if he has saved the situation. This is associated with obsessive compulsive disorders.

○   **What is the most familial of all psychiatric diseases?**

Idiopathic enuresis. If one parent had enuresis, there is a 44% chance that the child will have it. If both parents had enuresis then the likely hood increases to 77%.

○   **By what age do most children stop wetting their beds?**

By age 4. Bed wetting after this age is considered enuresis.

○   **What percentage of 4-year-olds still have nocturnal enuresis?**

30%. 10% of 6-year-olds still wet their beds.

○   **What is the medical treatment for idiopathic enuresis?**

Desmopressin nose drops or imipramine. Most cases eventually resolve spontaneously.

○   **What is folie a deux?**

An induced psychotic disorder. One patient who has a close relationship with another patient begins forming the same delusions as the other patient.

○   **How should a 12-year-old who snorts and shouts obscenities uncontrollably be treated?**

Neuroleptics are very good at controlling Gilles de la Tourette syndrome. It develops in childhood with facial twitches, uncontrollable arm movements, and tics. The condition worsens in adolescence.

○   **A 16-year-old male presents to your office complaining of pleuritic pain, palpitations, dyspnea, dizziness and tingling in his arms and legs. What is the diagnosis?**

Hyperventilation syndrome. This is frequently associated with anxiety. The tingling is due to decreased carbonate in the blood.

❍   **A 17-year-old male is brought to your office by a concerned friend. It appears the patient sleeps excessively, has been inhaling his food like there is no tomorrow, and is getting into fights at bars whenever he goes out. He also has been hypersexual, pursuing every female within a 5-mile radius. What is the diagnosis?**

No, this is not a description of every college guy you ever knew although the similarities are amazingly striking. This is the Kleine-Levin syndrome. It can be treated with stimulants.

❍   **Hallucinogens affect what neurotransmitter?**

Serotonin.

❍   **In olfactory hallucinations, is the olfactory sensation still intact?**

Yes. Patients remain responsive to normal odors. Hallucinations of foul odors are superfluous to normal smells.

❍   **Olfactory hallucinations are associated with lesions in what areas of the brain?**

The periuncal or in the inferior and medial surfaces of the temporal lobe.

❍   **A previously healthy patient who becomes suddenly and intensely excited, is in a delirious mania, and develops catatonic features and a high fever is most likely suffering from?**

Lethal catatonia. Such patients have a 50% death rate without treatment. Treatment is with ECT.

❍   **A 17-year-old male arrives somnolent with vitals of P: 130, R: 26, BP: 170/80, and T: 105°F. You note diffuse muscular rigidity and intermittent focal muscle twitching/jerking lasting 1–2 seconds. As you "work him up," your nurse returns from the waiting area with news from the family that the patient has had a progressive decline of mental status for 2 days after seeing his psychiatrist. The patient has had a history of 'psychosis' for almost one year. What process should be included in your differential diagnosis at this time?**

Neuroleptic malignant syndrome.

❍   **What labs would you expect to be elevated in this patient?**

CPK is usually elevated and correlates with increasing risk of fatality due to myoglobinuria. Serum alkaline phosphatase and serum aminotransferases are elevated. Leukocytosis with a left shift, hyponatremia, and hypokalemia are also present. Treatment for NMS is with dopaminergic agents, muscle relaxants, discontinuation of the neuroleptics, and supportive therapy. Mortality is 20%.

❍   **How is lethal catatonia differentiated from neuroleptic malignant syndrome (NMS)?**

They are differentiated by the timing of the hyperthermia. In lethal catatonia, severe hyperthermia occurs during the excitement phase before catatonic features develop. In neuroleptic malignant syndrome, hyperthermia develops later in the course of the disease with the onset of stupor.

❍   **What is the difference between the effects of low potency and high potency neuroleptics?**

Low potency neuroleptics have greater sedative, postural hypotensive, and anticholinergic effects. High potency neuroleptics have greater extra-pyramidal side-effects.

❍   **Neuroleptic medications come in three flavors: low, medium, and high potency. Can you name some of these meds and their category?**

Low potency: Chlorpromazine (Thorazine).

Medium potency: Perphenazine (Trilafon).
High potency: Haloperidol, droperidol (Inapsine), thiothixene (Navane), fluphenazine (Prolixin), trifluoperazine (Stelazine).

○   **Why is Haloperidol one of the preferred neuroleptics?**

It can be used IM in emergencies, and it has few side-effects. It does, however, have a high frequency of extra-pyramidal effects.

○   **What psychiatric disorder is associated with carcinoma of the pancreas?**

Depression.

○   **A non-pregnant women taking neuroleptics complains of breast engorgement and lactation. What is the diagnosis?**

Pseudolactation. This occurs due to an inverse relationship between prolactin and DA. Treatment is with amantadine.

○   **What is the treatment for a "bad trip" on LSD?**

Chlorpromazine can be used IM for severe or uncontrollable anxiety. Remind the patient of reality by constantly reminding him that his perceptions are only distortions due to the drug. This is called "talking down."

○   **What is the difference between malingering and factitious disorder?**

The goal of a malingerer is an external incentive such as workman's comp. The goal of a someone with factitious disorder is to enter into the sick role. Both involve voluntary faking of an illness.

○   **Who is at a greater risk for mood disorders, men or women?**

Women by a ratio of 7:3

○   **What is an extreme case of factitious disorder?**

Munchausen's syndrome. These patients may actually try to cause harm to themselves (i.e., by injecting feces into their veins) and are very accepting/seeking of invasive procedures. Munchausen by proxy is another example. In this disease the patient seeks medical care for another, usually a child.

○   **A patient has ingested a phenothiazine and arrives hypotensive. What intervention(s) may be considered?**

IV crystalloid boluses usually suffice. Severe cases are best managed with norepinephrine (Levophed), or metaraminol (Aramine). These pressors stimulate Σ-adrenergic receptors preferentially. Σ-agonists, such as isoproterenol (Isuprel), are contraindicated due to the risks of Σ-receptor stimulated vasodilation.

○   **What are extrapyramidal reactions?**

Dopamine receptor blockade within the nigrostriatal system results in involuntary and spontaneous motor responses including dystonia, akathisia, and Parkinson-like syndrome.

○   **What are some common obsessions?**

Dirt and contamination, order and symmetry, religion and philosophy, daily decisions. Unfortunately, compulsion does not relieve the anxiety of the obsession. Serotonin re-uptake inhibitors and exposure therapy have been found helpful.

❍   **A 6-year-old boy consistently wets his pants. You tell the mother to reward dry periods with treats and praise. This will help reinforce desired behavior. What kind of conditioning is this?**

Positive operant conditioning. This principle was defined by Pavlov.

❍   **A 14-year-old female comes to your office complaining of sudden episodes of palpitations, diaphoresis, lightheadedness, a fear of losing control, a sense of being choked, tremors, and paresthesias. What is the diagnosis?**

Panic disorder. Panic disorders need not be linked to any events. Though they are commonly associated with agoraphobia, social phobia, mitral prolapse, and late non-melancholic depression.

❍   **What percentage of patients with panic disorder also suffer from major depression?**

50%. Patients that suffer panic attacks generally have low self-esteem in addition to major depression.

❍   **What is the <u>most</u> <u>common</u> type of paraphilia?**

Pedophilia.

❍   **Paresis without clonus or anesthesia to midline are examples of what conversion disorder?**

Pseudoneurologic disorder. The findings do not match the medical neuropathophysiology.

❍   **Give an example for each of the following perceptual disturbances: illusion, complete auditory hallucination, functional hallucination, and extracampine hallucination.**

<u>Illusion</u>: A kitten is perceived as a dragon (the patient misinterprets reality).

<u>Complete auditory hallucination</u>: The patient claims to hear people talking to him when no one is around (clear voices are reportedly heard; they are perceived as being external to the patient).

<u>Functional hallucination</u>: The patient hears voices only when cars honk their horns (hallucinations occur only after sensory stimulus in the same category as the hallucination).

<u>Extracampine hallucination</u>: The patient can see people waving at him from the top of the Eiffel Tower—even though he is in Chicago (hallucinations that are external to the patients normal range of senses).

❍   **What is the <u>most</u> <u>common</u> specific phobia exhibited during childhood?**

Animal phobia.

❍   **At what age will a child understand concrete operations as defined by Piaget?**

6–12 years. By this age a child is able to tell that a line of 5 pennies all touching is equal to those same 5 pennies spread out into a much longer line.

❍   **Can a person get posttraumatic stress disorder (PTSD) if they did not actually witness a disturbing event?**

Yes. According to the DSM–IV, one can experience PTSD if an event, such as a violent personal assault, a serious accident, or the serious injury of a close friend or family member is learned of indirectly.

❍   **A 16-year-old female was raped 6 months ago. She has now suddenly developed recurrent, distressing flashbacks of the event; she is having nightmares and intense fear, is avoiding all males. She has a diminished memory of the rape, and an exaggerated startle response. Is this woman experiencing PTSD?**

Yes. This is delayed onset PTSD. The onset of symptoms can occur at least 6 months after the provoking event.

○   **What are the 5 criteria for brief reactive psychosis?**

1. Precipitating stressful event.
2. A rapid onset of the psychosis that develops temporally as a result of this event.
3. Affective liability and mood intensity.
4. The symptoms match the stress event.
5. Resolution of the symptoms once the stressor is removed (generally within 2 weeks).

○   **What are the signs and symptoms suggestive of an organic source of psychosis?**

Acute onset, disorientation, visual or tactile hallucinations, age less than 10, and evidence suggesting overdose or acute ingestion, such as abnormal vital signs, pupil size and reactivity, or nystagmus.

○   **When are females at their greatest risk for psychiatric illness?**

The first few weeks post partum. It most often occurs in patients who are primiparous, have poor social support, or have a history of depression.

○   **When does post partum psychosis begin?**

Within the first week to 10 days following childbirth. A second, though smaller, peak occurs 6–8 weeks post partum. This second peak correlates with the first menses post partum. Surprisingly, the risk of psychosis is lowest during pregnancy.

○   **What is the difference between schizophrenia and schizophreniform disorder?**

Schizophreniform disorder implies the same signs and symptoms as schizophrenia, yet these symptoms have been present for less than 6 months. The impaired functioning in schizophreniform disorder is not consistent. Schizophreniform disorder is generally a provisional diagnosis with schizophrenia following.

○   **What are the 5 criteria for a diagnosis of Schizophrenia?**

1. Psychosis.
2. Emotional blunting.
3. No affective features or episodes.
4. Clear consciousness.
5. The absence of coarse brain disease, systemic illness, and drug abuse.

○   **What percent of patients with schizophrenia become chronically ill?**

60–80%. Males are at a greater risk for chronic illness.

○   **The onset of schizophrenia generally occurs by what age?**

80% of schizophrenics develop the disease before their early twenties. The disease is very rare after 40.

○   **What are 5 causes of schizophrenia?**

1. Viral infection in the CNS.
2. Problem pregnancy that affects the neuronal development.
3. Head injury.
4. Seizure disorder.
5. Street drugs.

○ **Are first degree relatives of schizophrenics more likely to have schizoidia or schizophrenia?**

First degree relatives of schizophrenics are 3 times as likely to have schizoidia as schizophrenia.

○ **A patient who is unable to express his anger, has few close friends, is indifferent to praise from others, is absent-minded, and is emotionally cold and aloof most likely has what kind of personality disorder?**

Schizoidia.

○ **Separation anxiety has an average onset of what age?**

Age 9. These children fear leaving home, sleep, being alone, going to school and losing their parents. 75% develop somatic complaints in order to avoid attending school.

○ **What is the body's largest sex organ?**

Skin. The skin is also the body's largest overall organ.

○ **By what age are children aware of their own sex?**

18 months. By age 2–3, a child can answer the question as to whether he/she is a boy or a girl.

○ **Hyposexual sexual desire disorder is caused by one or more factors from the key triad. What is this triad?**

1. Relationship problems
2. Performance anxiety
3. Fear of the consequences (e.g., STD or pregnancy).

○ **Name 8 drugs that decrease sexual desire.**

1. Antidepressants
2. Antihypertensives
3. Anticonvulsants
4. Neuroleptics
5. Digitalis
6. Cimetidine
7. Clofibrate
8. High doses or chronic ingestion of alcohol or street drugs.

○ **What are four medical causes of sexual arousal disorder?**

1. Leriche syndrome
2. Diabetes
3. Perineal surgery
4. Transection of the spinal chord.

○ **A child reared by a homosexual couple will most likely have what sexual orientation?**

Heterosexual.

○ **How does the insomnia of a melancholic patient differ from that of a patient with dysthymia?**

Melancholics have a difficulty staying asleep often associated with early morning wakefulness. Dysthymics have trouble falling asleep and have a tendency to oversleep.

○ **In which stage of sleep do we spend most of our time?**

Stage 2, which accounts for 50% of our sleep time. This stage is characterized by sleep spindles and K complexes on EEG. REM, when we dream, accounts for only 25% of our sleep.

❍   **Is somnambulism more common in children or adults?**

15–30% of children sleepwalk, while only 1% of adults do. Sleepwalking begins around the age of 4 and generally resolves itself by age 15.

❍   **Sleepwalking and pavor nocturnus (night terrors) are disturbances of what stage in sleep?**

Stage 4. A stage 4 sleep depressant, such as a long-acting Benzodiazepine, is effective in curbing this behavior.

❍   **Narcolepsy is a disorder of which sleep cycle?**

REM. Attacks of sleep, dreams, and paralysis last anywhere from 10 minutes to 1 hour. Amphetamines and planned naps throughout the day can help.

❍   **A 15-year-old female complains of pain in her calf, headache, shooting pain when flexing her right wrist, random epigastric pain, bloating, and irregular menses, all of which cannot be explained following medical workup. What is the diagnosis?**

Somatization Disorder — multiple, unexplained medical symptoms involving multiple systems. In order to diagnose a patient with somatization disorder, one must have 4 or more unexplained pain symptoms. Symptoms generally begin in childhood and are full blown by the age of 30. This is more common in females than males.

❍   **Major depression and bipolar affective disorder account for what percentage of suicides?**

50%. Another 25% are due to substance abuse, and another 10% are attributed to schizophrenia.

❍   **What percentage of patients with melancholia attempt suicide?**

15%.

❍   **Give examples of the following thought disorders:**

Perseveration: "I've been wondering if the mechanical mechanisms of this machine are mechanically sound. Mechanically speaking, I must understand the mechanisms." (A repetition of certain words or phrases is found in the natural flow of speech.)

Non-sequiturs: Q: "Are you nervous about the upcoming boards? "A: "Why no, the king of France is an excellent king." (The patient's answers are totally unrelated to the questions he is asked.)

Derailment: "I first became interested in the study of medicine after mom bought me a toy ambulance. Toys can be very dangerous, especially if they are very small and can be swallowed. I've been having difficulty swallowing lately." (The patient suddenly switches lines of thought, though the second follows the first.)

Tangential speech: A: "Those are nice clothes you're wearing today." B: "Of course I'm wearing clothes today." A: "I mean, I like the outfit you have on." B: "I think everyone should wear clothes, except on Friday because Friday is casual day at my office." (Conversations are on the right subject matter; however, the responses are inappropriate to the previous questions or comments.)

Neologism: I'm going to explaphrase (explain by paraphrasing) the meaning of agnonoctaudiophobia (things that go bump in the night). (Neologisms are meaningless combinations of 2 or more words to invent a new word.)

Private word usage: "I can't believe the ectoplasm way he is formicating those tulips." (Words and or phrases used in unique ways.)

<u>Verbigeration</u>: "I have been studying, have been studying, have been studying, for hours for hours, hours, hours." (The patient repeats words, especially at the end of thoughts, thoughts, thoughts, thoughts.)

○   **What are some predictors of a potentially violent patient?**

Male gender, history of violence, and history of substance abuse are the only reliable predictors. Cultural, educational, economic, and language barriers to effective patient/staff communication, as well as trivializing a patient or family member's concerns can increase frustrations and lower the threshold for violent episodes.

○   **What are some important clinical considerations when handling intoxicated, violent, psychotic, or threatening patients?**

These patients require a careful history and physical with attention to the mental status exam. Look for evidence of trauma, toxic ingestion, or metabolic derangement. Historical sources, such as family, paramedics, mental health workers, police, or medical records may need to be accessed. The patient may need to be physically or chemically restrained to obtain an adequate examination and for the safety of the patient and hospital staff.

○   **What psychiatric problems are associated with violence?**

Acute schizophrenia, paranoid ideation, catatonic excitation, mania, borderline and antisocial personality disorders, delusional depression, posttraumatic stress disorder, and decompensating obsessive/compulsive disorder.

○   **What are the prodromes of violent behavior?**

Anxiety, defensiveness, volatility, and physical aggression.

○   **Define the following:**

<u>Akathisia</u>: Internal restlessness. The patient feels as if he is "jumping out of his skin." Treatment is with propranolol.

<u>Echolalia</u>: Meaningless automatic repetition of someone else's words. This may occur immediately or even months after hearing the words.

<u>Catalepsy</u>: The patient maintains the same posture over a long period of time.

<u>Waxy flexibility</u>: The patient offers resistance to anyone trying to change his position, then gradually allows himself to be moved to a new posture, much like a clay figure.

<u>Stereotypy</u>: Patient goes through repetitive motions that have no goal.

<u>Verbigeration</u>: Verbal stereotypy. The patient repeats words over and over.

<u>Gegenhalten</u>: The patient resists external manipulation with the same force being applied.

OBSTETRICS AND GYNECOLOGY PEARLS

❍　**What is the <u>most</u> <u>common</u> non-gynecologic condition that presents with lower abdominal pain?**

Appendicitis.

❍　**When is amniocentesis performed for prenatal diagnosis?**

16–18 weeks .

❍　**Which defects are suggested by elevated maternal serum Σ-fetoprotein?**

Neural tube defects (anencephalopathy), ventral abdominal wall defects, fetal demise, or more than one fetus. Down syndrome is associated with a low maternal serum Σ-fetoprotein.

❍　**What is secondary amenorrhea?**

No menstruation for 6 months or more in a women who previously had regular menses.

❍　**What is the <u>most</u> <u>common</u> cause of secondary amenorrhea?**

Yes, the obvious: pregnancy. The second most common cause is hypothalamic hypogonadism which can be due to weight loss, anorexia nervosa, stress, excessive exercise, or hypothalamic disease.

❍　**A 16-year-old with secondary amenorrhea and an essentially normal workup is given an IM injection of 100 mg of progesterone and responds with a normal menstrual period. What does this tell you?**

She has a functional endometrium and a normal production of estrogen. Patients producing less than 40 pg/ml of estrogen will not bleed.

❍　**What are the two major differential diagnostic possibilities in the above patient?**

Premature ovarian failure and hypothalamic dysfunction. Premature ovarian failure can be diagnosed if the serum LH level is greater than 25 mIU/ml; otherwise, the diagnosis is most likely hypothalamic dysfunction.

❍　**A patient with secondary amenorrhea fails the progestin challenge and has a high FSH level. What is the problem?**

Gonadal failure. If the FSH were low, it would be more indicative of hypothalamic dysfunction.

❍　**What is the <u>most</u> <u>common</u> cause of dysfunctional uterine bleeding in a child?**

Infection. For teenagers, it is most commonly due to anovulation.

❍　**Virtually all severe cases of dysfunctional uterine bleeding occur in what age group?**

Adolescent females shortly after the onset of menstruation.

❍ **What is the treatment of choice for a Bartholin gland abscess?**

Marsupialization. This prevents recurrences.

❍ **A patient presents complaining of pain in her eyes, canker sores in her mouth, and sores and scars in her genital area. What is the diagnosis?**

Behçet's disease. This is a very rare disease involving ocular inflammation, oral apthous ulcers, and destructive genital ulcers generally on the vulva. No cure is known, but remission may occur with high estrogen levels.

❍ **B-hCG is secreted by what and for what reason?**

B-hCG is secreted by placental trophoblasts; its purpose is to maintain the corpus luteum, which in turn maintains the uterine lining. The corpus luteum is maintained through the sixth to eighth week of pregnancy, by which time the placenta begins to produce its own progesterone for maintenance of the endometrium.

❍ **What is the most common benign breast tumor?**

Fibroadenoma. They are most common in young women (under 30). They are usually solitary, mobile masses with distinct borders.

❍ **What medicines are contraindicated in breast-feeding mothers?**

Tetracycline, warfarin, and chloramphenicol.

❍ **What is the most common invasive ductal tumor?**

Nonspecific infiltrating ductal carcinoma accounts for 80% of breast cancers. These tumors produce a fibrotic response and are hard nodules when they are palpable.

❍ **A 13-year-old female presents with a barely palpable hard lump in the upper, outer quadrant of her left breast. The lump is mobile and causes no pain. The patient has noted blood oozing from her nipple. What is the diagnosis?**

Benign intraductal papilloma. Intraductal papillomas are the most common cause of blood from the nipple. These growths usually develop just before or during menopause and are rarely palpable.

❍ **What is the American Cancer Society's 1996 recommendation for PAP smears?**

Annually for 3 years starting at age 18 or when the patient becomes sexually active, then every 1–3 years.

❍ **What percentage of cervical cancer is squamous cell?**

85%. 15% is adenocarcinoma.

❍ **What is the most common site of metastasis from cervical cancer?**

The liver.

❍ **What are the rates of pregnancy with the following forms of birth control: (1) surgical sterilization, IUDs, or oral contraceptives; (2) coitus interruptus and rhythm method; (3) condoms; and (4) foams, jellies, sponges, or diaphragms?**

1) .2–2%, 2) 10%, 3) 12%, and 4), 18–20%.

❍   **How long after the removal of Norplant capsules must patients wait to become pregnant?**

Ovulation usually occurs within 3 months.

❍   **A patient who is taking oral contraceptives is concerned about the added risk for gynecological cancers. What do you tell her?**

Combined (estrogen and progesterone) oral contraceptives are not associated with a significant risk for breast cancer. In fact, they decrease the risk of ovarian and endometrial cancer. It takes very large amounts of unopposed estrogen to cause a significant risk of breast cancer. Oral contraceptives do increase the risk for thromboembolism, MIs, CVAs, hypertension, amenorrhea, cholelithiasis, and benign hepatic tumors. In addition, oral contraceptives help regulate the menstrual cycle, decrease cramping, and curb the progression of endometriosis, ovarian cysts, and benign breast disease. They also decrease the incidence of ectopic pregnancy, salpingitis, and anemia, and they are therapeutic against rheumatoid arthritis.

❍   **The same patient is worried about weight gain with oral contraceptives. What chemical changes occur that might predispose the patient to weight gain?**

Increases in LDL, decreases in HDL, and sodium retention.

❍   **Oral contraceptives are contraindicated in which patients?**

Patients with DVTs, MIs, histories of smoking, liver tumors, breast cancer, or other estrogen-dependent tumors, heart disease, vascular disease, or prior thromboembolisms.

❍   **Failure of the hCG to increase by 66% over 48 hours in a pregnant females is indicative of what?**

An ectopic pregnancy or an intrauterine pregnancy that is about to abort.

❍   **What is the <u>most</u> <u>common</u> site of implantation in an ectopic pregnancy?**

The ampulla of the fallopian tube (95%).

❍   **What are the risk factors for ectopic pregnancy?**

Prior scarring of the fallopian tubes from infection (i.e., PID or salpingitis), IUDs, previous ectopic pregnancy, tubal ligation, and STDs.

❍   **When does an ectopic pregnancy <u>most</u> <u>commonly</u> present?**

6–8 weeks. Patients usually present with amenorrhea and sharp abdominal or pelvic pain. A mass can be felt in 1/2 of the patients. B-hCG confirms pregnancy; ultrasound generally confirms an ectopic pregnancy.

❍   **What percentage of pregnancies are ectopic?**

1.5%. Ectopic pregnancies are the leading cause of death in the first trimester.

❍   **What is the <u>most</u> <u>common</u> finding on pelvic exam in a patient with an ectopic pregnancy?**

Unilateral adnexal tenderness.

❍   **Who is eligible for methotrexate treatment of an ectopic pregnancy?**

Patients who are hemodynamically stable with unruptured gestations of < 4 cm in diameter by ultrasound.

❍   **Transient pelvic pain frequently occurs 3–7 days after methotrexate therapy for ectopic pregnancy. What is your concern?**

Pain from rupture may be difficult to differentiate from pain presumed to be due to tubal abortion, which typically lasts 4–12 hours.

❍   **What is the risk of a repeat ectopic pregnancy?**

10–15%.

❍   **For a gestational sac to be visible on ultrasound, what must the B-hCG be?**

At least 6,500 mIU/ml for a transabdominal ultrasound and 2,000 mIU/ml for a transvaginal ultrasound.

❍   **When can an abdominal ultrasound find an intrauterine gestational sac?**

In the fifth week. Fetal pole, sixth week. Embryonic mass with cardiac motion, seventh week.

❍   **What are the risk factors of endometrial cancer?**

Endometrial cancer correlates highly with estrogen levels. Early menarche, late menopause, obesity, nulliparity, anovulation in the reproductive years, and unopposed estrogen are all risk factors. Diabetes, gallbladder disease, and breast, colon, and ovarian cancer are additional risk factors.

❍   **Where do enteroceles most commonly occur due to a herniation?**

Herniation of the pouch of Douglas.

❍   **Matching—time to keep those "M"s straight:**

1. Menorrhagia.
2. Metrorrhagia (hypermenorrhea).
3. Menometrorrhagia.

a. Bleeding between menstrual periods.
b. Excessive amount of blood or duration.
c. Excessive amount of blood at irregular frequencies.

Answers: (1) b, (2) a, and (3) c.

❍   **Matching—more ways to describe menstrual bleeding:**

1. Hypermenorrhea.
2. Oligomenorrhea.
3. Polymenorrhea.

a. Menstrual periods > 35 days apart.
b. Menstrual periods < 21 days apart.
c. Menorrhagia.

Answers: (1) c, (2) a, and (3) b.

❍   **What is Meig's syndrome?**

Ascites and hydrothorax in the presence of an ovarian tumor.

❍   **The ovarian luteal phase corresponds to what phase of the uterus?**

The secretory phase. The luteal phase begins after ovulation. At this time, the expelled follicle is called the corpus luteum. The corpus luteum secretes estradiol and progesterone, which cause secretory ducts to develop in the endometrial lining.

❍   **What is indicated by a biphasic curve on a basal body temperature (BBT) chart of a 16-year-old woman?**

Normal ovulation and the effect of progesterone. A monophasic BBT curve would indicate an anovulatory cycle. A temperature that remained elevated following a normal biphasic curve would indicate pregnancy.

❍ **When are uterine myomas most common?**

Uterine myomas (nonmalignant smooth muscle growths) are responsive to hormones and grow primarily in the reproductive years. They are the most common type of gynecological pelvic neoplasm.

❍ **What type of myoma is symptomatic?**

Submucosal myomas, though small, can cause profuse bleeding, potentially requiring a hysterectomy. Most other myomas are asymptomatic.

❍ **What percentage of the population has supernumerary nipples?**

1–2%. The incidence is equal in males and females.

❍ **What is the most common complication of ovarian cysts?**

Torsion of the ovary. Torsion is more common with small to medium sized tumors. Emergency surgery is required.

❍ **What clinical findings will there be in a 7-year-old with an ovarian granulosa cell tumor?**

This girl will have pseudoprecocious puberty. She may have vaginal bleeding, axillary hair, and early breast budding.

❍ **Histologically speaking, what is the difference between adults and children in regards to ovarian cancer?**

In children, germ cells are affected; in adults, it is the epithelial cells that are affected.

❍ **What are the most common sites for metastasis of ovarian carcinoma?**

Peritoneum and omentum.

❍ **Most cases of PID are caused by what 2 organisms?**

Neisseria gonorrhea and *Chlamydia trachomatis*.

❍ **Which patients with PID should be admitted?**

Admit patients who are pregnant, have a temperature > 38°C (100.4°F), are nauseous or vomiting (which prohibits po antibiotics), have pyosalpinx or tubo-ovarian abscess peritoneal signs, have IUCD, show no response to oral antibiotics, or for whom diagnosis is uncertain.

❍ **What are the criteria for diagnosis of PID?**

All of the following must be present: (1) adnexal tenderness, (2) cervical and uterine tenderness, and (3) abdominal tenderness. In addition, one of the following must be present: (1) temperature > 38°C, (2) endocervix Gram's stain positive for Gram-negative intracellular diplococci, (3) leukocytosis > 10,000 /mm^3, (4) inflammatory mass on US or pelvic, or (5) WBCs and bacteria in the peritoneal fluid.

❍ **Teenage pregnancies are associated with increased risks of what disorders?**

Maternal complications, such as gonorrhea, syphilis, toxemia, anemia, malnutrition, low birth weight babies, and perinatal mortality.

○   **Why is Rh status important in a pregnant patient?**

If the mother is Rh negative and the fetus is Rh positive, fetal anemia, hydrops, and fetal loss can result. Rh immunoglobulin should be given to all Rh negative patients.

○   **What is Sheehan's syndrome?**

Anterior pituitary necrosis following post partum hemorrhage and hypotension. It results in amenorrhea, decreased breast size, and decreased pubic hair.

○   **What predisposes a female to yeast infections?**

Diabetes, oral contraceptives, and antibiotics.

○   **What organism is the most common cause of vaginitis?**

Candida albicans.

○   **A patient presents with a 2 day history of vaginal itching and burning. On exam, you note a thin yellowish–green bubbly discharge and petechiae on the cervix (also known as "strawberry cervix"). What test do you perform, and what results do you expect to find?**

Look at the discharge mixed with saline under a microscope. If you see a mobile and pear-shaped protozoa (*Trichomonas vaginalis*) with flagella, then the patient should be treated with Metronidazole (Flagyl).

○   **A 16-year-old sexually active female is complaining of a heavy but thin discharge with an unpleasant odor. When you add 10% KOH to the discharge, the combination emits a fishy odor. What would you expect to see on microscopic examination?**

"Clue cells"—epithelial cells with bacilli attached to their surfaces. This patient has Gardnerella vaginitis. The patient and her partner should both be treated with Metronidazole (Flagyl).

○   **When should you avoid using Flagyl to treat a female?**

If she is the first trimester of pregnancy. Metronidazole may have teratogenic effects. Clotrimazole (Gyne-Lotrimin) may be used instead. Flagyl has side-effects including nausea, vomiting, and metallic tastes. Most importantly, it acts similarly to disulfiram (Antabuse) and should, therefore, not be taken with alcohol.

○   **A 15-year-old female presents to your office complaining of a painful sore on her vulva that look like a pimple at first. On exam, you find an ulcer with vague borders and a gray base. What is the most likely diagnosis?**

Gram's stain, culture, and biopsy (used in combination because of the high false negative rates) should show that this woman has Haemophilus ducreyi, causing chancroid. Treatment is erythromycin or ceftriaxone.

○   **Condylomata acuminata frequently occur in combination with what other STD?**

Trichomonas vaginitis.

○   **What is the most common cause of septic arthritis in young adults?**

Disseminated gonococcal infection.

○   **What is the treatment for gonorrhea?**

Ceftriaxone and doxycycline. The latter is given because half of the patients infected with gonorrhea are simultaneously infected with chlamydia.

O   **What is the predominant organism in a healthy female's vaginal discharge?**

Lactobacilli (95%).

O   **A 16-year-old male presents to your office with a maculopapular rash on his palms and soles. He complains of headaches and general weakness. On exam, you find he has multiple condyloma lata and lymphadenopathy. What is the diagnosis?**

Secondary syphilis. This develops 6–9 weeks after the development of the syphilitic chancre, which resolves by this time. If it is allowed to progress untreated, tertiary syphilis develops. This can affect all the tissues in the body, including those of the CNS and the heart. Treatment is with penicillin G.

O   **Is the Stein-Leventhal syndrome a unilateral or bilateral phenomenon?**

Bilateral. Both ovaries are cystic and enlarged with a thickened and fibrosed tunica. These patients are often infertile, obese, and hirsute.

O   **What is the number one cause of urethritis in males?**

Chlamydia trachomatis.

O   **Female pseudohermaphroditism is most commonly due to what condition?**

Congenital adrenal hyperplasia. The defective adrenals cannot produce normal amounts of cortisol. These patients have normal XX chromosomes, but an excess of endogenous adrenal steroids has virilizing effects.

O   **What causes toxic shock syndrome (TSS)?**

An exotoxin elaborated by certain strains of *Staphylococcus aureus*. Other organisms causing toxic shock syndrome are group A Streptococcus, *Pseudomonas aeruginosa*, and *Streptococcus pneumoniae*. Tampons, IUDs, septic abortions, sponges, soft tissue abscesses, osteomyelitis, nasal packing, and post partum infections can all house these organisms.

O   **What dermatological changes occur with TSS?**

Initially, the patient will have a blanching erythematous rash that lasts for 3 days. 10 days after the start of the infection there will be a desquamation of the palms and soles.

O   **What criteria are necessary for the diagnosis of TSS?**

All of the following must be present: T > 38.9°C (102°F), rash, systolic BP < 90, and orthostasis, involvement of 3 organ systems (GI, renal, musculoskeletal, mucosal, hepatic, hematologic, or CNS), and negative serologic tests for diseases such as RMSF, hepatitis B, measles, leptospirosis, VDRL, etc.

O   **What is the treatment for TSS?**

Fluids, pressure support, FFP or transfusions, vaginal irrigation with iodine or saline (if the TSS was related to tampon use), and antistaphylococcal penicillin (nafcillin or oxacillin), or cephalosporin. Rifampin should be considered to eliminate the carrier state.

O   **What is the number one cause of UTIs?**

E. coli.

❍   **A 16-year-old female comes to you complaining of fever, aches and pains, and painful genital sores that looked like blisters 2 days ago until they popped and started hurting. What would you expect to find on culture of the vesicular fluid?**

This patient most likely has the herpes simplex virus, type 2. Tzanck smear or a culture will show multinucleated giant cells by Giemsa stain.

❍   **What subtypes of HPV are associated with cervical cancer?**

HPV types 16, 18 or 31 are risk factors for cervical dysplasia which can lead to cervical cancer. Multiple sex partners and early onset of sexual activity are also risk factors for cervical cancer.

❍   **What is the precursor of epidermoid carcinoma of the vulva?**

Leukoplakia.

❍   **Are fetal heart rate accelerations normal?**

Yes and no. Rapid heart rate can indicate fetal distress. 2 accelerations every 20 minutes is normal. An acceleration must last 15 seconds and be an elevation of at least 15 bpm above baseline.

❍   **What causes variable decelerations?**

Transient umbilical cord compression. These often change with maternal position.

❍   **Which anticoagulant should be used in pregnant patients?**

Heparin, as it does not cross the placenta.

❍   **Is appendicitis more common during pregnancy?**

No (1/850). However, the outcome is worse. The WBC count usually does not increase beyond the normal value of 12,000–15,000. In a pregnant patient, pyuria with no bacteria suggest appendicitis. Pregnant patients may lack GI distress, and fever may be absent or low grade.

❍   **How is the appendix displaced in pregnancy?**

Superiorly and laterally. Diagnosis of appendicitis in pregnant patients may be further complicated by the fact that normal pregnancy can itself cause an increased WBC. Prompt diagnosis is important because incidence of perforation increases from 10% in the first trimester to 40% in the third.

❍   **What are the 3 types of breech presentation?**

Frank breech: thighs flexed, legs extended.

Complete breech: at least one leg flexed.

Incomplete breech/footling breech: at least 1 foot below the buttocks with both thighs extended.

❍   **A 15-year-old, Tanner 5 girl presents with abdominal pain and dysuria; she has not yet started menses. Examination of the genitalia shows a mass at the introitus. What is the most likely diagnosis and cause?**

The most likely diagnosis is hematocolpos, which is due to either a transverse vaginal membrane or an imperforate hymen.

○   **A 3-year-old girl presents with painless vaginal bleeding; there is no history of trauma. Examination of the genitalia reveals a donut shaped, erythematous mass above the introitus. What is the diagnosis ?**

Urethral prolapse.

○   **What is the treatment of urethral prolapse?**

If there is no tissue necrosis, management consists of topical estrogen cream for 4-6 weeks. If there is tissue necrosis, excision under general anesthesia is necessary, which can be done as an outpatient.

○   **A mother comes to your office because she fears her 7 month old daughter's vagina is "closing up". Examination reveals midline fusion of the labia minora, obscuring the view of the introitus. What is the diagnosis ?**

Labial adhesions or acquired attachment of the labia minora. This is thought to occur because of low levels of endogenous estrogen in preadolescent girls, resulting in a thin epithelial surface of the labia minora. This thin epithelial surface is prone to maceration and inflammation, leading to fusion of the edges.

○   **What is the treatment for labial adhesions?**

Topical estrogen cream for 4-6 weeks, followed by application of an inert cream, such as zinc oxide, for an additional 2 weeks, to keep the healing surfaces apart. Expectant management is also acceptable, as this condition remits in early puberty; however, most caretakers will want their daughters treated.

○   **What is primary dysmenorrhea?**

Primary dysmenorrhea is painful menses that is not attributable to any other cause, such as endometriosis, PID or structural pelvic disorders.

○   **What is the etiology of primary dysmenorrhea?**

Primary dysmenorrhea is caused by endometrial prostaglandins that are secreted after ovulation, causing uterine contractions that can lead to myometrial ischemia and pain; this pain can last up to 48 hours after menses have begun.

○   **What are the treatment options for primary dysmenorrhea?**

First line therapy consists of prostaglandin inhibitors such as NSAIDS (aspirin, ibuprofen, naproxen sodium-the latter two are more potent prostaglandin inhibitors). For the sexually active teen, oral contraceptives, which will inhibit ovulation, are another alternative, especially if NSAIDS fail to work.

○   **What is the pathophysiology behind dysfunctional uterine bleeding (DUB)?**

DUB is due to anovulatory bleeding, caused by estrogen that is unopposed by progesterone. This causes the endometrium to undergo sporadic growth and sloughing without cyclic coordination. The amount of estrogen secreted by the ovaries varies and bleeding can occur because of a fall in estrogen (withdrawal bleeding) or when the endometrium outgrows its blood supply (breakthrough bleeding).

○   **What disorders need to be excluded before the diagnosis of dysfunctional uterine bleeding (DUB) can be made?**

Pregnancy, bleeding diathesis (such as von Willebrand's disease, thrombocytopenia), polycystic ovary syndrome (Stein-Leventhal syndrome), thyroid disease (most often hypothyroidism), aspirin use, and improper use of oral contraceptives.

○   **What is the most common cause of vaginitis in girls who are pubertal but not sexually active?**

C. albicans.

O **Among teenagers who are sexually active, what are the 3 most common causes of vaginitis?**

Gardnerella vaginalis (bacterial vaginosis), *C. albicans*, *Trichomonas vaginalis*.

O **How is the diagnosis of vaginitis by Trichomonas vaginalis made?**

Diagnosis is usually made by examination of a wet mount preparation of the vaginal discharge; one can see the movement of the flagellated protozoa.

O **How does an adolescent female acquire vaginitis due to Trichomonas vaginalis?**

Vaginitis due to *Trichomonas vaginalis* is primarily a sexually transmitted disease.

O **What is the treatment for vaginitis due to *Trichomonas vaginalis*?**

Metronidazole, which can be given orally as a single 2-gram dose.

O **When treating vaginitis due to Trichomonas vaginalis, what condition must be excluded before metronidazole is prescribed?**

Pregnancy, as metronidazole is teratogenic.

O **With what drugs does metronidazole interact?**

Ethanol, phenytoin, phenobarbital, warfarin and disulfiram.

O **A nine-week-old female infant has had a white, malodorous discharge for over seven weeks. Her physical examination is normal except for the aforementioned discharge. A wet prep of the discharge shows motile trichomonads. How did the infant acquire this infection?**

A small number of vaginally delivered female infants may acquire vaginitis due to *Trichomonas vaginalis* from their untreated mothers during delivery. This vaginal discharge may persist for several months if left untreated.

O **A 10-year-old girl presents with vaginal pain, pruritus and a yellow vaginal discharge. She also has a high fever and a sore throat. A gram stain of the vaginal discharge shows gram positive cocci in pairs. What is the most likely diagnosis, and what is the treatment?**

Group A beta hemolytic streptococcus (GABHS). Vaginitis can appear with or following acute GABHS pharyngitis. Penicillin therapy is curative. Also consider gonorrhea on an under-decolorized grain stain. The culture will be definitive.

O **What historical, clinical and laboratory findings are necessary to make the diagnosis of bacterial vaginosis (vaginitis due to *Gardnerella vaginalis*)?**

A whitish, adherent vaginal discharge; vaginal pH > 4.5; amine-like (fishy) odor generated after adding 10% KOH to a sample of the vaginal discharge; when examining the vaginal discharge under the microscope, > 20% of vaginal epithelial cells are studded with gram negative coccobacilli.

O **What are two treatment options for teenage girls with bacterial vaginosis?**

Oral metronidazole twice daily for 7 days. Topical clindamycin is an alternative for patients who are pregnant.

❍   **What is the most common bacteria isolated from a Bartholin's gland abscess?**

N. gonorrhoeae is isolated in up to 50% of cultures from Bartholin's gland abscesses. The remaining cases contain mixed growths of aerobic and anaerobic organisms, such as Bacteroides, and a smaller number will grow *C. trachomatis.* Up to 30% of cultures will be sterile.

❍   **What is the management of a Bartholin's gland abscess?**

Incision and drainage or aspiration is the usual treatment for the first episode of a Bartholin's gland abscess. All patients should also be treated for presumed gonococcal infection. Marsupialization of the gland is reserved for recurrent Bartholin's gland abscesses.

❍   **What is Fitz-Hugh Curtis syndrome?**

Fitz-Hugh Curtis syndrome is a peri-hepatitis, or inflammation of the liver capsule, in association with pelvic inflammatory disease (PID). In addition to the signs/symptoms of PID, patients will also complain of right upper quadrant pain and tenderness to palpation.

❍   **What other complications are seen in patients with PID and Fitz-Hugh Curtis syndrome?**

20% of patients will have tubo-ovarian abscesses.

❍   **What does "RPR" stand for and what does it detect in serum?**

RPR stands for "rapid plasma regain" and detects antibodies against a cardiolipin-cholesterol-lecithin complex. It is a "nonspecific" test for syphilis, as it does not directly detect *Treponema pallidum.*

❍   **Name five causes of a "false positive" RPR?**

1) Pregnancy
2) Collagen vascular disease
3) Drug addiction
4) Infection
5) Immunization

❍   **A 7-year-old girl presents with a greenish-brown, blood-streaked vaginal discharge. A gram stain of the discharge reveals gram-negative rods and polymorphonuclear cells. What is the most likely infectious cause of this discharge?**

Shigella species has been recently recognized as a cause of infectious vulvovaginitis. Only 30% of patients have associated diarrhea. The clinical appearance of the vaginal discharge closely resembles that of a vaginal foreign body. Vaginal culture is often diagnostic. If vaginal cultures are negative, then an examination under anesthesia to look for a vaginal foreign body is warranted.

❍   **What is the most prevalent sexually transmitted disease among adolescent females?**

Human papilloma virus.

❍   **What is the most likely causes of vaginal discharge in a neonate?**

Physiologic leukorrhea, which is due to the influence of maternal hormones during gestation. The vaginal discharge is clear, white and sticky. A gram stain will show white blood cells but no organisms; cultures will be sterile.

❍   **What pathogen is most often responsible for vaginal discharge immediately beyond the neonatal period?**

Trichomonas vaginalis, which is acquired during vaginal delivery of infants born to infected mothers.

❍   **A 10-year-old girl presents with chronic vaginal itching; there is no vaginal discharge. On examination her perineum has a hypopigmented, macular rash with telangiectasias in a "figure of 8" pattern. What is the diagnosis?**

Lichen sclerosus, which is a chronic idiopathic dermatitis characterized by atrophy, telangiectasias and hypopigmentation of the perineum, often in a "figure of 8" pattern.

❍   **What is the most common cause of abnormal vaginal discharge in sexually active adolescents?**

Trichomonas vaginalis.

❍   **What is the treatment for genital warts (condyloma acuminata)?**

Traditionally, the therapy was ablation of visible warts. Recently, because of the recognition of subclinical disease and the association of human papilloma virus (HPV) with cervical neoplasia, tissue ablation by podophyllin for localized warts and laser vaporization or cryotherapy for more extensive disease is now recommended.

❍   **What is the cause of condyloma acuminata (genital warts)?**

Human papilloma virus; types 6 and 11 are the most common subtype of virus grown from these lesions.

❍   **Cervical intraepithelial neoplasia (CIN) and cervical cancer are most often associated with what sexually transmitted disease?**

Human papilloma virus, which is the cause of genital warts (condyloma acuminata).

❍   **What is the most common etiology of genital ulcers in the United States?**

Herpes simplex, type 2.

❍   **How can one easily make the diagnosis of herpes simplex?**

By Tzanck smear, which will show multinucleated giant cells, or by viral culture.

❍   **How can one make the diagnosis of primary syphilis?**

1) Dark field microscopy of suspicious lesions, which will show the spirochete, 2) RPR, which is a good but nonspecific test, as it does not directly detect *Treponema pallidum*, or 3) fluorescent antibody testing (MHA-TP, FTA), which directly detect antibody response to *T. pallidum*.

❍   **What is the most common etiology of genital ulcers found in patients who reside in developing countries?**

Chancroid, which is caused by *Hemophilus ducreyi*.

❍   **What is the treatment for chancroid?**

Erythromycin or a third generation cephalosporin, like ceftriaxone.

❍   **An adolescent female presents with a fluctuant, tender breast mass and fever. What is the diagnosis and treatment?**

This patient has a breast abscess, which should be incised and drained; any loculated pockets should be broken up. Purulent fluid should be sent for culture. Anti-staphylococcal antibiotics should also be prescribed. Simple aspiration of the abscess is not sufficient.

❍   **A teenage girl presents with milky, non-bloody discharge from her nipples. She is not pregnant. What is the diagnosis and etiology of the discharge?**

This patient has galactorrhea, which is most often caused by a pituitary adenoma that secretes prolactin. Galactorrhea can also be caused by certain drugs, such as phenothiazine, antihistamines, diazepam, cimetidine, metoclopramide, opiates (codeine, morphine), antihypertensive agents (verapamil) and tricyclic antidepressants. If amenorrhea is also present, thyroid disease should be suspected.

❍   **What is oligomenorrhea?**

Oligomenorrhea is defined as an interval of more than 6 weeks between menses.

❍   **At what point does oligomenorrhea require evaluation?**

Adolescents with a pattern of oligomenorrhea that has continued more than 2 years after menarche or that began after the establishment of a regular menstrual cycle need evaluation.

❍   **What are some of the clinical features of polycystic ovary syndrome (Stein-Leventhal syndrome)?**

Hirsutism, obesity, amenorrhea or infertility, and ovarian enlargement are some of the principal features; acanthosis nigricans and insulin resistance are seen in a small percentage of patients. However, many patients may not have all of these features.

❍   **What are the clinical manifestations of secondary syphilis?**

Maculopapular rash of the trunk, soles, palms, that can resemble pityriasis rosea; mucous patches (white patches on the mucous membranes); condyloma lata, which are flat topped warts present in moist areas of the body, such as the perineum.

❍   **What is the treatment for sexually acquired syphilis?**

For primary and early (< 1 year duration of symptoms) syphilis, a single dose of IM benzathine penicillin is sufficient; for late (>1 year duration of symptoms) syphilis, 3 IM doses of benzathine penicillin separated by a weekly interval is required.

❍   **What is the most common cause of urethritis among sexually active adolescents in the United States?**

Chlamydia trachomatis.

❍   **A sexually active 16-year-old male complains of dysuria and a penile discharge. You suspect urethritis. What is the appropriate management of this patient?**

The two most common causes of urethritis in a sexually active male are *C. trachomatis* and *N. gonorrhoeae*: therefore, appropriate antibiotic therapy to cover both of these organisms, such as an IM dose of a third-generation cephalosporin (ceftriaxone) and an oral course of doxycycline, are needed. Test of cure urethral cultures are also suggested.

❍   **What if the patient in the above question is allergic to penicillin?**

Treat with IM spectinomycin, which is an alternative to IM ceftriaxone.

O   **What are the clinical manifestations of primary syphilis?**

A painless genital ulcer (chancre), which is the site of inoculation of the spirochete.

O   **Is Candida albicans a common cause of vulvovaginitis in pre-pubescent females?**

No, because estrogen promotes fungal growth by stimulating vaginal glycogen stores and acidity.

O   **What are some of the risk factors for developing vulvovaginitis from *C. albicans*?**

Estrogen, which increases vaginal stores of glycogen and increases vaginal acidity; impaired host immunity, due to systemic corticosteroids, diabetes mellitus; and broad spectrum antibiotics.

O   **What are the signs and symptoms of pelvic inflammatory disease (PID)?**

Classic PID, also known as acute salpingitis, is characterized by fever and lower abdominal pain. The patient may have just finished her menses. Physical examination reveals fever, lower abdominal tenderness and marked bilateral adnexal tenderness.

O   **What method of contraception is associated with a higher incidence of pelvic inflammatory disease (PID)?**

The risk of PID is twice as high in women who use intrauterine devices (IUD) when compared with women who use no contraceptive method.

O   **What is the organism most often isolated from patients with pelvic inflammatory disease (PID)?**

Nearly 50% of women with PID in the United States have coexisting gonococcal cervicitis.

O   **Which micro-organisms are responsible for pelvic inflammatory disease (PID)?**

N. gonorrhoeae, *C. trachomatis*, *Mycoplasma hominis*, and enteric anaerobes as *Bacteroides*.

O   **What is the appropriate antibiotic therapy for the treatment of an adolescent who has cervicitis?**

This patient may have cervicitis from *N. gonorrhoeae* and/or *C. trachomatis*. One strategy would be to give a single intramuscular dose of ceftriaxone and a 7-day course of oral doxycycline (provided the patient is not pregnant). To enhance compliance, a single oral dose of azithromycin may be substituted for the doxycycline. To avoid an intramuscular shot, a single oral dose of cefixime may be substituted for ceftriaxone.

O   **Would the treatment options change if the patient in the previous question were pregnant?**

Yes. If the patient is pregnant, a 7-day course of erythromycin should be substituted for doxycycline.

O   **A ten-year-old girl presents with a unilateral hematoma of the labia majora after a straddle injury. What is the appropriate treatment for this patient?**

Vulvar hematomas usually respond to ice-packs and bed rest. If there is mild urinary retention, voiding in a bathtub of warm water is helpful. If there is significant urinary retention, a urinary catheter may be necessary. Massive vulvar hematoma require evacuation.

O   **A teenage girl is treated for secondary syphilis with a single intramuscular dose of benzathine penicillin. Several days later, she develops fever and the maculopapular rash on her trunk becomes much more prominent. What is the cause of her symptoms?**

This patient has an acute systemic febrile reaction, the Jarisch-Herxheimer reaction, which can be seen in up to 20% of patients with acquired or congenital syphilis that are treated with penicillin. This reaction is self-limited and is not a reason to discontinue future therapy with penicillin.

○ **A sexually active teenage girl presents with fever, rash and pain of her knees and elbows. She just completed her menses. Examination reveals fever, a swollen, red, hot knee and erythematous macules of her hands and soles of her feet. What is the most likely diagnosis?**

Disseminated gonococcal infection.

○ **What are the clinical manifestations of disseminated gonococcal infection?**

Hematogenous dissemination of *N. gonorrhoeae* occurs in up to 3% of asymptomatic, primary infections in women. Symptoms start 7-28 days after infection and within 7 days of the last menstrual cycle. The most common signs are arthritis, polyarthralgia, tenosynovitis and a papular rash. Most patients do not have genitourinary symptoms; however, up to 80% of cervical cultures will be positive for *N. gonorrhoeae*.

○ **What is pseudocyesis?**

Pseudocyesis is a rare cause of amenorrhea in women who believe they are pregnant, when they are not. These patients exhibit many symptoms of pregnancy, such as nausea, vomiting, galactorrhea and abdominal distention. The diagnosis is made when the patient insists she is pregnant, despite the absence of fetal heart tones, fetal movement, uterine enlargement and a negative pregnancy test. All patients require psychiatric evaluation.

○ **What is the classic triad of symptoms seen in patients with ectopic pregnancies?**

Lower abdominal pain, vaginal bleeding and an abnormal menstrual history.

○ **A 16-year-old girl presents with a painless breast mass. You suspect a fibroadenoma. What is the management of this patient?**

Recommended management of a suspected fibroadenoma is observation of the mass as the patient goes through 3 menstrual cycles, as occasionally these masses will spontaneously regress. If the lesion persists, surgical excision is recommended.

○ **What is amastia?**

Amastia is a condition characterized by the unilateral absence of chest wall structures, such as ribs, intercostal muscles and mammary tissue.

○ **What is menorrhagia?**

Menorrhagia is abnormal menstrual bleeding that has a duration of greater than 8 days, or has an onset of less than 21 days between menstrual periods, or when the patient uses greater than 8 sanitary pads or 10 tampons per day.

○ **What is the management of a patient with dysfunctional uterine bleeding (DUB)?**

All patients should receive iron supplementation. If the bleeding is mild and the patient is not anemic, expectant management is all that is necessary, as this condition often remits. If the bleeding is moderate or severe and the patient is anemic, then hormonal therapy consisting of both estrogen and progesterone is needed. If the patient is hypovolemic, then intravenous estrogen followed by oral progesterone is needed; otherwise oral contraceptives are suitable, initially taken 4 times daily until the bleeding stops, and then once daily for one month. The patient should be counseled that the following menstrual period will be heavy.

○   **What are the mechanisms of action of oral contraceptives to prevent pregnancy?**

Suppression of ovulation; alteration of the cervical mucous, making it impermeable to sperm; and thinning of the endometrial lining, making it inhospitable to the implantation of the embryo.

○   **What are contraindications to prescribing oral contraceptives?**

Patients with a history of the following conditions: thrombophlebitis or thromboembolic disease; cerebrovascular accident; coronary artery disease; active liver disease; significant hypertension; estrogen dependent neoplasia; pregnancy.

○   **What is lymphogranuloma venereum (LGV)?**

Lymphogranuloma venereum (LGV) is an invasive lymphatic infection caused by *C. trachomatis*.

○   **What is the most common presentation of lymphogranuloma venereum (LGV)?**

The initial presentation is that of a local lesion on the genitalia accompanied by regional lymphadenitis.

○   **What is the treatment for lymphogranuloma venereum?**

Tetracycline (patients > 9 years of age), erythromycin, azithromycin or a sulfonamide for 3 to 6 weeks.

○   **How is the diagnosis of infection with *N. gonorrhoeae* made?**

By incubating infected secretions on selective media, such as chocolate agar impregnated with antibiotics, in a 5-10% CO_2 environment; this is the gold standard for diagnosing gonococcal infection.

○   **How soon, after conception, do serum pregnancy tests become positive?**

Within 7 days of conception, which is approximately 1 week before the first missed menstrual period.

○   **What is the recommended treatment for the first episode of genital herpes?**

If oral acyclovir is started within 6 days of the onset of lesions, the duration of the lesions may be shortened by 3-5 days.

○   **What is the recommended treatment for recurrent genital herpes?**

Oral acyclovir has minimal effect on the duration of recurrent episodes of genital herpes. If oral acyclovir is started within 48 hours of the onset of symptoms, the duration of the lesions may be shortened only by 1 day.

○   **A 13-year-old girl, Tanner stage 4, presents with yellow vaginal discharge. She has not started menstruating, and is not sexually active. There is no vaginal itching, pain or dysuria. What is the most likely diagnosis?**

Physiologic vaginal discharge, which is usually scant, yellow and without odor; there are no other associated symptoms. This occurs about 6 months prior to menarche.

○   **What are the typical symptoms of "mittelschmerz" (ovulatory pain)?**

1) Sudden onset of right or left lower quadrant pain that occurs 2 weeks after the last menses (mid-cycle).
2) No evidence of intrauterine pregnancy.
3) A pelvic examination that reveals unilateral adnexal tenderness with no mass, no cervical motion tenderness, and no vaginal bleeding.

4) Pain that lasts only 24-36 hours.

❍   **The majority of ovarian masses are of what histologic type?**

Teratomas.

❍   **What is the likelihood that an ovarian teratoma will become malignant?**

It depends on how much of the teratoma is cystic or solid. Primarily cystic teratomas have a low rate of malignancy, while solid teratomas have a much higher malignancy rate.

❍   **What factors make a young girl at risk for developing adenocarcinoma of the vagina?**

Maternal ingestion of diethylstilbestrol (DES) during pregnancy, which was previously used to prevent the progression of threatened abortions.

❍   **A 5-year-old girl has an uncomplicated urinary tract infection (UTI). What is the likelihood that an anatomic abnormality of the urinary tract will be discovered on voiding cystourethrogram (VCUG)?**

Approximately 30%.

❍   **If the patient in the question above does have an anatomic abnormality of the urinary tract, what is the most likely abnormality?**

Vesicoureteral reflux.

IMAGING PEARLS

❍   **An intrauterine gestational sac without a fetal pole, yolk sac or cardiac activity can be confused with what structure?**

The pseudosac of ectopic pregnancy (seen with 10-20% ectopics).

❍   **What is the incidence of allergic reaction to IV contrast materials?**

Severe allergic reactions occur in approximately 1/14,000 patients, whereas fatal reactions occur in about 1/40,000 cases.

❍   **What is the prevalence of adverse reactions to ionic and nonionic contrast materials?**

Ionic: 12.7%. Nonionic: 3.1%. Nonionic contrast causes hypotension, bronchospasm, arrhythmia, angioneurotic edema, urticaria, flushing, nausea, and vomiting less often than ionic contrast materials. Whether or not nonionic materials are less nephrotoxic is still controversial.

❍   **T/F: Oral contrast should be avoided in patients with marginal renal function.**

False. Little nephrotoxic iodine is absorbed with oral contrast administration. When barium is used, it is inert and not absorbed.

❍   **What are the contraindications to administration of oral iodine or barium contrast?**

Barium cannot be given when complete colon obstruction exists or intestinal perforation is suspected. Severe allergy to iodine is the only contraindication to oral iodine-containing preparations.

❍   **T/F: IV contrast material is contraindicated in chronic renal failure.**

False. The contrast material can be dialyzed, and the kidney is already maximally impaired.

❍   **The magnetic fields of a MRI can be detrimental to patients with what?**

Ferrous metal in their body or electrical equipment whose function can be disrupted by strong magnetic fields. Examples include pacemakers, metal foreign bodies in the eye (welders, sheet metal workers, artists who work with metal, etc.), ferromagnetic cerebral aneurysm clips (unless they are made of nonmagnetic steel), and cochlear implants. Relative contraindications for a MRI include: certain prosthetic heart valves, implantable defibrillators, bone growth, and neurostimulators. One might also include patients who are claustrophobic.

❍   **Technetium 99m-labeled studies of the gallbladder are viewed every 10 minutes for 1 hour. If the gallbladder is not visualized at 1 hour, what does this signify?**

Either complete obstruction of the cystic duct due to inflammation and stones (acute cholecystitis) or partial obstruction with a slow filling rate (due to scarring). Delayed images up to 4 hours are obtained to rule out the latter possibility (chronic cholecystitis).

❍   **Although bone scans are useful for detecting subtle fractures missed on x-ray, why is it not always useful in the emergent setting for recent fractures?**

Skeletal uptake is dependent on blood flow and osteoblastic activity; thus, a bone scan may not pick up the increased bone turnover until hours or days after trauma. A positive scan demonstrates asymmetric skeletal uptake.

O   **Which two studies can detect testicular torsion and differentiate it from epididymitis, orchitis, or torsion of the appendix testis?**

Technetium 99m nuclear studies and duplex ultrasound.

O   **What is the order of ossification centers in the elbow?**

Remember the acronym CRITOE. Capitellum, Radial Head, Internal (medial) epicondyle, Trochlea, Olecranon, External (lateral) epicondyle. These ossify ad 3-5-7-9-11-13 years, in that order. Considerable variation to these ages range, but the order of ossification is usually consistent.

O   **How much radiation exposure does a chest x-ray pose?**

5-10 rad.

O   **How much radiation exposure do we get per year from the environment (in rads)?**

Typically, between 300-360 rad/year.

O   **What are the radiographic clues to necrotizing enterocolitis (NEC)?**

Abdominal distention, pneumatosis intestinalis and hepatic portal venous gas. The latter two are felt to be pathognomonic for this entity.

STATISTICS AND PREVENTIVE PEARLS

○ **What infant immunization is most likely to cause a reaction in infants receiving standard immunizations?**

The pertussis component of the DTP. Minor reactions (local induration and pain, mild fever) occur in 75% of children who receive the vaccine. This is the most common reaction, though reactions can be as severe as shock, encephalopathy and convulsions.

○ **Differentiate between the Sabin and Salk vaccines.**

Both prevent polio; the Sabin (OPV) is a live, attenuated trivalent poliovirus. The Salk (IPV) is an inactivated trivalent vaccine.

○ **When is it appropriate to screen the population for a disease?**

When the disease is prevalent, when failure to catch the disease results in significant morbidity, when appropriate screening tests exist, and when therapy initiated due to the early detection will significantly alter the pattern of the disease.

○ **Matching:**

1. Sensitive.
2. Specific.
3. Positive predictive value.
4. Negative predictive value.

a. Actual positives/total number of positive test results.
b. Actual positives/total number with the disease.
c. Actual negatives/total number without the disease.
d. Actual negatives/total number of negative test results.

Answers: (1) b, (2) c, (3) a, and (4) d.
Sensitivity = $a/(a + c)$; Specificity = $d/(b + d)$; Positive predictive value = $a/(a + b)$; Negative predictive value = $d/(c + d)$.

○ **Give the equation for prevalence of a disease.**

Prevalence is the incidence of a disease multiplied by the duration of the disease.

○ **Define crude death rate.**

Crude death rate = (deaths in 1 year/population in same year) x 1,000.

○ **Define infant mortality rate.**

Infant mortality rate = (infant deaths in 1 year/live births in same year) x 1,000 (Infants = ≤ 1 year.).

○ **Define fetal mortality rate.**

Fetal mortality rate = (stillbirths in 1 year/live births in same year) x 1,000.

○ **Define neonatal death rate.**

Neonatal death rate = (the number of newborn deaths in 1 year/live births in same year) x 1,000. (Newborn = infant < 1 month.)

O   **If a population doubles in 35 years, what is its annual rate of increase?**

2%. An easy approximation for the annual rate of increase is the number of years it takes a population to double = 70 divided by the annual percentage increase of the population. The rate of population increase is the difference between the crude birth and death rates.

O   **Define Null hypothesis.**

The assumption that an inconsistency between two groups is due to chance instead of different conditions.

O   **Differentiate between type I and type II errors.**

Type I errors reject the Null hypothesis when it is true. Type II errors accept the null hypothesis when it is false.

O   **Define alternative hypothesis.**

The assumption that a real difference—that is, not one due to chance—exists. This is the hypothesis accepted when the Null hypothesis is rejected.

O   **What is variance, and how does it relate to standard deviation (SD)?**

Variance is the sum of the squares of the distance from the mean. SD = the square root of the variance.

O   **What is the difference between the standard error of the mean (SEM) and the standard deviation (SD)?**

SEM tells the uncertainty in the estimation of the mean. It represents the mean value of a collection of several sample means and is thus closer to the true mean of a population. The SD measures the variability in a given population.

O   **What test should be used to determine whether people who smoke are more likely to develop lung cancer than people who don't?**

Chi-square test would be most appropriate. A chi-square test is used to test qualitative data and tells how the frequencies of each group differ from the frequencies that we would expect to find if there were no relationship between the groups. The greater the difference between two groups, the lower the chi-square number.

O   **What is the equation for chi-square?**

$$X^2 = \Sigma \frac{(observed\ number\ -\ expected\ number)\ 2}{expected\ number}$$

O   **What is a retrospective study?**

A study in which people that have a disease are compared to those who don't.

O   **Three-hundred hypertensive patients are randomly assigned to 3 groups. Each group is given a separate treatment plan, and the results are recorded. What is the best statistical analysis method to use in this situation?**

Analysis of variance is the appropriate method when comparing two or more sample means.

○   **Fifty obese children are randomly divided into two groups. One group follows diet A for 3 months; the other group follows diet B for the same amount of time. What is the best statistical method for comparing the results of these two groups?**

The *t*-test. It is also good to use when dealing with small sample sizes.

○   **Why would you use a correlation coefficient?**

Correlation coefficient is best used when comparing the degree of linear relationship between two variables.

○   **Match the prevention with the example that fits.**

1. Primary prevention   a. Tetanus booster shots every 10 years
2. Secondary prevention   b. Controlling blood sugar with appropriate diet and insulin
3. Tertiary prevention   c. Identifying and treating a patient with asymptomatic
                                  diabetes mellitus.

Answers: (1) a, (2) c, and (3) b.

Primary prevention prevents a disease from ever occurring.

Secondary prevention prevents future problems if actions are taken during an asymptomatic period.

Tertiary prevention prevents further complications in a disease that is already present.

○   **What is the difference between Medicaid and Medicare?**

Medicaid is a need-based governmental entitlement that includes food stamps, Aid to Families with Dependent Children, Medicaid (financial assistance for medical bills), Medicare, Social Security, Disability, Supplemental Security Income, and Workers Compensation.

Medicare is the division of Medicaid based solely on age.

○   **What immunizations are recommended for a teenage patient with HIV?**

1. IPV and Td every 10 years.
2. Influenza vaccine yearly.
3. Pneumococcal vaccine once.
4. Hepatitis B vaccine for at risk patients.
5. Hib and MMR are optional.

○   **At what point should AZT treatment begin in an asymptomatic patient with HIV?**

When the CD-4+ count reaches 300 cells/mm^3 and 500 cells/mm^3, respectively.

○   **What is the prophylactic regime of choice for PCP in patients with AIDS?**

Trimethoprim-sulfamethoxazole DS should be started when the CD-4+ count reaches 200 cells/mm^3.

○   **At what point should prophylaxis treatment against Mycobacterium acium-intracellulare and toxoplasmosis be started in patients with AIDS?**

When the CD-4+ count reaches 100 cells/mm^3.

○   **What percentage of untreated group A *ß-hemolytic streptococcal* infections will progress to rheumatic fever?**

3%. Increased incidence of the disease is noted in lower socioeconomic areas.

❍   **In what age group is post streptococcal glomerulonephritis <u>most</u> <u>common</u>?**

Peak incidence is between ages 3 and 7.

❍   **What percentage of poisons have antidotes?**

5%.

❍   **In the US, what is the major source of typhoid fever?**

Overseas travel. 62% of the cases are contracted this way.

❍   **What must be checked in a patient with Down syndrome before medical clearance can be given for participation in sports?**

Atlantoaxial instability should be ruled out by means of cervical roentgenograms. 10–20% of children with Down syndrome have unstable atlantoaxial joints.

❍   **What is appropriate preventive immunization for a child with sickle cell anemia?**

Children with sickle-cell disease should receive all required immunizations, plus *Haemophilus B* conjugate, Hepatitis B immunization, and a pneumococcal vaccine. They should also take a folic acid supplements and prophylactic penicillin V until the age of 3.

❍   **When should you first check a child's blood lead level?**

At 1–2 years. By this age, children are mobile and can easily find tasty paint chips and other lead based objects.

❍   **What is used to control outbreaks of meningococcal meningitis?**

Rifampin and ceftriaxone are used as chemoprophylaxis for contacts. A vaccine for groups A, C, Y, and W-135 is available and widely used even though most outbreaks are caused by strains A, B, C, and W-135.

❍   **Geographically, where is multiple sclerosis most prevalent?**

In the northern US. Migration to warmer climates does not seem to affect the disease. People born in the north will still have a higher incidence of the disease.

❍   **A teenage girl is going on a summer trip to Benin, on the West Coast of Africa. What immunizations and prophylactic treatments must she receive before departing?**

1. Hepatitis A vaccine.
2. Oral polio vaccine.
3. Tetanus-diptheria vaccine.
4. Live oral typhoid vaccine.
5. Measles vaccine.
6. Yellow fever vaccine.
7. Mefloquine prophylaxis for malaria.

❍   **What is the incubation period of the Epstein–Barr virus?**

30–50 days.

❍   **Why is it important to identify food service workers with furunculosis?**

Furunculosis is most commonly caused by coagulase-positive Staphylococcus. Staphylococcal enterotoxin is a leading cause of food poisoning.

○ **How can ingestion of benzene—an ingredient in pesticides, detergent, and paint remover—be identified as a causative agent in illnesses such as dermatitis, leukemia, and aplastic anemia?**

Phenol, the metabolite, can be found in the urine.

○ **Which has a longer incubation period in food poisoning, Staphylococcus or Salmonella?**

Salmonella. It is generally ingested in small doses, then it multiplies in the GI tract. Symptoms occur 6–48 hours after ingestion. With Staphylococcus, the disease process is dependent not on the reproduction of the organism within the host, but rather on the enterotoxin it has already produced on the contaminated food.

○ **Name 7 risk factors for malignant melanoma.**

1. Fair skin
2. Sensitivity to sunlight
3. Excessive exposure to the sun
4. Dysplastic moles
5. 6 or more moles >.5 cm
6. Prior basal or squamous cell carcinoma
7. Parental history of skin cancer

Basal and squamous cell carcinomas are slow growing tumors that rarely metastasize.

○ **What percentage of melanomas occur in sun–exposed areas?**

Only 65%! A good screen of all surface area is important. In African–American, Hispanic, and Asian patients, acral lentiginous melanomas are more common. Careful examination of subungual, palmar, and plantar surfaces is important in these populations.

○ **What percentage of obesity can be attributed to genetic causes?**

25–30%.

○ **What percentage of obesity can be attributed to organic causes?**

1%.

○ **What disease is found only in obese individuals?**

Pickwickian syndrome. This syndrome involves hypoventilation, right ventricular failure, secondary polycythemia, and somnolence. Symptoms improve with weight loss.

○ **How high is the risk factor of sudden death in morbidly obese patients when compared to patients with normal body weight?**

15–30 times higher.

○ **What surgical procedures may be considered in the morbidly obese?**

A gastroplasty or gastric bypass may be considered to decrease obesity (conservative measures such as diet and exercise should, of course, be attempted before surgery is considered).

○ **When is the peak incidence of *H. influenzae* meningitis?**

6–7 months. 90% of *H. influenzae* cases occur before the age of 5.

○   **Immunocompromised patients can safely be given which vaccines?**

Killed or inactivated vaccines are safe for immunocompromised patients. The vaccines listed below all fit that criteria.

1. Diphtheria
2. *H. Influenzae*
3. Influenza
4. Pneumococcal
5. Enhanced inactivated polio
6. Hepatitis
7. Pertussis
8. Tetanus

○   **Which vaccines should immunocompromised patients avoid?**

Oral polio and MMR.

○   **Aside from those who are immunocompromised, which patients should not receive live vaccines?**

Pregnant women should not receive live viruses, especially MMR (due to the teratogenic potential). Oral polio should be avoided in anyone in close contact with an immunocompromised person because of the virus's ability to spread.

○   **Can you administer vaccinations to a patient who has a URI and a fever of 37.5°C?**

Yes. URI or gastrointestinal illness is not contraindications to vaccination. Fever may be as high as 38°C and the vaccine still administered. Likewise, use of antibiotics or recent exposure to illness is not a reason to delay vaccination.

○   **How many millimeters indicate a positive reaction to the Mantoux skin test in a person with HIV?**

≥ 5 mm. In individuals with risk factors for TB, induration must be ≥ 10 mm. For those with no risk factors, induration must be ≥ 15 mm to be positive.

○   **Influenza epidemics and pandemics are generally associated with which strain of influenza?**

Influenza A.

○   **Amantadine is 70–90% effective in preventing which strain of influenza?**

Influenza A. Amantadine should be prescribed as chemoprophylaxis in immunocompromised patients who are not vaccinated, or as a supplement to vaccination. It can also be given to healthy, unvaccinated people who want to avoid the flu.

○   **When should the influenza vaccine be given?**

In September or October, about 1–2 months before flu season begins. The vaccine, unlike amantadine, is protective against influenza A and B.

○   **What is a contraindication to the administration of the influenza vaccine?**

A history of anaphylactic hypersensitivity to eggs or their products.

○   **In which ethnic group is diabetes most common?**

Hispanics. The prevalence in Hispanics is 1.7–2.4 times higher than in non-Hispanics; the death rate is also twice as high. Reasons for the high rate of disease in this group is attributed to increased incidence of obesity and hyperinsulinemia.

O **What percentage of patients with gonococcal genital infections have concomitant *Chlamydia trachomatous* infections?**

45%. This is why treatment for gonorrhea includes ceftriaxone and doxycycline to cover both infections.

O **A female with condyloma acuminata is how many times more likely to develop cervical cancer than a female without this lesion?**

4 times more likely. These women should have yearly Pap smears and be screened for other STDs.

O **What are the risk factors for hernias?**

Conditions that chronically increase intraabdominal pressure, such as obesity, heavy lifting, chronic cough, constipation, tumors, pregnancy, and ascites.

O **Which nutritional deficiencies may lead to apthous ulcers?**

B12, folate, and iron deficiencies.

O **What is the ratio of attempted suicides to completed suicides?**

10:1.

O **What is the number one cause of death for African-American males between the ages of 10 and 24?**

Firearm injury. The overall homicide rate for young men in the US is over 7 times that of the next developed country. For Hispanic males, the rate is 10 times higher; for African-American males, the rate is over 30 times higher than in comparable countries.

O **Do intentional or unintentional causes account for more firearm-related deaths?**

Intentional, which account for 94% (with subcategories of suicide = 48%, and homicide = 46%). Unintentional firearm injuries account for about 5%. Only 1% of firearm deaths occur as a result of legal intervention. The number of firearm-related fatalities has more than doubled over the last 30 years.

O **What are some risk factors for homicide?**

Most homicide victims are killed by someone they know, someone of the same race, and usually during an argument or fight. Drugs and alcohol are important co-factors, as is the presence of a handgun.

O **What are the relative risks for suicide and homicide if a gun is kept in the home?**

If there is a gun in the home, a suicide is 5 times more likely to occur (9 times more likely if a loaded handgun is available). A homicide is 3 times more likely to occur, and the victim is 43% more likely to be a member of the family than an intruder. In the case of domestic violence, a gun at home increases the risk of homicide 20 fold.

O **What is the clinical significance of the increased availability of semi-automatic weapons?**

Between 1982 and 1992, the percentage of gunshot victims with multiple gunshot wounds increased from 5% to 20%. The rate of spinal cord injuries from GSWs quadrupled. This trend has resulted in an increased number of major organ injuries, complications, and surgeries, as well as in a greater severity of injury and a higher probability of death.

○   **In addition to the history, physical, laboratory tests, and collection of physical evidence, what else needs to be done in a case of sexual abuse of a child?**

File a report with child protective services and law enforcement agencies. Provide emotional support to the child and family. Give a return appointment for follow-up of STD cultures and testing for pregnancy, HIV, or syphilis, as indicated. Assure follow-up for psychological counseling by connecting the child/family to the appropriate services in your area.

○   **If the predictive value positive of a laboratory test for some infectious disease is 70%, what is the chance that a person with a positive test actually has the disease?**

70%.

○   **For a test with given sensitivity and specificity, what population parameter influences the predictive value of the test?**

Prevalence of the disease within the population. Increases in disease prevalence will increase the positive predictive value and decrease the negative predictive value.

○   **What is the negative predictive value of a test?**

The chance that a person with a negative test actually does not have the disease.

○   **What is the minimum recommended age for administration of measles, mumps and rubella (MMR) vaccine in the United States?**

12 months.

○   **There are two types of polio vaccine licensed for administration in the United States: oral and intramuscular. Which one carries a risk of vaccine-induced poliomyelitis?**

Oral polio vaccine, which is a live attenuated vaccine. The intramuscular vaccine is inactivated.

○   **What illnesses are more likely to occur among children exposed to second-hand tobacco smoke, compared to children not exposed?**

Asthma, pneumonia, bronchitis, otitis media, pharyngitis, and possibly meningitis.

○   **How many months must elapse between the third and fourth DPT immunizations in the recommended childhood immunization schedule?**

6 months.

○   **Children should ride in approved car seats until they are at least how many pounds?**

40 pounds.

○   **Which type of study design is least likely to produce biased results?**

Double blinded randomized prospective clinical trial.

○   **Which type of study design selects individuals with a disease and compares their exposures to individuals without the disease?**

Case-control study.

O   **Which type of study design selects individuals with some defined exposure and compares their outcomes with individuals who were not exposed?**

Cohort study.

O   **Consider two vaccines, one inactivated and one live attenuated. Which vaccine is more likely to cause fever and rash within 10 days after administration?**

The live attenuated vaccine. Most side effects of inactivated vaccines tend to occur 1-3 days after administration.

O   **To reduce the risk of neural tube defects in their offspring, prospective mothers should assure adequate periconceptional intake of what substance?**

Folic acid.

O   **Which of the following live vaccines should NOT be given to children with asymptomatic HIV infection: OPV or Measles?**

Oral polio virus vaccine is contraindicated. Routine measles vaccination is recommended for those with asymptomatic HIV infection.

O   **You are seeing an asymptomatic 12-year-old child who recently immigrated from a refugee camp in tropical Africa. The child's PPD skin test shows 8 mm induration. Should you order a chest radiograph?**

Yes. PPD reactions greater than 5 mm in duration are considered positive in recent immigrants from tuberculosis endemic countries, regardless of BCG vaccine history.

O   **You are seeing a child with recurrent episodes of otitis media and cough. What environmental exposure history should you elicit?**

Exposure to cigarette smoke in the household.

O   **What is the drug of choice for prophylaxis of most household contacts of a child with meningococcal meningitis?**

Rifampin or Zithromax.

O   **What is the principal vector for Lyme disease in the northeastern United States?**

The black-legged tick, also known as the "deer tick", Ixodes scapularis.

O   **The results of a double-blinded randomized clinical trial are reported as the risk of adverse events among treated patients divided by the risk of adverse events among patients who received placebo. What is this measure called?**

Relative risk.

O   **An asymptomatic one year-old child presents for her first health care maintenance visit since she was 2 months old. She has been living in a deteriorated apartment building in a small city in New England. What screening blood test should you order?**

Blood lead level.

○   An 8 year-old boy has recently acquired a pet iguana. This may place the household at increased risk of what disease?

Salmonellosis.

○   A 15 month-old child who has not yet received MMR vaccine recently received immunoglobulin to prevent hepatitis A (postexposure prophylaxis). What is the suggested interval before measles vaccination?

3 months.

○   Regular physical activity reduces risk of several diseases. Name three of these.

Cardiovascular disease, hypertension, non-insulin dependent diabetes.

○   You receive laboratory confirmation of hepatitis A infection in an 18 month old child who attends day care. What is recommended to prevent further spread of the infection?

Immune globulin .02 ml/kg to all susceptible day care contacts.

○   What is the minimum interval required between oral polio virus doses?

4 weeks, but preferably 6 weeks.

○   How many doses of varicella vaccine are recommended for adolescents 13 years and older?

2 doses at least 4 weeks apart.

○   What are three modifiable risk factors for sudden infant death syndrome (SIDS).

Prone sleeping position, maternal smoking, lack of breastfeeding.

○   What are three health consequences of iron deficiency anemia.

Reduced resistance to infection, fatigue, decreased intellectual performance.

○   What are four health consequences of childhood obesity.

Hypertension, hyperinsulinemia, low self-esteem, increased adult mortality.

○   What are six risk factors for perinatal Group B streptococcal disease.

Prematurity, prolonged rupture of membranes, maternal GBS colonization, intrapartum fever, maternal black race, maternal age < 20 years.

○   What type of study compares the costs of different interventions with the health outcomes of each intervention?

Cost-effectiveness study.

○   What type of study compares the net monetary costs with net monetary savings of different interventions?

Cost-benefit study.

○   Perinatal administration of zidovudine (ZDV) to HIV-infected mothers and their newborns has been shown to reduce risk of perinatal HIV transmission by how much?

About two-thirds (from 24% down to about 8%).

○ **Bicycle helmets appear to reduce the risk of bicycle-related head injury by about how much?**

80%.

○ **From 1970 to 1990, have suicide rates among adolescents aged 15-19 in the United States increased, decreased, or stayed the same?**

Increased. From 5.9 to 11.1 per 100,000.

○ **Give two characteristics of news stories about suicide that might increase suicide contagion.**

Simplistic explanations of suicide, describing technical details of suicide, glorifying the person that committed suicide.

○ **What proportion of high-school aged adolescents in the United States smoke or use smokeless tobacco?**

About 33%.

○ **What intervention at a national and state level has significantly reduced cigarette smoking?**

The increase of cigarette price.

○ **What is the principle vector for malaria?**

Anopheles mosquitoes.

○ **What is the principal vector for yellow fever and dengue fever?**

Aedes aegypti mosquitoes.

○ **Which of the above two types of mosquitoes are more likely to breed in swamps?**

Anopheles breed in swamps. Aedes aegypti breed primarily in peridomestic water containers.

○ **What is the principal route of transmission of schistosomiasis?**

Skin contact with lakes or rivers that are infested with schistosomes.

○ **What are three clinical manifestations of kwashiorkor (severe protein malnutrition)?**

Fatigue, edema, dermatitis, sparse and reddened or grayish hair.

○ **Should MMR vaccine be given intramuscularly, subcutaneously, or intradermally?**

Subcutaneously.

○ **You are seeing a two-month old child whose 5 year-old brother is immunodeficient. Should you administer OPV (oral poliovirus vaccine) to the two-month old?**

No. Administer IPV.

○ **Can MMR vaccine be safely administered to a child who has developed a non-anaphylactic mild red rash after eating eggs?**

Yes.

❍   **What approximate proportion of American 16 year-olds are sexually active?**

50%

❍   **In the United States, can a minor be treated for a sexually transmitted disease without parental consent?**

Yes.

❍   **You have just diagnosed syphilis in a 17 year-old girl. After assuring appropriate patient education and treatment, what should you do next?**

Notify public health department for contact tracing and treatment.

❍   **To conduct a survey, a sample of high school students is obtained by selecting every 10th student from an alphabetically ordered school enrollment list. Is this a random sample?**

No. It is a systematic sample.

❍   **You are considering ordering a diagnostic test for some disease. You determine the probability of a positive test among individuals with the disease and the probability of a positive test among those without the disease. What is the ratio of these probabilities called?**

The likelihood ratio.

❍   **For a given test, you determine that the pretest probability of the disease is exactly the same as the posttest probability of disease. What is the likelihood ratio for this test?**

LR = 1

❍   **You obtain a positive result of a test that has a likelihood ratio greater than 1. Is the posttest probability of the disease higher or lower than the pretest probability?**

Higher.

❍   **What is the leading cause of death among infants (less than one year of age) in the United States?**

Congenital anomalies.

❍   **Injuries accounted for 4% of infant deaths in the United States in 1995. What was the leading cause of injury deaths among these infants?**

Suffocation.

❍   **What is the leading cause of death among children aged 1 - 14 years in the United States?**

Motor vehicle traffic injuries.

❍   **What is the most important factor for reducing infectious disease transmission in day care centers?**

Hand-washing.

○ **You have diagnosed an E coli O157:H7 infection in an 18 month old child who attends day care. When should you allow the child to return to day care?**

After diarrhea resolves and two stool cultures are negative.

○ **A 4-year-old child who attends day care has impetigo. When should the child be allowed to return to day care?**

24 hours after treatment has been initiated.

○ **A 4-year-old child who attends day care has streptococcal pharyngitis. When should this child be allowed to return to day care?**

24 hours after treatment has been initiated and after the child has been afebrile for 24 hours.

○ **A three-year-old girl has varicella. When should she be allowed to return to day care?**

6 days after the onset of the rash or sooner if all lesions have dried and crusted.

○ **A 15-month-old boy has a mild case of hepatitis A. When should he be allowed to return to day care?**

1 week after onset of illness or jaundice.

○ **Should an immunocompetent child with erythema infectiosum (Parvovirus B19 infection) be excluded from day care?**

No. Little or no virus is present in respiratory secretions by the time that the erythema infectiosum rash appears.

○ **Can a PPD skin test for tuberculosis infection be planted the same day that you administer measles vaccine?**

Yes.

○ **If a PPD skin test and measles vaccine are not administered on the same day, how long after measles vaccination should you wait before administering the PPD skin test?**

4 to 6 weeks.

○ **A friend of yours tells you his wife has caught "a bad case of the flu", with all the typical signs and symptoms. He is concerned that he and their children will catch it, and they want to avoid that. What can they do to prevent catching it?**

Wash your hands frequently, avoid toughing your face, and maintain a healthy diet.

○ **What medications can help prevent the "flu"?**

The new flu drugs oseltamivir (Tamiflu) and zanamivir (Relenza) have recently been approved for preventing, as well as treating, the flu. Other health remedies, such as Zinc, Echinacea, and vitamin C may help decrease the duration of symptoms.

LEGAL PEARLS

○   **In general, do minors have the right to give consent for their own treatment?**

No--this right belongs to their parents or guardians.

○   **In an emergency, is it necessary to obtain consent in order to treat a child?**

No.

○   **May a child who lives away from home, is no longer subject to parental control, is economically self-supporting, is married, or is a member of the armed forces give or refuse consent to treatment?**

In general, yes. Such children are considered *emancipated minors.*

○   **May a child who is sufficiently mature to understand the nature of his/her illness and the potential risks and benefits of proposed therapy give or refuse consent to treatment?**

In general, yes. Such children are considered *mature minors.*

○   **Are there other circumstances in which a child has the right to give informed consent to treatment?**

Yes--many states have laws giving children such rights for treatment of sexually transmitted or other communicable diseases, crisis counseling, or substance abuse.

○   **What are the physician's legal obligations where a minor child requests that information obtained in the course of treatment not be communicated to the child's parents?**

In the absence of circumstances such as those outlined in the preceding questions, the physician may not legally honor such a request.

○   **Does an adolescent have the right to obtain an abortion without parental consent?**

This varies by state.

○   **May a child less than 18 years of age donate blood?**

No, except in Delaware where the age requirement is 17 years.

○   **May a physician become directly involved in the private placement of a child with adoptive parents?**

This depends on the state.

○   **May a physician inform an adopted child of the identity of its natural parents?**

In general, no--such information is confidential.

○   **May a minor serve as an organ donor without parental consent?**

No.

○   **If parental consent exists, may a child serve as an organ donor if there is an alternative adult donor?**

In general, no.

○   **If there is parental consent, and no alternative adult donor, may a child serve as an organ donor if the transplant is not necessary to save the life of the recipient?**

In general, no.

○   **Are there any other requirements that must be met for a child to serve as an organ donor?**

Yes--it must be determined that the child will not suffer as a result of the procedure.

○   **Does this include only physical suffering?**

No--the likelihood of either physical or psychological harm is sufficient to preclude a child's organ donation.

○   **May Jehovah's Witness parents refuse blood transfusions for their minor children?**

No.

○   **May parents be criminally prosecuted if their child dies because they treated the child with prayer rather than with medicine?**

Yes, in some jurisdictions.

○   **May treatment be withheld from severely defective neonates?**

It varies by state.

○   **May parents authorize removal of life support for a minor child in a persistent vegetative state?**

Yes.

○   **Is it legally mandatory to screen newborns for PKU?**

It varies by state.

○   **Under what circumstances might this be possible?**

First of all, an IRB must determine that the risk is justified by the potential benefit.

○   **What if there is an existing available treatment that poses a lesser risk to the child?**

The child may not serve as a research subject.

○   **From whom must consent be obtained in order for a child to serve as a research subject?**

From the child and at least one parent.

❍   **Must an initial adversary hearing be provided when a minor is committed involuntarily by his/her parents to a mental institution?**

This is not constitutionally required, but some states provide for an administrative hearing for minors over a certain age if they object to being institutionalized.

❍   **Do adult brain death criteria apply to children?**

Yes, except for premature newborns and all infants less than seven days old.

❍   **Is it legally required for a physician who suspects child abuse or neglect to report it?**

Yes.

❍   **Is reporting required only for suspected physical abuse?**

No--emotional abuse, sexual abuse, and other forms of abuse are covered by reporting statutes.

❍   **May a parent's refusal to authorize indicated medical treatment be considered child neglect for purposes of the reporting statute?**

Yes.

❍   **May a physician suffer a penalty for failure to report suspected abuse, neglect, or endangerment?**

Yes.

❍   **May a physician be sued by a child or family for failing to report suspected abuse, neglect, or endangerment?**

Yes.

❍   **What would it take for the child or family to win such a suit?**

They must show that the failure to report contributed significantly to a subsequent injury that might have been averted.

❍   **May a physician be sued for defamation based on her/his report of suspected abuse, neglect, or endangerment?**

No, if the report was made in good faith.

❍   **May mothers who engage in substance abuse while pregnant be the subject of criminal prosecution?**

No--such prosecutions have been brought but not upheld.

❍   **May a child bring suit for injuries that were sustained *in utero*?**

Yes.

❍   **In order for a physician to be guilty of malpractice, must the existence of a physician-patient relationship be proven?**

Yes.

❍ **What is medical negligence?**

Acting below the accepted standard of care.

❍ **Is a physician legally required to do what the best specialist in the field would do?**

No--only what a typical reasonable competent physician would do under the circumstances.

❍ **In order for a physician to be found guilty of malpractice, must it be shown that the patient was injured?**

Yes.

❍ **In order for a physician to be found guilty of malpractice, must it be shown that the patient's injury was caused by the physician's act or omission?**

Yes.

❍ **May a physician be held legally liable for the negligence of workers whom the physician employs?**

Yes.

❍ **May a physician disclose the content of a medical record to someone other than a patient (or, in the case of a minor or ward, to the patient's parent or guardian)?**

In general, no--but there are exceptions.

❍ **May a physician disclose the content of a medical record to another health care professional in the regular course of treatment?**

Yes.

❍ **May a physician disclose the content of a medical record under a court order?**

Yes--indeed, the physician is required to do so.

❍ **May a physician disclose the content of a child's medical record to school officials who request it?**

In general, no.

❍ **Does a physician-patient relationship exist where the physician is employed by a school, juvenile court, or other agency?**

No.

❍ **What are the consequences for confidentiality of the absence of a physician-patient relationship?**

Where such a relationship does not exist, information the physician obtains is not confidential.

❍ **In artificial insemination by donor (AID), where the mother is married, who is considered the legal father?**

The mother's husband.

❍ **May a physician be found liable for a child's reaction to a vaccine he administers?**

Only if a typical reasonable competent physician would not have acted as the physician did.

RANDOM PEARLS

○   **What signs should be charted when performing a neurological exam on a patient with a suspected anterior dislocation of the shoulder?**

Sensation over the lateral deltoid. In anterior dislocations of the shoulder, the radial nerve may be easily torn. Intact sensation to the lateral deltoid will indicate an intact radial nerve.

○   **What condition does boggy blue turbinates and eosinophils indicate?**

Allergic rhinitis.

○   **What are the major distant sequelae of untreated streptococcal infections?**

Acute glomerulonephritis and rheumatic heart disease.

○   **A patient treated with cyclophosphamide should be monitored every 2–4 weeks for what condition?**

Bone marrow toxicity. Leukopenia is the most common. CBCs should be obtained every 2–4 weeks. Urinalysis is also important for screening hemorrhagic cystitis (cyclophosphamide should be administered in the morning to reduce the amount present in the bladder over night).

○   **Which antibiotic most commonly produces the diarrhea associated with *clostridium difficile*?**

Ampicillin, because it is the most frequently used. Vancomycin and metronidazole are the antibiotic treatments of choice.

○   **Which malignant neoplasm has the highest rate of spontaneous regression?**

Neuroblastoma. This neoplasm occurs predominantly before age six. Although spontaneous rate of regression is high; the overall survival rate is only 30%, due to the spread of the disease before it is detected.

○   **What is the first line of therapy for a migraine headache?**

Ergotamine derivatives. Second line therapies include Sumatriptan (Imitrex), phenothiazine, NSAIDs, and opiates.

○   **What kinds of exercise will most likely trigger an asthma attack in patients with exercise-induced asthma?**

High intensity exercise for more than 5–6 minutes.

○   **A patient recently hit in the eye during a brawl has diplopia when looking up. The injured eye does not appear able to look up. What is the diagnosis?**

Orbital blowout fracture with entrapment of inferior rectus or inferior oblique.

○   **What is the most common joint dislocation?**

Anterior shoulder dislocation. This condition accounts for 1/2 of all joint dislocations. Anterior shoulder dislocations occur with abduction and external rotation.

○ **When estimating vaginal blood loss in the gynecological patient, sanitary pads are often used as a means of measurement. How much blood loss can be estimated per pad?**

20-30 ml.

○ **Which organism is typically associated with CNS involvement in an AIDS patient?**

Toxoplasmosis.

○ **Where are Kaposi's sarcoma lesions usually found?**

Everywhere—both inside and out. This type of lesion typically occurs on the face, neck, arms, back, thighs, and in the lungs, lymphatic system, and the GI system.

○ **How is jaundice diagnosed in an African-American patient?**

African-American patients often have subconjunctival fat that results in a yellowing sclera. In patients where icterus is suspected, it is imperative to examine the edges of the cornea and the posterior hard palate.

○ **How does pallor appear in an African-American patient?**

Yellow/brown or gray skin. This is due to the loss of the underlying red tones. The conjunctiva will appear pale.

○ **What is the most common cause of hypercalcemia?**

Hyperparathyroidism. This condition accounts for 60% of ambulatory hypercalcemics.

○ **What is the most common cause of nongonococcal urethritis?**

Chlamydia trachomatis. Ureaplasma urealyticum is another common cause.

○ **What is the most common clinical manifestation of disseminated gonococcal infection?**

Gonococcal arthritis-dermatitis syndrome. Arthritis, a pustular or papular rash, and tenosynovitis are exhibited with this syndrome.

○ **What is the most common cause of epididymitis?**

Chlamydia trachomatis.

○ **Which bacterial organism most commonly causes epididymitis?**

E. coli.

○ **What is the Jarisch-Herxheimer reaction?**

A reaction of headache, fever, myalgia, hypotension, and increased severity of syphilis symptoms (which occur after taking benzathine penicillin G for the treatment of syphilis). The reaction may also result in neurological, auditory, or visual changes.

○ **Which strain of influenza is more common in adults, and which is more common in children?**

Adults: Influenza A.

Children: Influenza B.

O   **Which strain of influenza is most virulent?**

Influenza A.

O   **What are the four degrees of frostbite?**

First degree: Erythema and edema.
Second degree: Blister formation.
Third degree: Necrosis.
Fourth degree: Gangrene.

O   **A patient with polyuria, a low urine osmolality, and a high serum osmolality is given vasopressin. No change in osmolality is noted. Which type of diabetes insipidus (DI) does she have?**

Nephrogenic.   The distal renal tubules are refractory to antidiuretic hormone; thus, vasopressin will not help either.

O   **Which organism is typically responsible for causing bacterial conjunctivitis?**

Staphylococcus.   The second most common organism is Streptococcus.

O   **A patient presents with a painful eye, blurred vision, and conjunctivitis. On a slit lamp exam, you detect a dendritic ulcer. What is the most likely cause of the patient's symptoms?**

Herpes.   This type of infection probably occurs secondary to corneal abrasions or corticosteroid eye drops. Treatment entails the administration of idoxuridine. If the eye has a bacterial super-infection, then topical antibiotics should be prescribed.

O   **What is the most common cause of portal hypertension in children?**

Extrahepatic portal vein occlusion.

O   **Which virus causes herpangina?**

Coxsackievirus Group A. A sore throat, fever, malaise, and vesicular lesions on the posterior pharynx or the soft palate are often seen with this disease.

O   **A complication of central sleep apnea in a child is:**

Sudden infant death syndrome (SIDS).   Affected children develop morning cyanosis. However, children can be treated with theophylline.

O   **A patient presents with arms extended and fingers spread apart. Her extremities are flexing and extending in a static-kinetic tremor. What disease is this tremor associated with?**

Hyperthyroidism.

O   **Hypovolemia is a major concern when treating a patient with hypernatremia. What is the calculation for determining water deficit?**

$(0.6 \times wt) \times (Na-140)$

O   **Which organisms most often induce lymphedema?**

Staphylococcus or Σ-hemolytic *Streptococcus.*

O   **Cricothyroidotomy is not recommended in children of less than what age?**

10 years.

O   **What is the most common opportunistic infection associated with AIDS?**

PCP. It is the initial opportunistic infection in 60% of AIDS patients, and eventually affects 80%.

O   **What is the most common cause of focal encephalitis in AIDS patients?**

Toxoplasma gondii.

O   **In what part of the airway are foreign bodies usually lodged in children older than 1 year?**

The lower airway.

O   **What is the most probable age of presentation of malrotation in children? What is a common complication, and what signs and symptoms are usually present?**

1) Malrotation usually occurs in children under 12 months of age. Volvulus is a common complication. The signs and symptoms typically include vomiting, blood streaked stools, and abdominal pain.

O   **Name two causes of toxic epidermal necrolysis.**

1. Drug or chemical. The onset of this condition by drug and chemical-related causes typically occurs in adults and is characterized by cleavage at the derma-epidermal junction.
2. Staphylococcal. Bacterial-related SSSS is usually contracted by children < 5 years and results in the an intraepidermal cleavage beneath the stratum granulosum.

O   **Describe the presentation of SSSS.**

This disease begins after URI or purulent conjunctivitis. Initially, the lesions are tender, erythematous, and scarlatiniform and they are usually found on the face, neck, axillae, and groin. Later, the skin peels off in sheets with lateral pressure, and a + Nikolsky's sign is displayed.

O   **Which of the following drugs may not be effective for treating bullous impetigo: erythromycin, amoxicillin, or cefaclor?**

Amoxicillin.

O   **Which nerve is usually injured in glenohumeral dislocation?**

Axillary nerve (numb area over lateral deltoid).

O   **Describe the mechanism and cause of a boutonniere deformity.**

A Boutonniere deformity is secondary to rupture of the extensor apparatus of the PIP joint. The cause of the injury is a PIP joint which is flexed and a DIP joint which is hyperextended. Treat by splinting the PIP joint in full extension.

O   **A cyanotic patient has a low oxygen saturation as measured by ABG. What type of cyanosis does this patient have, central or peripheral?**

Central.

O   **What is a peripheral cyanosis?**

ABG reveals normal oxygen saturation (i.e., shunting or increased O_2 extraction is occurring).

○   **Name the 2 primary types of peripheral cyanosis which have a normal SaO_2?**

Decreased cardiac output and redistribution (may be $2°$ to shock, DIC, hypothermia, vascular obstruction).

○   **What are the 4 causes of central cyanosis with decreased SaO_2?**

1. Decreased PaO_2 or decreased O_2 diffusion.
2. Hypoventilation.
3. V-Q mismatch, pulmonary shunting.
4. Dysfunctional hemoglobin, which includes sickle cell crisis and drug-induced hemoglobinopathies.

N.B. Hb-CO does not cause cyanosis, although the cherry red appearance of skin and mucous membranes can suggest cyanosis.

○   **What is a positive Chvostek's sign?**

Chvostek's sign is characterized by a twitch in the corner of the mouth that occurs when the examiner taps the facial nerve located in front of the ear. It is present in approximately 10–30% of normal individuals. Eyelid muscle contraction resulting from the Chvostek's maneuver is generally indicative of hypocalcemia.

○   **What is Trousseau's sign and when is it exhibited?**

Trousseau's sign is a carpal spasm that is induced when a blood pressure cuff on the upper arm maintains a pressure above systolic for approximately 3 minutes. Fingers become spastically extended at the interphalangeal joints and flexed at the metacarpophalangeal joints. Trousseau's is generally a more reliable indicator of hypocalcemia than the Chvostek's sign.

○   **What is the most common form of anorectal abscess?**

Perianal abscess. Anorectal abscesses are usually mixed infections (i.e., both Gram-negative and anaerobic organisms). Fistula formation is a frequent complication.

○   **What is the most common rhythm disturbance in a pediatric arrest?**

Bradycardia.

○   **How long does it take to prepare type-specific saline cross-matched blood?**

Ten minutes.

○   **Describe the common features of a slipped femoral capital epiphysis.**

Injury usually occurs in adolescence. The rupture typically presents with an insidious development of knee or thigh pain and a painful limp. Frequently hip motion is limited, particularly that of internal rotation. Anteroposterior and frog-leg lateral films of both hips aid evaluation.

○   **Dobutamine administered in moderate doses induces what cardiovascular effects?**

Decreased peripheral resistance, pulmonary occlusive pressure, and inotropic stimulation of the heart.

○   **What are the two most common causes of fatal anaphylaxis?**

1. Drug reactions (95% of which are due to penicillin). Parenteral administration results in the deaths of approximately 300 people/year.
2. Hymenopteran stings cause fatal anaphylaxis in 100 people/year.

❍   **Which type of hypersensitivity reaction is responsible for anaphylaxis?**

Type I (IgE mediated) hypersensitivity reaction. Immediate IgE binds allergen, and stimulate mast cells and basophils. Examples include food allergy and asthma.

❍   **Which organisms produce focal nervous system pathology via an exotoxin?**

Clostridium diphtheria, Clostridium botulinum, Clostridium tetani, Wood and dog tick (Dermacentor A and B), and Staphylococcus aureus.

❍   **Describe botulism intoxication.**

Botulism exotoxin is elaborated by Clostridium botulinum. It affects the myoneural junction and prevents the release of acetylcholine. In the US, it is caused principally by the ingestion of foods that were inadequately prepared. The most common neurologic complaints are related to the bulbar musculature. Neurologic symptoms usually occur within 24–48 hours of ingestion of contaminated foods. Muscle paralysis and weakness typically spread rapidly to involve all muscles of the trunk and extremities. It is important to distinguish between botulism poisoning and myasthenia gravis. Using the edrophonium (Tensilon) test, usually performed by a neurologist, can make this distinction.

❍   **Which test is considered to be the gold standard for determining acute cholecystitis?**

Radionuclide scan of the biliary tree.

❍   **Which test should be performed to confirm the diagnosis of Boerhaave's syndrome?**

An esophagram. A water soluble contrast medium should be used in place of barium to confirm the diagnosis.

❍   **What four pseudonyms are associated with regional enteritis?**

1. Crohn's disease.
2. Terminal ileitis.
3. Regional enteritis.
4. Granulomatous ileocolitis.

❍   **What are the signs and symptoms of Boerhaave's syndrome?**

Substernal and left sided chest pain with a history of forceful vomiting leading to spontaneous esophageal rupture.

❍   **What is the single most common cause of upper GI tract hemorrhage?**

Duodenal ulcers.

❍   **Which layers of the bowel wall and mesentery are affected by regional enteritis?**

Inflammatory reaction of regional enteritis involves all layers of the bowel wall.

❍   **What are Kanavel's four cardinal signs of infectious digital flexor tenosynovitis?**

1. Tenderness along the tendon sheath.
2. Finger held in flexion.
3. Pain on passive extension of the finger.
4. Finger swelling.

○   **What symptoms are associated with presentation of regional enteritis?**

Fever, abdominal pain, weight loss, and diarrhea. Fistulas, fissures, and abscesses may also be noted. Ulcerative colitis, on the other hand, usually presents with bloody diarrhea.

○   **Which organism most commonly causes subacute infectious endocarditis?**

Viridans Streptococcus.

○   **Which valve does subacute bacterial endocarditis (SBE) most commonly affect?**

SBE usually involves the left side of the heart, specifically the mitral valve. The aortic valve is the second most commonly involved valve. Rheumatic fever is the most probable underlying cause of valvular damage associated with SBE. Mitral stenosis is a very common predisposing factor in SBE. Drug addicts tend to develop right-sided SBE, usually involving the tricuspid valve.

○   **Which organism most commonly causes acute infectious endocarditis?**

Staphylococcus aureus.

○   **Describe the skin lesions found in a patient with disseminated gonococcemia.**

Umbilicated pustule with a red halo.

○   **Describe the skin lesions associated with a *Pseudomonas aeruginosa* infection.**

Pseudomonas aeruginosa typically produces pale, erythematous skin lesions that are approximately 1 cm in size with an ulcerated necrotic center (ecthyma gangrenosum).

○   **What is the fundamental cause of sickle cell disease?**

Valine is substituted for glutamic acid in the sixth amino acid of the ß-chain.

○   **Describe the intracorporeal travel of the rabies virus.**

The virus is spread centripetally up the peripheral nerve into the CNS. The incubation period for rabies is usually 30–60 days with a range of 10 days to 1 year. The route of transmission usually occurs via infected secretions, saliva, or by infected tissue. Stages of the disease include upper respiratory tract infection symptomatology, followed by encephalitis. The brainstem is affected last.

○   **A septic appearing child has multiple skin lesions 1 cm in diameter with necrotic, ulcerated centers and erythematous surrounding regions. What is the likely pathogen?**

Pseudomonas aeruginosa.

○   **What is the IM treatment for acute streptococcal pharyngitis?**

1.2 million units of benzathine penicillin G. Use 0.6 million units of benzathine penicillin-G for children weighing less than 27 kg.

○   **What is the most common initial symptom in botulism poisoning?**

Visual disturbances are reported in up to 90% of the cases. Abducent nerve (CN VI) palsy is common, and severe cases may show third cranial nerve involvement with dilated and fixed pupils. Other common initial symptoms include headache, dizziness, weakness, malaise, and a dry mouth. Nausea and vomiting are found in about 35% of the cases. Symptoms usually appear within 24–72 hours after exposure.

O **Describe the signs and symptoms of spinal shock.**

Spinal shock represents complete loss of spinal cord function below the level of injury. Patients have flaccid paralysis, complete sensory loss, areflexia, and loss of autonomic function. Such patients are usually bradycardic, hypotensive, hypothermic, and vasodilated.

O **Active adduction of the thumb tests which nerve?**

Ulnar nerve.

O **Describe the rash that is present with exanthem subitum (roseola).**

The rash is usually found on the trunk and the neck and is maculopapular.

O **What is the most common cause of death among children between 1–12 month(s) old?**

Congenital anomalies.

O **Is GI bleeding common with a perforated ulcer?**

No.

O **What is the most common site of Crohn's disease?**

The ileum. Crohn's disease can actually involve any part of the GI tract from the social end to the antisocial end. It is segmental, often involving granuloma formation along with inflammatory reactions. Crohn's disease has two incidence peaks, one in the 15–22 year old age group and a second in the 55–60 year old age group.

O **What are the signs and symptoms of Crohn's disease?**

Fever, diarrhea, right lower quadrant pain with mass possible, fistulas, rectal prolapse, perianal fissures, and abscesses. Arthritis, uveitis, and liver disease are also associated with this condition.

O **What systemic diseases are associated with Crohn's disease?**

Pyoderma gangrenosum, uveitis, episclerosis, scleritis, arthritis, erythema nodosum, and nephrolithiasis.

O **What contrast x-ray findings are associated with Crohn's disease?**

The segmental involvement in the colon with an abnormal mucosal pattern and fistulas, often without involvement of the rectum. A narrowing of the small intestine may also be displayed.

O **What are the principal signs and symptoms of ulcerative colitis?**

Fever, weight loss, tachycardia, panniculitis, and six bloody bowel movements per day.

O **Does toxic megacolon commonly occur with ulcerative colitis or with Crohn's disease?**

Toxic megacolon is a very common, serious complication of ulcerative colitis.

O **Which medications may be used in the treatment of Crohn's disease but are absolutely contraindicated in the treatment of ulcerative colitis?**

Antidiarrheal agents.

O   **Does cancer more often develop with ulcerative colitis or with Crohn's disease?**

Ulcerative colitis. Think of toxic megacolon and cancer. Avoid antidiarrheal agents.

O   **What are the two most common causes of acute diarrhea?**

Rotavirus and Norwalk agent.

O   **What is the most common cause of diarrhea in a child less than one year old?**

Rotavirus.

O   **Which cause of diarrhea is most commonly associated with seizures?**

Shigella.

O   **What induces rose spots and watery diarrhea, as well as high fever and relative bradycardia?**

Salmonella. This condition is particularly common in IV drug abusers with new pet turtles! .

O   **What is the treatment for individuals infected with *Salmonella*?**

Supportive care without antibiotics. However, if a severe fever is exhibited, antibiotic therapy may be warranted.

O   **Which microbial agents are associated with mesenteric adenitis and pseudoappendicitis?**

Yersinia.

O   **What is the most common food–borne pathogen?**

Staphylococcus. This pathogen produces diarrhea and vomiting within 6–12 hours after ingestion.

O   **Which type of infectious gastroenteritis is associated with the consumption of seafood?**

Vibrio parahaemolyticus.

O   **Which type of diarrhea is perfuse and bloody, but does not involve vomiting?**

Entamoeba histolytica. Diarrhea that is not necessarily bloody and that is associated with contaminated meat may be due to *Clostridium perfringens.*

O   **What is the most common parasitic cause of diarrhea in the US?**

Giardia. Infected individuals presents with foul-smelling, floating stools; abdominal pain; and profuse diarrhea. The parasite may be identified with a positive string test or duodenal aspiration for trophozoites.

O   **What causes the diarrhea commonly seen in AIDS patients?**

Cryptosporidiosis. A positive acid fast stain diagnoses this agent. Patients with this condition present with profuse, watery diarrhea that is not bloody.

O   **What types of defects cause left to right shunt murmurs?**

ASD, VSD, and PDA.

O   **What type of defect produces diminished pulses in the lower extremities of a pediatric patient?**

Coarctation of the aorta.

❍   **Which fairly common conditions produce cardiac syncope in pediatrics?**

Aortic stenosis, which is not cyanotic, and tetralogy of Fallot, which is.

❍   **What are the signs and symptoms of aortic stenosis in a child?**

Exercise intolerance, chest pain, and a systolic ejection click with a crescendo, decrescendo murmur
radiating to the neck with a suprasternal thrill. No cyanosis!

❍   **What are the signs of left-sided heart failure in an infant?**

Increased respiratory rate, shortness of breath, and sweating during feeding.

❍   **What is the single most common cause of CHF in the second week of life?**

Coarctation of the aorta.

❍   **What is the most common cause of impetigo?**

Group A *ß-hemolytic streptococcus.*

❍   **What is the most common cause of bullous impetigo?**

Staphylococcus aureus.

❍   **What is the most common cause of orbital infections?**

Staphylococcus aureus. Periorbital infections are usually caused by *H. influenzae.*

❍   **What is the most common cause of pediatric bacteremia?**

Streptococcus pneumonia.

❍   **A patient presents with a staccato cough and a history of conjunctivitis in the first few weeks
after birth. What causes this type of pneumonia?**

Chlamydia trachomatis.

❍   **What is the most common cause of viral pneumonia in the pediatric patient?**

RSV.

❍   **What is the most common type of asthma in children?**

Extrinsic asthma which is a type I. An immediate hypersensitivity reaction mediated by IgE is induced by
this condition. Common causes include molds and pet dander.

❍   **How do steroids function in the treatment of asthma?**

Steroids increase cAMP, decrease inflammation, and aid in restoring the function of ß-adrenergic
responsiveness to adrenergic drugs.

❍   **Which two viral illnesses are prodromes for Reye syndrome?**

Varicella (chicken pox) and influenzae B.

○   **What are the signs and symptoms of Reye syndrome?**

Irritability, combativeness, and lethargy, right upper quadrant tenderness, history of influenzae B or recent chicken pox, papilledema, hypoglycemia, and seizures. Lab results reveal hypoglycemia, an ammonia level greater than 20 times normal, and a bilirubin level that is normal.

○   **Describe the five stages of Reye syndrome.**

Stage I: Vomiting, lethargy, and liver dysfunction.
Stage II: Disorientation, combativeness, delirium, hyperventilation, increased deep tendon reflexes, liver dysfunction, hyperexcitable, tachypnea, fever, tachycardia, sweating, and pupillary dilatation.
Stage III: Coma, decorticate rigidity, increased respiratory rate, and a mortality rate of 50%.
Stage IV: Coma, decerebrate posturing, no ocular reflexes, loss of corneal reflexes, and liver damage.
Stage V: Loss of deep tendon reflexes, seizures, flaccidity, respiratory arrest, and 95% mortality.

○   **What are the first, second, and third drugs of choice for the treatment of seizures in children?**

First: Phenobarbital
Second: Phenytoin
Third: Carbamazepine.

○   **What hormones are produced by the adrenal cortex?**

Mineralocorticoids, glucocorticoids, and androgenic steroids. Remember: salt, sugar, and sex.

○   **What is the major mineralocorticoid?**

Aldosterone. Aldosterone is regulated by the renin angiotensin system; it increases sodium reabsorption and K^+ excretion.

○   **What is the major glucocorticoid?**

Cortisol.

○   **What hormones are produced by the medulla of the adrenal gland?**

Epinephrine and norepinephrine.

○   **What are the typical ECG results of patients with Addison's disease?**

Because of the hyperkalemia, expect peaked T-waves.

○   **What key lab results are expected with SIADH?**

Low serum sodium levels and high urine sodium levels (i.e., > 30).

○   **If a lesion is in the right hemisphere, which way will the eyes deviate?**

The eyes will deviate toward the lesion.

○   **If there is a lesion in the brain stem, which way will the eyes deviate?**

Away from the lesion in the brain stem.

○   **Where is the most common intraparenchymal site of intracranial bleeding?**

The putamen.

○   **In the pediatric esophagus, where is a foreign body <u>most</u> <u>commonly</u> lodged.**

The cricopharyngeal narrowing.

○   **Do household pets transmit *Yersinia*?**

Yes, especially puppies.

○   **What is the most common cause of an urinary tract infection in a female child?**

E. coli.

○   **What is the first line of treatment for a seizing five year old?**

Phenobarbital.

○   **What is the most common cause of intrinsic renal failure?**

Acute tubular necrosis.

○   **What is the most common cause of cardiac arrest in an uremic patient?**

Hyperkalemia.

○   **What is the most common cause of right sided endocarditis in IV drug addicts?**

Staphylococcus aureus.

○   **Which valve is the usually affected in IV drug addicts?**

The tricuspid.

○   **What is the most common cause of osteomyelitis or septic arthritis in an IV drug addict?**

Serratia marcescens.

○   **What is the most common cause of chronic heavy metal poisoning?**

Lead. Arsenic is the most common acute heavy metal poisoning.

○   **Are steroids effective in treatment of toxic epidermal necrolysis?**

No.

○   **Erythema nodosa is associated with which type of gastroenteritis?**

Yersinia.

○   **A baby boy is brought to the emergency department with vomiting and persistent crying for two hours. On exam, a testicle is tender and enlarged. What is the most common cause?**

A testicular torsion.

○   **A child presents with bluish discoloration of the gingiva. What diagnosis should you suspect?**

Chronic lead poisoning. Expect the erythrocyte protoporphyrin level to be elevated with this condition.

○   **What is the anatomical weakness of the esophagus?**

Lack of a serosa.

○   **What disorder is most likely to be confused with erythema nodosum?**

Cellulitis.

○   **What is erythema nodosum?**

An inflammatory disease of the skin and subcutaneous tissue which is characterized by tender red nodules. The nodules are usually found in the pretibial area. This condition typically affects young adults; primary causes are streptococcal infections and sarcoidosis. The most common cause in children is UTI, especially with Streptococci. Other causes include leprosy, TB, psittacosis, ulcerative colitis, and drug reaction.

○   **What is the most common dysrhythmia in a child?**

Paroxysmal atrial tachycardia.

○   **On an upright chest x-ray, what is the earliest radiographic sign of left ventricular failure?**

An apical redistribution of the pulmonary vasculature.

○   **What is the most common cause of hyponatremia?**

Dilution.

○   **A fracture of the acetabulum may be associated with damage to what nerve?**

The sciatic nerve.

○   **What are the causes of normal anion gap metabolic acidosis?**

Diarrhea, ammonium chloride, renal tubular acidosis, renal interstitial disease, hypoadrenalism, ureterosigmoidostomy, and acetazolamide.

○   **What are some common causes of respiratory alkalosis?**

Respiratory alkalosis is defined as a pH above 7.45 and a pCO_2 less than 35. Common causes of respiratory alkalosis include any process that may induce hyperventilation, such as shock, sepsis, trauma, asthma, PE, anemia, hepatic failure, heat stroke, and exhaustion, emotion, salicylate poisoning, hypoxemia, pregnancy, and inappropriate mechanical ventilation. Alkalosis shifts the O_2 disassociation curve to the left. It also causes cerebrovascular constriction. Kidneys compensate for respiratory alkalosis by excreting HCO_3^-.

○   **How should neurogenic shock be managed?**

With the replacement of volume deficit followed by vasopressors.

○   **What is the order of appearance of a CHF on a chest x-ray?**

Initially cephalization and the redistribution of blood flow is observed, with the subsequent appearance interstitial edema with evident Kerley B lines, as well as a perihilar haze. These findings are followed by alveolar infiltrates in the typical butterfly appearance. Finally, flagrant pulmonary edema and effusions become evident.

O   **What is the most common cause of sporadic encephalitis?**

Herpes simplex virus.

O   **What is the classic EKG for Wolff-Parkinson-White syndrome?**

A change in the upstroke of QRS, the delta wave.

O   **Which agent is usually responsible for the onset of endemic encephalitis?**

Arbovirus.

O   **What is the best treatment for an unstable patient with Wolff-Parkinson-White syndrome presenting with rapid atrial fibrillation?**

Shock.

O   **What are the most common dysrhythmias associated with digitalis?**

PVC's are the most common. AV block and PSVT with block are next. V-tach and junctional tachycardia arrhythmias are usually not associated with digitalis.

O   **Describe the signs, symptoms, and ECG findings associated with lithium toxicity.**

Tremor, weakness, and flattening of the T-waves, respectively.

O   **How many days after a measles vaccine could a fever and a rash be expected to develop?**

7–10 days.

O   **What is the most common complication of acute otitis media?**

Tympanic membrane perforation. Other complications include mastoiditis, cholesteatoma, and intracranial infections.

O   **Describe a mallet finger deformity.**

A mallet finger deformity is produced by forced flexion of the DIP joint when the finger is in full extension. The deformity is a result of either a rupture of the distal extensor tendon, or an avulsion fraction of the tendon insertion on the distal phalanx with a dorsal plate avulsion.

O   **What agents commonly induce the onset of laryngotracheitis?**

Parainfluenza virus type I.

O   **What gynecological infection presents with a malodorous, itchy, white to grayish, and sometimes frothy vaginal discharge?**

Trichomoniasis.

O   **What are the signs of an upper motor neuron lesion?**

Upper motor neuron lesion involves the corticospinal tract. The lesion usually induces paralysis with:

1) The initial loss of muscle tone and then increased tone, resulting in spasticity.
2) Babinski sign.
3) The loss of superficial reflexes.
4) Increased deep tendon reflexes.

A lower motor neuron lesion is associated with the anterior horn cells' axons. These lesions cause paralysis with decreased muscle tone and prompt atrophy.

○ **What condition frequently presents with ocular bulbar deficits?**

Botulism poisoning. Patients with myasthenia gravis may present similarly. The diphtheria toxin rarely produces ocular bulbar deficits.

○ **Describe the symptoms and signs of myasthenia gravis.**

Weakness and fatigability with ptosis, diplopia, and blurred vision are the initial symptoms in 40–70% of the patients. Bulbar muscle weakness is also prevalent with dysarthria and dysphagia.

○ **Describe the symptoms of botulism poisoning.**

Botulism poisoning often presents with ocular bulbar deficits. Symmetrical descending weakness, usually with no sensory abnormalities, also develops. Other classical symptoms include dysphagia, dry mouth, diplopia, dysarthria, and the deep tendon reflexes may be decreased or absent.

○ **Describe the signs and symptoms of Guillain-Barré disease.**

Guillain-Barré disease classically presents with symmetrical weakness in the legs, which ascends to include the arms or trunk. Distal weakness is usually greater than proximal. The onset of the disease rarely involves the cranial nerves.

○ **Which nerve provides sensations to both dorsum and volar aspects of hand?**

Ulnar. Radial is primarily dorsum, and median is primarily volar.

○ **What are the key features of viral labyrinthitis or vestibular neuritis?**

Vertigo is severe, usually lasting 3–5 days, with nausea and vomiting. Symptoms generally regress over 3–6 weeks. Nystagmus may be spontaneous during the severe stage.

○ **Describe signs and symptoms of acoustic neuroma.**

Signs and symptoms may include an unilateral high tone sensorineural hearing loss and tinnitus. Decreased corneal sensitivity, diplopia, headache, facial weakness, and positive radiographic findings may also be displayed. Vertigo usually appears late, is more often exhibited as a progressive feeling of imbalance, and can be provoked by changes in head movement. Nystagmus is frequently present and is usually spontaneous. The CSF may have elevated protein.

○ **What's that little bone seen behind the tympanic membrane?**

The malleus.

○ **What disease should be suspected in a patient with a 2 week history of lower limb weakness?**

Guillain-Barré usually causes an ascending weakness which begins in the lower extremities. Conversely, the weakness is descending with botulism poisoning. Cranial nerves are typically affected first with myasthenia gravis.

❍   **Deep tendon reflexes are usually maintained in which of the following diseases: Myasthenia gravis, Guillain-Barré, or Eaton-Lambert syndrome?**

Myasthenia gravis. Reflexes are usually depressed in Eaton-Lambert syndrome and absent in Guillain-Barré.

❍   **What is the most common cause of pain with an odontogenic origin?**

Dental caries.

❍   **What is the most serious complication of abscessed anterior maxillary teeth?**

Septic cavernous sinus thrombosis. This condition results from an infection extending into the canine space and facial venous system.

❍   **What electrolyte abnormality is commonly associated with the transfusion of packed red blood cells?**

Hypocalcemia secondary to citrate toxicity. Citrate, when rapidly infused, binds ionized calcium and therefore decreases the calcium level. Hyperkalemia may also develop with rapidly packed red blood cell transfusion, especially if the patient is in renal failure or if the blood products are old.

❍   **What invasive measurement should be performed to evaluate a patient with swelling of the face, neck, and arms?**

CVP. Swelling of the face, neck and arms suggests a superior vena cava syndrome. To confirm superior vena cava syndrome, an increased CVP pressure in the upper body and abnormal pressure in the lower extremities must be documented. A chest x-ray will detect only about 10% of the masses causing superior vena cava syndrome.

❍   **Describe a typical patient with intussusception.**

Intussusception usually occurs in children between the ages of 3 months to 2 years. The majority are 5-10 months old, and it is more common in boys. The area of the ileocecal valve is typically the source of the problem.

❍   **What are the common symptoms and signs of hyperthyroidism?**

Symptoms include weight loss, palpitations, dyspnea, edema, chest pain, nervousness, weakness, tremor, psychosis, diarrhea, hyperdefecation, abdominal pain, myalgias, and disorientation. Signs such as fever, tachycardia, wide pulse pressure, CHF, shock, thyromegaly, tremor, weakness, liver tenderness, jaundice, stare, and hyperkinesis are evident. Mental status changes include somnolence, obtundation, coma, or psychosis. Pretibial myxedema may also be found—a true misnomer!

❍   **A patient suffers a rotational knee injury and hears a pop. Within 90 minutes a hemarthrosis develops. Where is the suspected location of the injury?**

The anterior cruciate.

❍   **What drugs should be avoided in G-6-PD deficiency?**

ASA, phenacetin, primaquine, quinine, quinacrine, nitrofurans, sulfamethoxazole, sulfacetamide, and methylene blue.

❍   **What is the current therapeutic regimen for treatment of meningitis in a neonate?**

Initially, ampicillin and aminoglycoside were favored for treating the neonate with meningitis. However, today recommendations include ampicillin and cefotaxime. A combination of these two antibiotics should be used infants up to 2 months of age to cover coliform, Group B *Streptococci*, *Listeria*, and *Enterococcus*. In children older than 2 months and up to 6 years, cefotaxime alone is indicated.

○ **What is the formula for calculating changes in potassium as a function of pH?**

For a pH increase of 0.1, expect the potassium to drop by 0.5 mmol/L.

○ **Describe the symptoms of optic neuritis.**

The patient suffers a variable loss of central visual acuity with a central scotoma and change in color perception. The patient also has a painful eye. The disk margins are blurred from hemorrhage, and the blind spot is increased.

○ **What are the signs and symptoms of acute pericardial tamponade?**

Triad of hypotension, elevated CVP, and tachycardia are usually indicative of either acute pericardial tamponade or a tension pneumothorax in a traumatized patient. Muffled heart tones may be auscultated.

○ **What EKG result is pathognomonic of pericardial tamponade?**

Total electrical alternans. Pulsus paradoxus is nonspecific. Muffled heart tones are subjective findings and are difficult to appreciate.

○ **Define sensitivity and specificity.**

Sensitivity is true positives divided by true positives plus false negatives. It represents how well a test identifies people who have a condition from among all the people who have the condition.

Specificity is true negatives divided by true negatives plus false positives. It is the percentage of people who do not have a disease and are thus correctly classified as negative by the test.

○ **What cause of death is secondary to an untreated tension pneumothorax?**

Decreased cardiac output. The vena cava is compressed, which lowers the right heart blood return and severely compromises stroke volume, blood pressure and cardiac output.

Ed. Note: 2° arrhythmias can also occur. V-tach in a young, apparently healthy person is 2° to a tension pneumothorax until proven otherwise. (JNA)

○ **How does a chronic pericardial effusion appear on a chest x-ray?**

A gradual pericardial sac distention results in a "water bottle" appearance of the heart.

○ **What are the symptoms and signs of adrenal insufficiency?**

Fatigue, nausea, anorexia, abdominal pain, change in bowel habits, and syncope are frequently reported symptoms. Hyperpigmentation, hypertension, vitiligo, and weight loss may be noted. Laboratory abnormalities are possible, including hypoglycemia, hyperkalemia, hyponatremia, and azotemia.

○ **The treatment for myxedema coma includes:**

IV thyroid replacement with thyroxine, IV glucose, hydrocortisone. Water restriction may also be considered.

○ **What are the signs and symptoms of thyrotoxicosis?**

Weight loss and weakness may be reported. Tachycardia and fever are common abnormal vital signs with hypotension and shock occurring less frequently. Mental status changes of decreased consciousness or psychosis may be present. Signs of CHF, thyromegaly, tremor, and eye signs, including lid lag and proptosis, should also be sought.

○   **Which type of streptococci causes acute post streptococcal glomerulonephritis?**

Group A ß-hemolytic *Streptococci*.

○   **What signs and symptoms are prevalent with post streptococcal glomerulonephritis?**

A physical exam may reveal facial edema and decreased urinary output; these are the most common findings. Urine may also be dark. Other laboratory results include normochromic anemia due to hemodilution, increased sedimentation rate, numerous RBC's and WBC's in the urine with casts, and hyperkalemia. Hospitalization is advised.

○   **What disorder is present when the modified Jones criteria are met?**

Rheumatic fever.

○   **Describe the symptoms and signs of varicella (chicken pox).**

The onset of varicella rash is 1–2 days after prodromal symptoms of slight malaise, anorexia, and fever. The rash begins on the trunk and scalp, appearing as faint macules and later becoming vesicles.

○   **Describe the signs of roseola infantum.**

Roseola infantum usually affects children ages 6 months to 3 years. It is characterized by a high fever that begins abruptly and lasts 3–5 days, possibly precipitating febrile seizures. A rash appears as the temperature drops to normal.

○   **What dose of sodium bicarbonate should be initially administered to a child who is in cardiopulmonary arrest?**

1 mEq/kg.

○   **How is the normal systolic blood pressure (SBP) for pediatric patients (toddlers and up) calculated?**

Average SBP (mm Hg) = (patient's Age x 2) + 90.
Low normal limit SBP (mm Hg) = (patient's Age x 2) + 70.
SBP for a term newborn is about 60 mm Hg.

○   **How does a patient older than 12 months present with sickle cell disease?**

Initial symptoms are often pain in the joints, bones, and abdomen. The child may have abdominal tenderness and even rigidity. Mild icterus and anemia may be present.

○   **How does a child present with erythema infectiosum (fifth disease or slapcheek syndrome)?**

Fifth disease typically does not infect infants or adults. There are no prodromal symptoms. The illness usually begins with the sudden appearance of erythema of the cheeks, followed by a maculopapular rash on the trunk and extremities that evolve into a lacy pattern.

○   **Which organism typically causes paronychia?**

Staphylococcus.

O   **How does myasthenia gravis present?**

Weakness of the voluntary muscles, usually the extraocular muscles. Diagnostic confirmation is dependent on the edrophonium (Tensilon) test. Treatment includes neurologic consultation, anticholinesterases, steroids, and thymectomy.

O   **What visual deficit is typically associated with lesions at the optic chiasm?**

Bitemporal hemianopsia.

O   **Describe the signs and symptoms of neuroleptic malignant syndrome.**

Muscle rigidity, autonomic disturbances, and acute organic brain syndrome. Blood pressure and pulse fluctuate wildly, and a fever as high as 42°C (108°F) may be evident. Muscle necrosis may occur with resultant myoglobinuria.

O   **Which organism commonly induces a septic joint in a child?**

Staphylococcus aureus.

O   **What organism commonly causes a septic joint in an adolescent?**

Neisseria gonorrhoeae.

O   **What are the signs of tension pneumothorax on a physical exam?**

Tachypnea, unilateral absent breath sounds, tachycardia, pallor, diaphoresis, cyanosis, tracheal deviation, hypotension, and neck vein distention.

O   **Which organism most commonly causes bacterial pneumonia, except for in the first week of life?**

Streptococcus pneumoniae.

O   **What is the most common cause of abdominal pain in children?**

Constipation.

O   **What is the most common cause of an intestinal obstruction in children under 2 years of age?**

Intussusception.

O   **Do local anesthetics freely cross the blood brain barrier?**

Yes. Most systemic toxic reactions to local anesthetics involve the CNS or cardiovascular system.

O   **Where is the most common site of thrombophlebitis?**

The deep muscles of the calves, particularly the soleus muscle.

O   **What are the most common causes of aortic stenosis?**

Rheumatic fever and congenital bicuspid valve disease.

O   **What is the most common cause of pulsus paradoxus in a child?**
Asthma.

○   **What is the most common dysrhythmia associated with Wolff-Parkinson-White syndrome?**

A paroxysmal atrial tachycardia.

○   **Which gender is more apt to develop symptomatic gallstones?**

Females.

○   **What type of ulcer is the most common?**

Duodenal ulcers occur more frequently than gastric ulcers.

○   **A patient has a non-red, painful eye with decreased visual acuity. What is the diagnosis?**

Optic neuritis.

○   **What disease is associated with retrobulbar optic neuritis?**

Multiple sclerosis.

○   **How can the mydriasis caused by third cranial nerve compression be distinguished from the mydriasis induced by anticholinergic drugs or mydriatics?**

Mydriasis caused by third cranial nerve compression is reversible with pilocarpine; other causes are not.

○   **At what child's age is a cuffed ET tube preferred?**

6 years.

○   **What is the correct ET tube size for a 6 month old?**

3.5–4.5 mm.

○   **What is the correct ET tube size for a newborn?**

3.0–3.5 mm. For a premature newborn, use a 2.5–3.0 mm ET tube.

○   **How should hypercalcemia be treated?**

By administering furosemide and normal saline. Mithramycin may be used, especially in hypercalcemia secondary to bone cancer. Other treatments include calcitonin, hydrocortisone, and indomethacin.

○   **What is the treatment for multifocal atrial tachycardia?**

1. Treat underlying disorder.
2. Administer magnesium sulfate, 2 grams over 60 seconds, with supplemental potassium to maintain serum K^+ above 4 mEq/L.
3. Consider verapamil, 10 mg IV, as a second treatment

○   **What is the treatment for ectopic SVT due to digitalis toxicity?**

1. Stop digitalis.
2. Correct hypokalemia.
3. Consider digoxin specific Fab, magnesium IV, lidocaine IV, or phenytoin IV.

○   **What is the treatment for ectopic SVT not due to digitalis toxicity?**

1. Digitalis, verapamil, or ß-blocker to slow rate.
2. Quinidine, procainamide, or magnesium to decrease ectopy.

❍ **What is the treatment for verapamil-induced hypotension?**

Calcium gluconate IV over several minutes.

❍ **Discuss the treatment of digitalis toxicity.**

1. Charcoal.
2. Phenytoin (Dilantin) or lidocaine for ventricular arrhythmias (increases AV node conduction).
3. Atropine or pace for bradyarrhythmias.
4. Digoxin specific Fab (Digibind).

❍ **What "hypos" can lower the seizure threshold?**

Hypoglycemia, hyponatremia, and hypocarbia.

❍ **What motor function is spared in locked-in syndrome?**

Upward gaze.

❍ **What are the signs and symptoms of a middle cerebral artery lesion?**

Hemiplegia or hemiparesthesia, homonymous hemianopsia, and speech disturbance.

❍ **Describe the symptoms and signs of pressure on the first sacral root (S1).**

Symptoms of S1 injury include pain radiating to the mid-gluteal region, posterior thigh, posterior calf, and down to the heel and sole of the foot. Sensory signs are localized to the lateral toes. S1 root compression would typically involve the plantar flexor muscles of the foot and toes. The ankle reflex is decreased or absent.

❍ **What drug should be used to treat a patient in cardiac arrest secondary to hyperkalemia?**

Calcium chloride—IV acts fastest. Also provide $NaHCO_3$.

❍ **What are the effects of dopamine at various doses?**

At 1–10 mg/kg, dopamine causes renal, mesenteric, coronary, and cerebral vasodilation.
At 10–20 mg/kg, both Σ- and ß-adrenergic effects are present.
At 20 mg/kg, effects are primarily Σ-adrenergic.

❍ **What is the effect on serum sodium as glucose increases by 100?**

Serum sodium decreases by 5 mEq/l.

❍ **In addition to phenytoin, what traditional anti-arrhythmic agents can be used to treat digitalis induced ventricular arrhythmias.**

Lidocaine and bretylium. Procainamide and quinidine are contraindicated in digitalis toxicity.

❍ **What is an anaphylactoid reaction?**

An anaphylactoid reaction is very similar to anaphylaxis; however, it does not require prior exposure to the reaction product. Cases may occur from a radiopaque contrast media or from medications, such as NSAIDs.

❍   **What is the universal donor blood?**

Type Rh-negative blood with anti-A and anti-B titers of less than 1:200 in saline.

❍   **What are the common presentations of a transfusion reaction?**

Myalgia, dyspnea, fever associated with hypocalcemia, hemolysis, allergic reactions, hyperkalemia, citrate toxicity, hypothermia, coagulopathies, and altered hemoglobin function.

❍   **What are the signs of the Cushing reflex?**

Increased systolic blood pressure and bradycardia, as a result of cerebral edema.

❍   **What are normal results in the oculocephalic reflex?**

Conjugate eye movement is opposite to the direction of head rotation.

❍   **In a comatose patient, what does tonic eye movement towards an irrigated ear in response to caloric testing signify?**

Life.

❍   **Define strabismus.**

Strabismus is defined as a lack of parallelism of the visual axis of the eyes.
Esotropia = medially deviated. Exotropia = laterally deviated.

❍   **Which drugs commonly cause bradycardia?**

ß-blockers, cardiac glycosides, pilocarpine, and cholinesterase inhibitors (such as organophosphates) are responsible for bradycardia. Sympathomimetics, such as amphetamines and cocaine, and anticholinergics, such as atropine and cyclic antidepressants, commonly cause tachycardia.

❍   **What drug commonly causes both horizontal and vertical nystagmus?**

Phencyclidine (PCP).

❍   **Name 5 drugs or conditions that cause hypertension and/or tachycardia.**

<u>S</u>ympathomimetics,
<u>W</u>ithdrawal,
<u>A</u>nticholinergics,
<u>M</u>AO Inhibitors,
<u>P</u>hencyclidine (PCP).
A mnemonic for this is SWAMP.

❍   **Name six common drugs that can cause hyperthermia.**

<u>S</u>alicylates
<u>A</u>nticholinergics
<u>N</u>euroleptics
<u>D</u>initrophenols
<u>S</u>ympathomimetics and <u>PCP</u>.

The mnemonic for this one is SANDS-PCP.

○ **Which drugs or environmental exposures can induce bullous lesion formation?**

Sedative hypnotics, carbon monoxide, snake bite, spider bite, caustic agents, and hydrocarbons.

○ **What is a mnemonic for remembering the drugs that cause nystagmus?**

MALES TIP

M= methanol.
A = alcohol.
L = lithium.
E = ethylene glycol.
S = sedative hypnotics and solvents.

T = thiamine depletion and Tegretol (carbamazepine).
I = isopropanol.
P = PCP and phenytoin.

○ **What is a mnemonic for remembering drugs that are radiopaque?**

BAT CHIPS
B = barium.
A = antihistamines.
T = tricyclic antidepressants.
C = chloral hydrate, calcium, cocaine.
H = heavy metals.
I = iodine.
P = phenothiazine, potassium.
S = slow-release (enteric coated).

○ **Name some side-effects of alkalization of the urine.**

Hypernatremia and hyperosmolality.

○ **Can theophylline be dialyzed?**

Yes.

○ **When does acetaminophen become toxic?**

When there is no glutathione to detoxify its toxic intermediate.

○ **Which type of acid base disturbance initially occurs with a salicylate overdose?**

Respiratory alkalosis. Approximately 12 hours later, an anion gap metabolic acidosis or mixed acid base picture may occur.

○ **Is hyperglycemia or is hypoglycemia expected with a salicylate overdose?**

Expect either hyperglycemia or hypoglycemia.

○ **What are the common signs and symptoms of chronic salicylism?**

Fever, tachypnea, CNS alterations, acid base abnormalities, electrolyte abnormalities, chronic pain, ketonuria, and noncariogenic pulmonary edema.

❍   **A patient presents with an acute salicylate ingestion. What symptoms are expected with a mild, a moderate, and a severe overdose?**

1. Mild: Lethargy, vomiting, hyperventilation, and hyperthermia.
2. Moderate: Severe hyperventilation and compensated metabolic acidosis.
3. Severe: Coma, seizures, and uncompensated metabolic acidosis.

❍   **What is the treatment for a salicylate overdose?**

Decontaminate, lavage and charcoal, replace fluids, supplement with potassium, alkalize the urine with bicarbonate, cool for hyperthermia, administer glucose for hypoglycemia, place on oxygen and PEEP for pulmonary edema, prescribe multiple dose activated charcoal, and initiate dialysis.

❍   **A patient presents with vomiting, hematemesis, diarrhea, lethargy, coma, and shock. What is the suspected cause?**

Iron intoxication. Order a flat plate of the abdomen to exam for concretions.

❍   **What drugs can cause methemoglobinemia?**

Nitrites, local anesthetics, silver nitrate, amyl nitrite and nitrites, benzocaine, commercial marking crayons, aniline dyes, sulfonamides, and phenacetin.

❍   **When evaluating a pediatric cervical spine film, what are the normal values?**

The predental space in a child is < 5 mm; in an adult, it is < 3 mm. The posterior cervical line attaching the base of the spinous process of C1 to C3 should be considered. If the base of C2 spinous process lies > 2 mm behind the posterior cervical line, a hangman's fracture should be suspected. The anterior border of C2 to the posterior wall of the fornix distance is < 7 mm. Finally, the anterior border of C6 to the posterior wall of the trachea distance is 14 mm in children younger than 15 years of age; it is < 22 mm in an adult.

❍   **The most common adverse effect of AZT is:**

Granulocytopenia and anemia.

❍   **What local anesthetics may cause anaphylaxis?**

The ester derivatives that contain para-aminobenzoic acid (PABA) are known to stimulate IgE antibody formation and thereby cause anaphylaxis. Such anesthetics include procaine and tetracaine.

❍   **Which test best discriminates between functional and organic blindness?**

Optokinetic nystagmus.

❍   **Red blood cell basophilic stippling occurs with what 2 disorders?**

Thalassemia and lead poisoning.

❍   **What triad is associated with Reiter's syndrome?**

Non-gonococcal urethritis, polyarthritis, and conjunctivitis. The conjunctivitis is the least common and occurs in only 30% of the patients. Acute attacks respond well to NSAIDs.

❍   **Which drugs can induce a lupus reaction?**

Procainamide, hydralazine, isoniazid, and phenytoin.

○   **What is the most serious complication associated with dental infections, besides possible respiratory compromise from Ludwig's angina?**

Septic cavernous sinus thrombosis.

○   **What are the complications of impetigo?**

Streptococcal-induced impetigo can result in post streptococcal glomerulonephritis. However, it has not been shown to be associated with rheumatic fever. Treat with erythromycin, dicloxacillin, or cephalexin to help eliminate the skin lesions. There is no conclusive proof that treatment prevents glomerulonephritis.

○   **Describe the key features of the Rocky Mountain Spotted Fever (RMSF) rash.**

RMSF is caused by *Rickettsia rickettsii* and is transmitted by Ixodidae ticks. Patients become sick with a high fever, headache, chills, and muscular pain. Around the fourth day of fever, a rash begins on the wrists and ankles and spreads centripetally.

○   **Describe the scarlet fever rash.**

The rash has a sandpaper type texture and begins on the face, neck, chest, and abdomen. It then spreads to extremities. Patients may also have strawberry tongue.

○   **Syncope is a characteristic symptom of what valvular disease?**

Aortic stenosis.

○   **Which complications may develop in a patient with a sickle cell trait?**

Hematuria and decreased urine concentrating ability.

○   **How does an infant with botulism present?**

Lethargy, failure to thrive, paralysis, and then death. Raw honey is generally the source of botulism.

○   **What is the pathophysiology of myasthenia gravis?**

Circulatory antibody against ACh receptor which binds at the motor end plate. In myasthenics, ACh receptors are in short supply, resulting in fatigable weakness.

○   **What is the most serious transfusion reaction?**

Hemolytic. Treat with aggressive fluid replacement and Lasix.

○   **What is the most common transfusion reaction?**

Febrile.

○   **What diseases are associated with myasthenia gravis?**

Rheumatoid arthritis, pernicious anemia, SLE, sarcoidosis, and thyroiditis. 10–25% of patients with this condition are also afflicted with thymoma.

○   **A patient presents with ocular, bulbar, and limb weakness which worsens during the day and decreases with rest. What is the diagnosis?**

Myasthenia gravis.

❍   **What are some factors commonly associated with meningitis?**

Age less than 5, low socioeconomic status, male sex, crowding, black race, sickle cell disease, splenectomy, alcoholism, diabetes, cirrhosis, immunologic defects, dural defect from congenital, surgical or traumatic source, contiguous infections such as sinusitis, household contacts, malignancy, bacterial endocarditis, intravenous drug abuse, and thalassemia major.

❍   **A patient has xanthochromic CSF with a high protein count (> 150 mg/dl). What is the most likely cause?**

Traumatic tap.

❍   **Explain how methylene blue functions as an antidote for methemoglobinemia.**

A NADPH-dependent enzyme usually maintains a normal level of 3% methemoglobin. This enzyme capacity can be exceeded with oxidant poisoning. Methylene blue enhances NADPH-dependent hemoglobin reduction by acting as a cofactor. Methylene blue is usually only needed for metHb levels > 30%; its dose is 1–2 mg/kg IV over 5 minutes.

❍   **Does botulism produce fever?**

No. This can be important in differentiating neurologic symptoms in a sick patient who could have diphtheria.

❍   **Describe a patient with Chlamydial pneumonia.**

Chlamydial pneumonia is usually seen in children 2–6 weeks of age. The patient is afebrile and does not appear toxic.

❍   **A patient has had 3 days of diarrhea which was abrupt in onset. The patient reports slimy green, malodorous stools that contain blood. In addition, the patient is febrile. What is the most likely cause?**

Salmonella.

❍   **What is the drug treatment for Campylobacter?**

Erythromycin or tetracycline.

❍   **In a child, does coarctation of the aorta typically cause cyanosis?**

No.

❍   **What is the drug treatment for persistent *E. coli*?**

Trimethoprim with sulfamethoxazole (TMP/SMX).

❍   **What is the drug treatment for *Giardia lamblia*?**

Quinacrine or metronidazole or furazolidone.

❍   **What is the drug treatment for Salmonella?**

Ampicillin, TMP/SMX, Chloramphenicol (Adults.)

❍   **What is the drug treatment for Yersinia?**

TMP/SMX, tetracycline, third generation cephalosporin.

○ **What are the 8 common clinical presentations of pediatric heart disease?**

1. Cyanosis.
2. Pathologic murmur.
3. Abnormal pulses.
4. CHF.
5. HTN.
6. Cardiogenic shock.
7. Syncope.
8. Tachyarrhythmias.

○ **Complications of the use of sodium bicarbonate in severe metabolic acidosis include:**

Hypernatremia, paradoxical CSF acidosis, decreased oxygen unloading at the tissue level, hyperosmolality, dysrhythmias, and hypokalemia.

○ **What is the function of aldosterone?**

Aldosterone causes sodium conservation and K^+ excretion. As a result, it causes increased reabsorption of sodium and fluid.

○ **What drug will most rapidly decrease K^+?**

Calcium chloride IV (1–3 minutes).

○ **What is a potential side-effect of the use of Kayexalate?**

Kayexalate exchanges sodium for K^+. As a result, sodium overload and CHF may occur.

○ **What is Addison's disease?**

Deficiency or absence of mineralocorticoid (aldosterone). This results in increased sodium excretion. Potassium is retained. The urine cannot concentrate, which can lead to severe dehydration, hypotension, and circulatory collapse. Deficiency of cortisol (also produced in the adrenal cortex) leads to metabolic disturbances, weakness, hypoglycemia, and deceased resistance to infection.

○ **What conditions lead to hypocalcemia?**

Shock, impaired production, pancreatitis, hypomagnesemia, alkalosis, decreased serum albumin, hypoparathyroidism, osteoblastic metus, and fat embolism syndrome.

○ **What vital sign might be affected with hypermagnesemia?**

Hypermagnesemia causes hypotension because it relaxes vascular smooth muscle. Deep tendon reflexes may disappear.

○ **Name the common causes of hypercalcemia:**

PAM P SCHMIDT.

P = Parathormone.
A = Addison's.
M = Multiple Myeloma.

P = Paget's.

S = Sarcoidosis.
C = Cancer.
H = Hyperthyroidism.
M = Milk-alkali Syndrome.
I = Immobilization.
D = Vitamin D Excess.
T = Thiazides.

○ **What dose of ASA will cause mild to moderate toxicity?**

200–300 mg/kg. Greater than 500 mg/kg is potentially lethal.

○ **What is the ferric chloride test and what toxic ingestion does it detect?**

Add a few drops of 10% ferric chloride solution to a few drops of urine. A purple color indicates presence of salicylic acid. Ketones or phenothiazine can lead to falsely positive results.

○ **What electrolyte abnormality may mimic the signs and symptoms of hypocalcemia?**

Hypomagnesemia.

○ **What are some signs and symptoms of Thrombotic Thrombocytopenic Purpura (TTP)?**

Thrombocytopenia, purpura, and microangiopathic hemolytic anemia. Patient with TTP presents with fever, fluctuating neurologic signs, and renal complications. If the disease goes untreated, it is almost uniformly fatal. Therapy includes steroids, splenectomy, plasmapheresis and exchange, and antiplatelet agents, such as dipyridamole and aspirin.

○ **In what type of patients is Staphylococcal pneumonia likely?**

Patients that are in hospital, debilitated, or abusing drugs.

○ **How low does the platelet count drop before spontaneous bleeding occurs?**

Below 50,000/mm^3 spontaneous bleeding may occur. CNS bleeds usually do not occur until counts drop below 10,000/mm^3.

○ **What effect will heparin or warfarin overdose have on the prothrombin time (PT) the partial thromboplastin time (PTT)?**

When administered in excessive doses, both cause increases in PT and PTT.

○ **What are the 5 key lab findings in DIC?**

1. Increased PT.
2. Increased PTT.
3. Increased fibrin degradation products.
4. Decreased fibrinogen.
5. Decreased platelet levels.

○ **What are the classic findings of shaken baby syndrome?**

1. Failure to thrive.
2. Lethargy.

3. Seizures.
4. Retinal hemorrhages.
5. CT may show subarachnoid hemorrhage or subdural hematoma from torn bridging veins.

○   **Define spondylolysis.**

Spondylolysis is a defect in the pars interarticularis.

○   **T/F: High fever in neonates with bacterial pneumonia usually follows a period of general fussiness and decreased feeding.**

True.

○   **Chlamydia pneumonia is more likely to occur in the neonate after how many weeks of age?**

Three weeks.

○   **Conjunctivitis is an associated finding in about what percentage of neonates with chlamydia pneumonia?**

About 50%.

○   **Neonates with chlamydia pneumonia are usually tachypneic with a bad cough. Are they febrile?**

Usually not.

○   **What is the most common bacterium causing septic arthritis of the hip?**

Staphylococcus aureus.

○   **Newborns should stop losing weight how many days after birth?**

About 6 days.

○   **T/F: A neonate's stool color can be an important sign.**

False. Unless blood is evident, stool color is insignificant.

○   **What is the difference between vomiting and regurgitation?**

Very little once it's on you! Vomiting is caused by forceful diaphragmatic and abdominal muscle contraction. Regurgitation occurs without effort.

○   **Is regurgitation dangerous in an otherwise thriving neonate?**

No. However, it can be dangerous for newborns with failure to thrive or respiratory problems, and it may be associated with chronic aspiration.

○   **Projectile vomiting in the neonate is often associated with pyloric stenosis. When this is the case, such vomiting becomes a prominent sign at what age?**

2–3 weeks.

○   **What is the name for diarrhea associated with sepsis, otitis media, UTI or any other systemic disease?**

Parenteral diarrhea.

❍   **T/F: Bacterial and parasitic etiologies of diarrhea in the neonate are rare.**

True.

❍   **What are some entities in the differential diagnosis of bloody diarrhea in the neonate?**

Necrotizing enterocolitis, bacterial enteritis, allergic reactions to milk, and iatrogenic causes secondary to antibiotics.

❍   **Neonates with necrotizing enterocolitis are sick; what are some of the signs of sepsis to look for?**

Poor feeding, lethargy, fever, jaundice, abdominal distention, and poor color.

❍   **What should be considered in the case of a neonate who has never passed stool?**

Meconium ileus or plug, Hirschsprung's disease, intestinal stenosis, or atresia.

❍   **Anal stenosis, hypothyroidism, and Hirschsprung's disease can all present with what clinical sign?**

Constipation that was not present at birth but which began before the infant was 1 month old.

❍   **Describe the signs and symptoms of a slipped capital femoral epiphysis. What x-ray tests are necessary for its diagnosis?**

Gradual onset of hip pain and stiffness with restriction of internal rotation; patient may walk with a limp. X-ray analysis should include both the anterior-posterior and lateral views of both hips. The slip of the epiphyseal plate posteriorly is best seen on the lateral view.

❍   **Describe the signs and symptoms of a patient with chondromalacia patellae.**

Chondromalacia patellae typically occurs in young, active females. The pain is localized to the knee. There is no effusion and no history of trauma. Patella compression tests are usually positive.

❍   **Describe the signs and symptoms of tarsal tunnel syndrome.**

Insidious onset of paresthesia, as well as burning pain and numbness on the plantar surface of the foot. Pain radiates superiorly along the medial side of the calf. Rest decreases pain.

❍   **What causes swimmer's itch (schistosome dermatitis)?**

An invading cercariae.

❍   **What is the vector of malaria?**

Anopheles mosquito.

❍   **What is the vector of trypanosomiasis?**

Tsetse fly.

❍   **What is the infectious agent of elephantiasis?**

Nematode microfilaria.

❍   **What vector transmits Chagas' disease (trypanosoma Cruzi)?**

Reduviid (assassin or kissing bug).

○ **Hookworm is associated with what sort of anemia?**

Iron deficiency anemia.

○ **Fish tapeworm (*Diphyllobothrium latum*) is associated with what clinical entity?**

Pernicious anemia.

○ **Onchocerciasis (from *Onchocerca volvulus*) is associated with what visual deficit?**

Blindness. The name "river blindness".

○ **Chagas' disease is associated with what clinical entity?**

Acute myocarditis. Trypanosoma Cruzi invades the myocardium resulting in myocarditis. Conduction defects may occur.

○ **Roundworm is associated with what clinical entity?**

Small bowel obstruction.

○ **Describe the presentation of a patient with post extraction alveolitis.**

"Dry socket" pain occurs on the second or third day after extraction.

○ **Ludwig's angina typically involves what spaces in the head?**

The submental, sublingual, and submandibular spaces.

○ **What are the signs and symptoms of a peritonsillar abscess?**

Sore throat, dysarthria (hot potato voice), odynophagia, ipsilateral otalgia, low grade fever, trismus, and uvular displacement.

○ **What is the presentation of a patient with diphtheria?**

Sore throat, dysphagia, fever, and tachycardia. A dirty, tough gray fibrinous membrane so firmly adherent that removal causes bleeding may be present in the oropharynx. Corynebacterium diphtheriae exotoxin acts directly on cardiac, renal, and nervous systems. It can cause ocular bulbar paralysis that may suggest botulism or myasthenia gravis. The exotoxin may also cause flaccid limb weakness. Of note, such weakness may also include decreased or absent DTRs, a finding suggestive of Guillain-Barré or tick paralysis.

○ **Magnesium containing antacids may cause:**

Diarrhea.

○ **Aluminum containing antacids may cause:**

Constipation.

○ **When does an elevation of HBsAg occur in relation to symptoms of hepatitis B?**

HBsAg always rises before clinical symptoms of hepatitis B.

O   **Is hepatitis A associated with jaundice?**

Typically not, as more than 50% of the population has serologic evidence for hepatitis and do not recall being symptomatic.

O   **Describe a patient with intussusception.**

Patients are most likely very young. 70% of patients have intussusception within the first year of life. In children, the cause is thought to be secondary to lymphoid tissue at the ileocecal valve; in adults, it is thought to be caused by local lesions, Meckel's diverticulum, or tumor. On exam, bowel sounds are usually normal. Intussusception typically involves the terminal ileum. Meckel's diverticulum is the single most common intrinsic bowel lesion involved.

O   **Should salmonella be treated?**

Only if symptomatic infection persists. Treat with ampicillin, TMP/SMX, or Chloramphenicol.

O   **What is the most common cause of acute food-borne disease?**

Staphylococcus aureus and the enterotoxins it produces.

O   **What are the common features of *Vibrio parahaemolyticus*?**

This condition is caused by organisms associated with oysters, clams, and crabs. Symptoms include cramps, vomiting, dysentery, and explosive diarrhea. Severe infections are treated with tetracycline and Chloramphenicol.

O   **Painful, bright red rectal bleeding is most often due to:**

Anal fissure. External hemorrhoids present with acute painful thrombosis and are not typically associated with constant, bright red bleeding. Internal hemorrhoids present with painless bright red bleeding, usually with defecation.

O   **Where is the narrowest part of the ureter?**

The ureterovesical junction.

O   **What is the drug of choice for treating urinary tract infection due to *Proteus mirabilis*?**

Ampicillin. This condition is common in young boys.

O   **As pCO_2 increases, pH will decrease. How much is the pH expected to decrease for every 10 mm Hg increase in pCO_2?**

pH decreases by 0.08 units for each 10 mm increase Hg in pCO_2.

O   **How much protamine is required to neutralize 100 units of heparin?**

1 mg of protamine will neutralize $\approx$ 100 units of heparin. The maximum dose of protamine is 100 mg.

O   **What organisms are most commonly present in a pulmonary abscess?**

Mixed anaerobes.

❍ **What are some causes of thoracic outlet syndrome?**

The most common cause is a cervical rib. Compression of the subclavian artery by an anomalous cervical rib, compression of the neurovascular bundle as it passes through the interscalene triangle, and compression of the neurovascular bundle in the retroclavicular space anterior to the first rib when the arms are hyperabducted are also causes. Symptoms are typically produced when the shoulders are moved backward and downward.

❍ **What are the classic signs and symptoms of aortic stenosis?**

Left heart failure, angina, and exertional syncope.

❍ **What patient position will enhance the murmur of mitral stenosis?**

Left lateral decubitus.

❍ **What is the optimal patient position and maneuver for auscultation of aortic insufficiency?**

Have the patient sit up and lean forward with his or her hands tightly clasped. During exhalation, listen at the left sternal border.

❍ **What murmurs will the Valsalva maneuver increase?**

Only IHSS. All other murmurs are diminished.

❍ **What are the symptoms of endocarditis?**

Fever, chills, malaise, anorexia, weight loss, back pain, myalgia, arthralgia, chest pain, dyspnea, edema, headache, stiff neck, mental status changes, focal neurologic complaints, extremity pain, paresthesia, hematuria, and abdominal pain.

❍ **What are the key diagnostic features of coarctation of the aorta?**

Rib notching seen on x-ray and significant differences in the blood pressure between the upper and lower extremities.

❍ **What is an interesting diagnostic feature of aortic regurgitation?**

Head bobbing.

❍ **What is the most common arrhythmia associated with digitalis?**

PVC (60%), ectopic SVT (25%), and AV Block (20%).

❍ **What effect does furosemide have on calcium excretion?**

Furosemide causes increased calcium excretion in the urine.

❍ **What is the most common arrhythmia in mitral stenosis?**

Atrial fibrillation.

❍ **What is the differential diagnosis of pulmonary edema with a normal size heart?**

Constrictive pericarditis, massive MI, non-cardiogenic pulmonary edema, and mitral stenosis (not mitral regurgitation).

○   **How does dobutamine differ from dopamine?**

Dobutamine decreases afterload with less tendency to cause tachycardia.

○   **Describe Kerley A and B lines.**

Kerley A lines are straight, non-branching lines in the upper lung fields. Kerley B lines are horizontal, non-branching lines at the periphery of the lower lung fields.

○   **What effect does the Valsalva maneuver have on the heart?**

Valsalva decreases blood return to both the right and left ventricles. All murmurs decrease in intensity except IHSS.

○   **A 15 year old female presents with altered mental status and a temperature of 105°F. The patient's muscles are rigid. She feels very hot in the trunk, but her extremities are cool. What diagnosis is likely?**

Neuroleptic malignant syndrome. Check the CPK.

○   **How should a patient with neuroleptic malignant syndrome be treated?**

1. Ice packs to the groin and axilla.
2. Cooling blankets.
3. Fan.
4. Water mist evaporation.
5. Dantrolene at an IV rate of 0.8 to 3 mg/kg IV q 6 hours to a total of 10 mg/kg.

○   **Why should the use of atropine be considered in a pediatric patient prior to intubation?**

Many pediatric patients develop bradycardia associated with intubation, which can be prevented by pre-treatment with atropine (0.01 mg/kg).

○   **What are the effects of using ketamine in a pediatric patient?**

The child's eyes will be wide open with a glassy stare. He or she will have nystagmus, hyperemic flush, and hypersalivation. There will also be a slight rise in the heart rate. A very rare complication of ketamine use is laryngospasm. Hallucinations are a common side-effect in children over the age of 10; as a consequence, ketamine should be restricted to use only in patients under the age of 10.

N.B. Ketamine may also cause sympathetic stimulation, which increases intracranial pressure and may cause random movements of the head and extremities. Thus, it is not a good sedative for children going to CT scan.

○   **What are the contraindications to TAC?**

Mucus membranes, burns, and large abrasions. TAC used on the tongue and mucus membranes has led to status epilepticus and patient death.

○   **Why are quinolones contraindicated in children?**

Quinolones impair cartilage growth.

○   **A patient presents with a symmetric weakness that has progressed over several days and associated paresthesia. Diminished reflexes are noted. What is the diagnosis?**

Guillain-Barré syndrome. Other signs and symptoms are diminished reflexes, minimal loss of sensation, paresthesias, and leg weakness.

○ **How is Guillain-Barré syndrome diagnosed in the ED?**

Suspect the diagnosis based on signs and symptoms, but confirmation requires nerve conduction studies performed as an inpatient.

○ **What conditions may make the end tidal CO_2 monitor inaccurate?**

Monitor may be falsely yellow due to contamination from acid dilutants and drugs, such as lidocaine-HCl and epinephrine-HCl. Contamination with vomit or acid dilutants may also produce false readings.

○ **Under what conditions does neurogenic pulmonary edema occur?**

Neurogenic pulmonary edema is commonly associated with increased intracranial pressure. It is commonly seen with head trauma, subarachnoid hemorrhage, and even with seizures.

○ **You are having a hard time remembering which anesthetics are amides and which anesthetics are esters. What is a fairly easy way of telling these two classifications apart?**

With the exception of the suffix "ca_ine," only the anesthetics in the am_ide classification include the letter "I."

Am_ides:
L_idocaine (Xylocaine).
Bup_ivacaine (Marcaine).
Mep_ivacaine (Carbocaine).

Esters:
Procaine (Novocain).
Cocaine.
Tetracaine (Pontocaine).
Benzocaine.

○ **What are the classic signs and symptoms of adrenal insufficiency?**

Fatigue, weakness, GI symptoms, anorexia, hypotension, and dehydration. The classic clue is history of chronic steroid use. Order plasma cortisol level. Remember: cortisol level should be drawn prior to giving steroid therapy.

○ **What is the initial treatment for adrenal insufficiency?**

Fluids and hydrocortisone IV in a typical dose of 100–200 mg.

○ **A young competitive figure skater complains of generalized weakness following practice. What might be the cause?**

Hypokalemic "paralysis" is a cause of acute weakness.

○ **What is the most commonly missed fracture in the elbow region?**

A radial head fracture. Like the navicular fracture, radiographic signs of a radial head fracture may not show up for days after the injury. A positive fat pad sign may be the only finding suggestive of this injury.

○   **What are the two most common errors made in the intubation of a neonate?**

1) Placing the neck in hyperextension; this moves the cords even more anteriorly.
2) Inserting the laryngoscope too far.

○   **What is the most common cause of food-borne viral gastroenteritis?**

Norwalk virus commonly found in shell fish.

○   **What are some common entities in the differential diagnosis of a limp or gait abnormality in a child?**

Legg-Calvé-Perthes disease (avascular necrosis of the femoral head), Osgood-Schlatter disease, avulsion of the tibial tubercle, infection, toxic transient tenosynovitis, patellofemoral subluxation, chondromalacia patella, slipped capital femoral epiphysis, septic arthritis, metatarsal fracture, proximal stress fracture, and toddler fracture (spiral tibia fracture).

○   **What signs indicate an HIV positive patient is at increased risk for opportunistic infections like PCP?**

An absolute CD-4 count of less than 200 and a CD-4 lymphocytic percentage of less than 20.

○   **What is the most common cause of small bowel obstruction in the surgically virgin abdomen?**

Incarcerated hernia.

○   **A patient with a temperature of 29°C develops V-fib. Is defibrillation likely to be successful?**

Defibrillation should be attempted but is unlikely to be successful at temperatures less than 29°C.

○   **T/F: The presentation of infectious endocarditis in an IV drug abusing patient does not usually include a murmur.**

True. Less than 1/2 present with a murmur.

○   **How is a retropharyngeal abscess diagnosed on the plain films of an infant?**

Look for prevertebral thickening of the soft tissues. More than 3 mm suggests the possibility of a retropharyngeal abscess.

○   **A straight (Miller) blade is preferred for intubating children of less than what age?**

4 years.

○   **What is the Parkland formula for treating a pediatric burn victim?**

Ringer's lactate 4 ml/% BSA/kg over 24 hours with 1/2 given in first 8 hours.

○   **Large burns in children less than 5 years old may require:**

Colloid (5% Albumin or FFP) at 1 ml/ % BSA/kg/day.

○   **A burned pediatric patient is receiving fluids per the Parkland formula. How much additional fluid should be given for maintenance requirements?**

100 ml/kg/day for each kg up to 10 kg + 50 ml/kg/day for each kg from 10-20 kg + 20 ml/kg/day for each kg thereafter.

❍   **In the evaluation of retropharyngeal abscess, what is the usual age of the patients, how do they present, what diagnostic tests are used in their evaluation, and what treatment modalities are recommended?**

Retropharyngeal abscess is most commonly seen in children less than 4 years old. Usual presentation is with dysphagia, a muffled voice, stridor, and a sensation of a lump in the throat. Patients usually prefer to lie supine. Diagnosis is made with a soft tissue lateral neck film which may demonstrate edema and air/fluid levels. CT may be useful. Treatment includes airway, IV antibiotics, and admission to the ICU. Intubation may rupture the abscess.

❍   **What is the usual cause of facial cellulitis in children less than 3 years of age?**

H. influenzae.

❍   **An asthmatic patient suddenly develops a supraventricular tachycardia. Blood pressure is normal and the QRS complex is also narrow. What therapy is most appropriate?**

Verapamil. Avoid the use of adenosine as it is relatively contraindicated and may exacerbate bronchospasm in asthmatic patients. Also avoid ß-blockers.

❍   **A patient's blood gases reflect a mixed metabolic acidosis and respiratory alkalosis; what cause immediately comes to mind?**

Salicylate intoxication.

❍   **What is the appropriate paralyzing agent to use when intubation is required in a seizing patient?**

Use pancuronium (Pavulon) because succinylcholine has a greater tendency to increase serum potassium and ICP.

❍   **What neurologic disorder presents similarly to symptoms caused by the wood tick's bite?**

Guillain-Barré. Recall that tick paralysis may have decreased or absent DTRs as a clinical finding, which may also be associated with diphtheria exotoxin.

❍   **What nerve supplies taste to the anterior two-thirds of the tongue and the lacrimal and salivary glands?**

Cranial nerve VII.

❍   **What antibiotics should be avoided in myasthenia gravis patients?**

Polymyxin and aminoglycoside have curare-like properties that may cause paralysis in these patients.

❍   **A patient complains of pronounced weakness when attempting to climb stairs and even becomes tired when she does such simple tasks as brushing their teeth. What is the diagnosis?**

Myasthenia gravis.

❍   **What is the treatment for myasthenia gravis?**

Steroids, thymectomy, immunosuppressive drugs, plasmapheresis, and cholinergic agents such as pyridostigmine.

❍   **What is a chalazion?**

This is a Meibomian gland granuloma, a complication of conjunctivitis. A chalazion can deform the eyelid which can lead to blindness.

O   **How should a chalazion be treated?**

Surgical curettage.

O   **Patient presents with eye pain. She has a constricted pupil, ciliary flush, and red injected sclera at the limbus. What is the diagnosis?**

Acute iritis.

O   **A patient presents with loss of central vision. Likely, what is the diagnosis?**

A retrobulbar neuritis is likely. MS is associated with about 25% of retrobulbar neuritis cases. Macular degeneration and central retinal vein occlusion can also lead to loss of central vision.

O   **A patient presents with fever, neck pain or neck stiffness, and trismus. Exam reveals pharyngeal edema with tonsil displacement and edema of the parotid area. What is the diagnosis?**

Parapharyngeal abscess.

O   **A patient presents with hearing loss, nystagmus, complaint of facial weakness, and diplopia. Vertigo is provoked with sudden movement. A lumbar puncture reveals elevated CNS protein. What diagnosis is suspected?**

An acoustic neuroma.

O   **Can a parapharyngeal abscess present with an associated finding of edema in the area of the parotid gland?**

Yes.

O   **Describe Stevens-Johnson syndrome?**

It is a bullous form of erythema multiforme that involves mucous membranes. It may cause corneal ulcerations, anterior uveitis, or blindness.

O   **What are the most common drugs causing TEN?**

Phenylbutazone, barbiturates, sulfa drugs, anti-epileptics, and antibiotics.

O   **What is the most common site of aseptic necrosis?**

The hip.

O   **Which epicondyle is involved in tennis elbow?**

The lateral epicondyle.

O   **What is the most common site of infectious arthritis?**

The knee, followed by the hip. Staphylococcus is the most common cause.

O   **What nerve is located in the tarsal tunnel?**

The tibial nerve.

❍ **A patient has difficulty squatting and standing. What is the most likely spinal pathology?**

L4 root compression with involvement of quadriceps.

❍ **Describe the leg position associated with an obturator hip dislocation.**

External rotation, flexion, and abduction.

❍ **A positive TB test is what type of reaction?**

Type 4—cellular mediated, hypersensitivity is delayed, and neither complement nor antibodies are involved.

❍ **What drugs commonly cause erythema multiforme?**

Carbamazepine, penicillin, sulfa, pyrazolone, phenytoin, and barbiturates.

❍ **What aerobe is most commonly found in cutaneous abscesses?**

Staphylococcus aureus.

❍ **What is the most common Gram-negative aerobe found in cutaneous abscesses?**

Proteus mirabilis.

❍ **Describe the Gram's stain appearance of *Staphylococcus aureus*.**

Gram-positive cocci in grape-like clusters.

❍ **How is erysipelas treated?**

With penicillin—or erythromycin for allergic patients.

❍ **A child presents to the ED with a history of fever, conjunctival hyperemia, and erythema of the mucus membranes with desquamation. What is the diagnosis?**

Kawasaki's Disease. Remember: Kawasaki's disease may have lesions resembling erythema multiforme.

❍ ***Clostridium tetanus*, a Gram and anaerobe, produces a neurotoxin. Is it an endotoxin or an exotoxin?**

Tetanospasmin is an exotoxin. It prevents transmission of inhibitory neurons in anterior horn cells, resulting in motor system disinhibition.

❍ **What findings mark the presentation of a patient with rapidly progressive glomerulonephritis?**

Hematuria (most common), edema (periorbital), HTN, ascites, pleural effusion, rales, and anuria.

❍ **What arrhythmia is frequently encountered during renal dialysis?**

Hypokalemia induced ventricular fibrillation.

❍ **What are causes of priapism?**

Prolonged sex, leukemia, sickle cell trait and disease, blood dyscrasias, pelvic hematoma or neoplasm, syphilis, urethritis, and drugs including phenothiazine, prazosin, tolbutamide, anticoagulants, and corticosteroids.

○   **What causes a greenish-gray frothy vaginal discharge with mild itching?**

Trichomonas vaginitis. On physical exam, the cervix will have a strawberry appearance 20% of the time.

○   **Describe the presentation of a patient with Gardnerella vaginitis?**

On physical exam, note a frothy, grayish-white, fishy smelling vaginal discharge. Wet mount may show clue cells (clusters of bacilli on the surface of epithelial cells). Remember: Sherlock Holmes always uses his magnifying lens to look for "clues" in the "garden."

○   **Sulfamethoxazole may lead to hemolysis in a patient with:**

G6PD deficiency.

○   **When can one auscultate the fetal heart?**

Ultrasound: 6 weeks.
Doppler: 10–12 weeks.
Stethoscope: 18–20 weeks.

○   **Describe a Brudzinski sign.**

Flexion of the neck produces flexion of the knees.

○   **Describe Kernig's sign.**

Extension of the knees from the flexed thigh position results in strong passive resistance.

○   **Is phenobarbital more quickly metabolized by children or by adults?**

Adults. Neonates are especially slow at metabolizing phenobarbital.

○   **What hypersensitivity skin rashes are noted with phenytoin use?**

Lupus-like and Stevens-Johnson syndrome.

○   **What are the cardiac effects of phenytoin?**

Inhibits sodium channels, decreases the effective refractory period and automaticity in the Purkinje fibers. It has little effect on QRS width or action potential duration.

○   **In endocarditis, what is the most commonly involved cardiac valve?**

Mitral > Aortic > Tricuspid > Pulmonic.

○   **What is the most common causative bacterium associated with right-sided endocarditis in IV drug abusers?**

Staphylococcus aureus. Left- sided endocarditis in IV drug abusers is usually due to *E. coli*, streptococcus, Klebsiella, Pseudomonas, or Candida.

○   **A heroin addict presents with pulmonary edema. What is the best treatment?**

Naloxone, O_2, and ventilatory support. Don't bother using diuretics.

O   **What is the most common neurologic complication of IV drug abuse?**

Nontraumatic mononeuritis (i.e., painless weakness 2–3 hours after injection).

O   **Salicylate levels should ideally be checked how long after an ingestion?**

6 hours.

O   **What is the minimum toxic dose of salicylates?**

150 mg/kg.

O   **What salicylate level, measured 6 hours after ingestion, is associated with toxicity?**

45 mg/dl.

O   **What Acetaminophen level, measured 4 hours after ingestion, is associated with toxicity?**

150 μg/ml.

O   **What are the signs of salicylate poisoning?**

Hyperventilation, hyperthermia, mental status change, nausea, vomiting, abdominal pain, dehydration, diaphoresis, ketonuria, metabolic acidosis, and respiratory alkalosis.

O   **A child presents with lethargy, seizures, and hypoglycemia. She has had viral syndrome symptoms for several days. Name two disorders that should be considered.**

Reye's syndrome and salicylate intoxication.

O   **What is the most reliable site for detecting central cyanosis?**

The tongue.

O   **What is a common complication of pancuronium?**

Tachycardia from its vagolytic action

O   **What is the most common cause of hypermagnesemia in a patient with renal failure?**

Patient use of compounds high in magnesium, such as antacids. This can result in neuromuscular paralysis. Consider IV calcium. Saline and furosemide assisted diuresis may not help a patient with renal failure, so consider dialysis as well.

O   **How much energy should be used to cardiovert an unstable infant with a wide complex tachycardia?**

0.5–1.0 J/kg.

O   **How much energy should be used to cardiovert unstable VF in an infant?**

2 J/kg.

O   **What are the three most common presenting signs of aortic stenosis?**

Syncope, angina, and heart failure.

○ What are the potential, though often rare, complications of Mycoplasma pneumonia?

Non-pulmonary: Hemolytic anemia, aseptic meningitis, encephalitis, Guillain-Barré syndrome, pericarditis, and myocarditis.

Pulmonary: ARDS, atelectasis, mediastinal adenopathy, pneumothorax, pleural effusion, and abscess.

○ Under what conditions should Staphylococcal pneumonia be considered as a possible diagnosis?

Although it only accounts for 1% of bacterial pneumonias, it should be considered in patients with sudden chills, hectic fever, pleurisy, and cough—especially following a viral illness, such as measles or influenza.

○ Differential diagnosis of a ring lesion on CT scan:

Toxoplasmosis, lymphoma, fungal infection, TB, CMV, Kaposi's, and hemorrhage.

○ Does erythema multiforme itch?

Not typically. It may be tender.

○ A patient presents with granuloma inguinale. What does it look like?

Papular, nodular, or vesicular painless lesions. These can result in extensive destruction of local tissues. Cause is *Calymmatobacterium granulomatis.*

○ What causes chancroid?

Hemophilus ducreyi.

○ Describe lesions associated with Chlamydia.

Painless, shallow ulcerations, papular or nodular lesions, and herpetiform vesicles that wax and wane.

○ What state is associated with akinetic mutism?

North Dakota is a bucolic state. Akinetic mutism is an abulic state, which is like a coma vigil. Patients seem awake and may have their eyes open. They respond to questions very slowly. The cause is typically due to depressed frontal lobe function.

○ What is normal blood pressure in a newborn?

60 mmHg.

○ What is the initial drug of choice to treat SVT in a pediatric patient?

Adenosine 0.1 mg/kg is drug of choice. Digoxin 0.02 mg/kg may take ≈ 4 hours for conversion. Verapamil may be used in children > 2 years of age; however, it is has caused several deaths in children younger than 2. Synchronized cardioversion at 0.5–1.0 J/kg.

○ After the first month of life, what is the # 1 cause of meningitis and the # 1 cause of pneumonia in children?

Meningitis: *H. influenzae,* though this should change with widespread use of Hib vaccine.
Pneumonia: *Streptococcus pneumoniae. H. influenzae* is the second most common cause.

○   **Discuss infantile spasms.**

Onset is by 3–9 months of age. It typically lasts seconds, and may occur in single episodes or bursts. The EEG is often abnormal. 85% of these patients will be mentally handicapped.

○   **Erythema multiforme can be associated with which anticonvulsants?**

Phenobarbital, phenytoin, and carbamazepine.

○   **Hepatic failure is commonly associated with what anticonvulsant?**

Valproic acid.

○   **What drugs, activities, and cooking habits are associated with an increased clearance of theophylline (decreasing the theophylline level)?**

Phenytoin, phenobarbital, cigarette smoking, and charcoal barbecuing.

○   **Anaphylaxis is a common cause of what type of renal failure?**

Prerenal.

○   **When does ECM show up in Lyme disease?**

Stage I: 3–32 days after the bite.

○   **What pathogen is suggested by a pneumonia with a single rigor?**

Pneumococcus.

○   **What pathogen does a strawberry cervix suggest?**

Trichomonas.

○   **What is the vector and causative organism of Lyme disease?**

The vector is *Ixodes dammini*, and the organism is *Borrelia burgdorferi*. It is the most frequently transmitted tick-borne disease.

○   **What causes Q fever?**

Coxiella burnetii, also known as *Rickettsia burnetii*. It is found in *Dermacentor andersoni* tick.

○   **A hordeolum is:**

A Meibomian gland infection, usually of the upper lid.

○   **Ludwig's angina pathology:**

Hemolytic streptococci, staphylococcus, mixed aerobes and anaerobes.

○   **What are the 3 most common locations of malignant melanomas?**

The skin, eyes, and anal canal.

○   **What is the initial dose of blood given to children?**

10 ml/kg of packed RBC's.

○ **What is achalasia?**

Disorder of esophageal motility and incomplete relaxation of the lower esophagus.

○ **Name four enterotoxin-producing organisms that can cause food poisoning.**

Clostridium, *Staphylococcus aureus*, vibrio cholerae, and *E. coli*.

○ **Antibiotics should be avoided with what infectious diarrhea?**

Salmonella. Exceptions include severe cases of diarrhea in the very young, the immunocompromised, or those with enteric fever (where the infecting strain is *S. typhi* or is otherwise in the bloodstream).

○ **Name 3 disorders associated with decreased DTRs.**

Guillain-Barré, tic paralysis due to *Dermacentor andersoni* (Wood Tick) bite, and diphtheria exotoxin.

○ **What is the most likely cause of CHF in a premature infant?**

PDA.

○ **What is the most likely cause of CHF in the first 3 days of life?**

Transposition of the great vessels which leads to cyanosis and failure.

○ **What is the most likely cause of CHF in the first week of life?**

Hypoplastic left ventricle.

○ **What is the most likely cause of CHF in the second week of life?**

Coarctation of the aorta.

○ **Do you treat Shigella with antibiotics?**

In general, yes.

○ **What is a pinguecula?**

It is a yellowish nodule, particularly on the nasal aspect of the eye, but it may be lateral. It is often caused by wind and dust.

○ **What is a pterygium?**

It is a chronic growth over the medial or lateral aspect of the cornea approaching the pupil. It is much thicker than pingueculae.

○ **What is the most common cause of painless upper GI bleeding in an infant or child?**

Varices from portal hypertension.

○ **What is the most common cause of major painless lower GI bleeding in an infant or child?**

Meckel's diverticulum.

❍   **Common cause of orbital cellulitis:**

Staphylococcus aureus.

❍   **What would you expect to find in the hippocampus of a patient with rabies?**

Negri bodies. Incubation for rabies is 30–60 days. Treatment includes cleaning of the wound, rabies immune globulin, and human diploid cell vaccine.

❍   **What kind of tick transmits Rocky Mountain Spotted Fever (RMSF)?**

The female andersoni tick. It transmits rickettsia rickettsii.

❍   **What is the most common symptom in RMSF?**

Headache occurs in 90% of patients.

❍   **Describe the rash of RMSF.**

It is a macular rash, 2–6 mm in diameter, located on the wrists and palms and spreading to the soles and trunk.

❍   **What tick transmits Lyme disease?**

The *Ixodes dammini* tick.
Spirochete *Borrelia burgdorferi* is diagnosed by culture on Kelly's medium.

❍   **Describe the skin lesion seen in Lyme disease.**

A large distinct circular skin lesion called erythema chronicum migrans. It is an annular erythematous lesion with central clearing.

❍   **Describe a patient with tick paralysis.**

Bulbar paralysis, ascending flaccid paralysis, paresthesias of hands and feet, symmetric loss of deep tendon reflexes, and respiratory paralysis.

❍   **What is the causative organism of otitis externa?**

Pseudomonas.

❍   **What are the signs and symptoms of Lyme Disease, stages I–III?**

Stage I: Erythema Chronicum Migrans, malaise, fatigue, headache, arthralgias, fever, and chills.
Stage II: Neurologic and cardiac symptoms include headache, meningoencephalitis, facial nerve palsy, radiculoneuropathy, ophthalmitis, and 1°, 2° and 3° AV blocks.
Stage III: Arthritis (knee > shoulder > elbow > TMJ > ankle > wrist > hip > hands > feet).

❍   **With brain stem herniation, is decorticate or decerebrate posturing expected?**

Decerebrate posturing (hyperextension). Decorticate posturing is flexion of the upper extremities and extension of the lower extremities.

❍   **A patient presents after experiencing trauma to the head. He has an elevated systolic blood pressure and bradycardia. What is the diagnosis?**

Cushing reflex.

O   **Describe the corneal reflex.**

The ophthalmic branch of the fifth nerve and the afferent branch of the facial (seventh) nerve conduct it.

O   **What is a frequent complication of ethmoid sinusitis?**

Orbital cellulitis.

O   **What is the most common site of aspiration pneumonitis?**

Right lower lobe.

O   **A patient presents with a history of hearing a "pop" in his knee and ankle as he fell. What is the diagnosis?**

Tear of the anterior cruciate and Achilles tendon rupture.

O   **What nerve may be injured with a knee dislocation?**

The peroneal nerve.

O   **What are the most common sites of stress fractures in the foot?**

Second and third metatarsals.

O   **What is the most common cause of subarachnoid hemorrhage in teenagers?**

AV malformations.

O   **A patient presents with a painful, red eye and a decrease in visual acuity. What is the differential?**

Central corneal lesions, glaucoma, and iritis.

O   **What is the most common cause of acute aortic regurgitation?**

Infectious endocarditis.

O   **What is the most common congenital valvular disease?**

Bicuspid aortic valve.

O   **What metabolic abnormality is commonly associated with hypercalcemia?**

Up to 1/3 will have hypokalemia.

O   **What is the most common cause of retrobulbar optic neuritis,?**

Multiple sclerosis.

O   **What are the initial symptoms of a patient with hypocalcemia?**

Paresthesias around the mouth and fingertips, irritability, hyperactive deep tendon reflexes, and seizures.

O   **What ECG change is associated with hypocalcemia?**

Prolonged T waves.

O   **A patient is digitalis toxic. What electrolytes will need to be replaced?**

Potassium and magnesium.

O   **What is the most common arrhythmia associated with Wolff-Parkinson-White syndrome?**

PAT. The patient presents with angina, syncope, and shortness of breath.

O   **How may mydriasis caused by mydriatics and anticholinergic drugs be distinguished from mydriasis caused by third cranial nerve compression?**

Pilocarpine will reverse cranial nerve compression, but it won't have any effect on anticholinergic drugs or mydriatics.

O   **During CPR, the mean cardiac index is what percentage of normal?**

25%.

O   **Why is verapamil a bad choice to treat ventricular tachycardia?**

Verapamil could increase the heart rate and decrease the blood pressure without converting the rhythm.

O   **What drugs should never be used in atrial fibrillation with Wolff-Parkinson-White?**

Digitalis, verapamil, and phenytoin. Atrial fibrillation with Wolff-Parkinson-White should be treated with cardioversion or procainamide. SVT with Wolff-Parkinson-White should be treated with verapamil or adenosine.

O   **Name the drug of choice for Wolff-Parkinson-White with atrial flutter or fibrillation?**

Procainamide.

O   **What makes the first heart sound?**

Closure of the mitral valve and left ventricular contraction.

O   **The second heart sound?**

Closure of the pulmonary and aortic valves.

O   **The third heart sound?**

This is caused by the deceleration of blood flowing into the ventricle when the ventricle reaches its final stages of filling.

O   **The fourth heart sound?**

Vibrations of the left ventricular muscle, the mitral valve, and the left ventricular flow tract cause this.

O   **What is a common pathological cause of an S_3?**

Congestive heart failure.

O   **What are the pathological causes of an S_4?**

Decreased left ventricular compliance due to acute ischemia is the most common cause. Others include aortic stenosis, subaortic stenosis, HTN, coronary artery disease, myocardiopathy, anemia, and hyperthyroidism.

○   **What is the chief benefit of dopamine, and what is its chief complication?**

The chief benefit is prompt elevation of blood pressure with ß-adrenergic effects at low doses and Σ-adrenergic effects at high doses. The chief complication is tachycardia, which unfortunately increases myocardial oxygen demand.

○   **What is the chief effect of dobutamine?**

Dobutamine increases the cardiac contractility. It has only minor effects on peripheral Σ-receptors. It can increase cardiac output without increasing blood pressure.

○   **What effect does morphine have on preload and afterload?**

Morphine decreases both preload and afterload.

○   **Does furosemide affect preload or afterload?**

Furosemide decreases preload.

○   **What is the most common cause of post splenectomy (post splenic) sepsis?**

Streptococcus pneumonia.

○   **What is the most common cause of tricuspid regurgitation?**

Right heart failure secondary to left heart failure, typically caused by mitral stenosis.

○   **What two diseases does the deer tick, *Ixodes dammini*, transmit?**

Lyme disease and Babesia.

○   **How do patients present with Babesia infection?**

Intermittent fever, splenomegaly, jaundice, and hemolysis. The disease may be fatal in patients without spleens. The disease can simulate rickettsial diseases like Rocky Mountain spotted fever. Treat with clindamycin and quinine.

○   **Time for a food question! There are 9 questions in this book that deal with either strawberry tongue, strawberry cervix, currant jelly sputum, or currant jelly stool. Describe the pathology associated with each of these.**

Strawberry tongue: Scarlet fever and Kawasaki's disease.
Strawberry cervix: Trichomonas.
Currant jelly sputum: Klebsiella and (less commonly) type 3 Pneumococcus.
Currant jelly stool: Intussusception.

MEDICAL MNEMONICS

Abdominal pain
("red flags" for medical attention)

Fever persistent
Loss of weight
Anal diseases (perianal findings)
Away from midline
Growth retardation
Stool Guaiac positive

Achondroplasia

Autosomal dominant
Cervical spine stenosis
Hydrocephalus
Orthopedic (tibial bowing)
Nasal bridge (low/flat)
Developmental delay (hypotonia)
Respiratory distress (b/c small chest or airway
   obstruction due to bony anomaly)
Old paternal age usually are related to it

Acne (causes or irritants)

Androgen
Bacteria
Cosmetics
Drugs
Emotional stress
Free fatty acid (in the skin)

Acne (topical treatment)

A-retin
Benzoyl peroxide
Clindamycin/erythromycin

Acute glomerulonephritis
(clinical features)

Normal (IgA) or low C3
Edema
Proteinuria
Hypertension
RBC or RBC cast
Oliguria (renal insufficiency)

Acute lymphoblastic leukemia
(poor prognostic factors)

Lymphoblast high
Younger than one year old
Male
Philadelphia marker
Hb>10
Older than ten
Blood cells > 50,000
Lymph node enlarged
Anterior mediastinum masses
Spleen enlarged
T-cells
Induction > 4 weeks
Chromosome < 46

Addison's disease (clinical features)

Anorexia
Diarrhea
Dehydration
Increased K+
Skin pigmentation
Orthostatic hypotension
Na level is abnormal

ADHD (causes or associations)

Diet (malnutrition)
Exposed to toxin (lead poisoning)
Fetal alcohol syndrome
Iron deficiency
Congenital (genetics or metabolic)
Infection (brain or ears)
Traumatic brain injuries

Adolescent anticipatory guidance

Avoid abusing drugs/alcohol
Belt (seat belts)
Condoms
Don't drive drunk
Exercise
Fruit; not fat
Gangs/guns; conflict resolution
Help each other

Aicardi syndrome

Agenesis of corpus callosum
Infantile spasms
Chorioretinal lacunae
Abnormal vertebrates
Rib anomaly
Dandy-Walker malformation
IQ impaired

AIDS (maternal HIV)

(management of infant)
AZT (antiviral therapy)
Bottle-feeding
C-section
Diagnosis on baby (PCR)

Albinism (key features)

Physical health is normal
Interaction (social life) is fair
Growth is fine
Mental health is normal
Eyes are involved
Night trouble
Tumor potential (but melanoma is very rare)
Skin vulnerable to sunburn

Alcohol Withdrawal

(clinical features)
Epileptic activity
Tremors
Hallucination
Anxiety/anorexia
Nausea/vomiting
Organic brain changes (delirium)
Loss of memory/orientation

Allergic child (allergens)

Animals
Basement
Cigarette
Dust
Encased Bedding
Floors carpeting

Allergic Rhinitis (complications)

Adenoidal hypertrophy
Loss of hearing
Loss of smell sensation
Ear infection
Red eyes
Gum/teeth anomaly
Itching
Chronic sinusitis
Speech delay

Allergy to milk protein

(clinical features)
Albumin is low
Blood loss (bloody stool)
Chronic diarrhea
Distended abdomen
Emesis
Failure to thrive

Alopecia (hair loss-etiologies)

Alopecia Areata
Lesion/Trauma
Oral Contraceptive Pills
Poisons/Drugs
Endocrine/Metabolic
Congenital
Infections (tinea capitis)
Anorexia Nervosa

Anemia (important historical data)

Age/Sex
Nutrition/Pica/Picky
Ethnicity
Medication (rifampin, antimalarials)
Infection
Congenital/Family HX
Stools (Occult bleeding, also Urine/Jaundice)

Angelman syndrome

Abnormal EEG
Neural-seizure d/o
Gait anomaly (puppet-like)
Epidermal hypopigmentation
Laughter
MR
Absent speech
Nystagmus
Sleep disorder

Anorexia nervosa

(poor prognostic factors)

Non-responsive to intervention
Education poor
Relative's similar condition
Vomiting
Obesity (premorbid)
Social dysfunction
Aged (old at onset)

Aortic aneurysms (risk factors)

It present with pulsatile abdominal mass (remember this mass)

Marfan syndrome
Atherosclerosis
Syphilis
Smoking
Injury/infection
Vascular diseases
Elevated blood pressure

Apert syndrome

Apnea (choanal stenosis)
Premature closure of cranial sutures (craniosynostosis)
Extremity (syndactyly, thumb anomalies)
Retarded
Tall forehead

Asthma (etiologies/triggers)

Allergens
Stress
Tobacco smoke
Hereditary
Medications
Animals
Thyroid dysfunction
Infection
Cold air

Asthma (factors in asthma scores)

Sound (breath sounds)
CNS function/mental status
O2 requirement/cyanosis
Retraction
Expiratory wheeze

Atherosclerosis (risk factors)

Smoking
Cholesterol
Low HDL
Elevated blood pressure
Relatives (positive family history)
Obesity
Stress/sex (male >female)
Inactivity
Sugar (diabetes)

Autism (evaluation)

Audiology
UA and CBC
Thyroids
Infection (TORCH)
Seizure (CT/MRI/EEG)
Toxin (lead)
Inborn errors
Chromosome and fragile X
Speech

Beckwith-Wiedemann syndrome

Weight >90th% at birth
Insulin-like growth factor-2 involved
Ear creases or dysplasia
Defected Umbilicus (omphalocele)
Enlarged liver
Macroglossia
Asymmetric extremities
Neonatal hypoglycemia
Neoplasm (Wilms tumor or hepatoblastoma)

Beta-blockers (contraindications for use)

Bradycardia
Low blood pressure
Obstructive lung diseases
CHF
Ketoacidosis (DKA)
Edema of lung
RAD/Raynaud phenomenon

Bloom syndrome

Breakage of chromosomes
Low birth weight
Over-pigmented (café-au-lait spots)
Ocular/otic/odontic anomalies
Malignancy potential
Skin erythema of face

Breast cancer (risk factors)

<u>F</u>ibrocystic disease
<u>O</u>pposite breast with cancer
<u>R</u>elatives with breast cancer

<u>W</u>hite
<u>O</u>lder
<u>M</u>utations of BRCA genes
<u>E</u>ndometrial cancer
<u>N</u>ulliparous

Carpenter syndrome

<u>C</u>raniosynostosis
<u>A</u>crocephaly
<u>R</u>etarded
<u>P</u>oly/syndactyly
<u>E</u>picanthal folds
<u>N</u>arrow palate
<u>T</u>horax (CHD)
<u>E</u>xtremity anomaly
<u>R</u>enal/genital anomalies

Cat-eye syndrome

<u>C</u>oloboma of iris
<u>A</u>nal atresia
<u>T</u>APVR
<u>E</u>motional retardation with mild MR
<u>Y</u>ellow(Jaundice) due to biliary atresia
<u>E</u>ar anomalies

Chaga's disease (clinical features)

<u>C</u>ardiomyopathy
<u>H</u>epatosplenomegaly
<u>A</u>denopathy
<u>G</u>astrointestinal
<u>A</u>nemia
<u>S</u>kin

Chest pain (etiologies)

<u>C</u>hest wall
<u>H</u>eart
<u>E</u>sophagus
<u>S</u>houlder
<u>T</u>rachea
<u>P</u>leuritis
<u>A</u>ortic
<u>I</u>ntraabdominal/diaphragmatic pain
<u>N</u>euromuscular

Child syndrome

<u>C</u>ardiac (VSD)
<u>H</u>ypotonia
<u>I</u>UGR
<u>L</u>imb anomaly
<u>D</u>ermal anomaly

Cholelithiasis (etiologies)

<u>C</u>ystic fibrosis
<u>H</u>emolysis
<u>O</u>besity
<u>L</u>asix(diuretics) usage
<u>E</u>arly birth (prematurity)
<u>S</u>hort gut syndrome
<u>T</u>PN
<u>E</u>nterocolitis (NEC)
<u>R</u>esection of ileum
<u>O</u>CP
<u>L</u>eukocytosis

Cholestasis (medication etiologies)

<u>C</u>imetidine
<u>H</u>yperalimentation
<u>O</u>CP
<u>L</u>-asparaginase
<u>E</u>rythromycin
<u>S</u>ulfonamides
<u>T</u>etracycline
<u>A</u>cetaminophen
<u>S</u>alicylates
<u>I</u>NH, Iron
<u>S</u>eizure medications

Chondrodysplasia punctata

<u>P</u>roximal shortening of extremity
<u>U</u>pper pelvis dysplasia
<u>N</u>euro (MR)
<u>C</u>oronal cleft of spine
<u>T</u>one (hypertonia or spasticity)

Chronic cough (etiologies)

<u>C</u>ystic fibrosis
<u>H</u>abit
<u>R</u>eactive airways (asthma)
<u>O</u>bstructive lung disease
<u>N</u>eoplastic
<u>I</u>mmune deficiency (HIV)
<u>C</u>hronic bronchitis
<u>I</u>rritation (FB, GERD, Sinusitis)
<u>T</u>uberculosis
<u>Y</u>oung syndrome

Chronic cough (evaluation)

Sputum
Serum Ig profile
Sweat
Swallow of Barium
Scope (endoscope)

Cirrhosis of Liver (etiology)

Chronic active hepatitis
Inborn errors (Wilson's, Alpha-antitrypsin
    deficiency)
Recent infection by HBV, HCV or HDV
Repeated alcohol intake
Heart failure
Outflow obstruction (Budd-Chiari syndrome)
Syphilis
Intoxication/medication (methotrexate)
Sclerosing cholangitis

Coffin-Lowry syndrome

CNS (MR)
Ocular (down-slanting)
Finger (tapering)
Facial coarseness
Incisor (teeth) anomaly
Nose (bulbous)
Skeletal anomaly/Short stature

Coma (etiologies)

Carbon monoxide
Overdose of medications
Metabolic
Alcohol
Trauma
Oxygen deficit
Seizure
Encephalitis

Coma (evaluation)

Ammonia
Blood Gas
CBC
Drug Screening
Electrolytes
Fluids
Glucose
Hepatic function
Imaging (EKG, CT, MRI)

Congenital infections

(clinical features)
Conjugated hyperbilirubinemia
Osteochondritis
Neonatal myocarditis
Growth retardation
Eye abnormality
Neurologic
Intracranial calcification
Thrombocytopenia
Anemia
Lung (pneumonitis)

Constipation (etiologies)

Congenital
Obstruction
Neuromuscular
Surgical Conditions
Tumor
Infection (Botulism)
Poison
Anal Anomalies
Thyroid Function
Electrolytes
Drugs

Contraception

(absolute contraindication to use)
Coronary disease
Obesity/Hyperlipidemia Type II
Neoplasm of liver
Cerebrovascular disease
Estrogen-dependent tumors
Pregnancy
Thrombophlebitis
IDDM
Vaginal bleeding undiagnosed
Enzymes of liver increasing

Croup (five factors of "croup score")

Stridor
Cough
Oxygenation/color
Retraction
Entry of air (air movement)

Cushing syndrome (clinical features)

Cutaneous atrophy/pigmentation
Upper body obesity (face, back, trunk)
Skeletal (osteoporosis)
Hirsutism
Intolerance of glucose
Neoplastic effects
Growth arrest

Cystic fibrosis (clinical presentations)

Chronic sinusitis
Hyponatremic dehydration
Lung
Obstruction-colonic;
Retarded growth
Infertility
Digital clubbing
Endocrine (pancreas insufficiency)

Dehydration (assessment)

Decreased weight
Eyes sunken
Heart rate increased
Yucky skin (tenting, doughy)
Dry mucous membranes
Refill of capillary slow
Appearance (alert, awake, active)
Tears
Intake
Output (urine/diarrhea/emesis)
Na level

Depression (dysfunctional behaviors)

Decision-making
Esteem (hopeless)
Psychomotor
Reluctant (distress)
Energy
Sleep
Suicidal
Interest
Oddity/Occupational dysfunction
Nutrition (anorexia)

Diarrhea (etiologies)

Allergy
Bacterial/viral
Congenital (microvillus atrophy, CF)
Drugs
Endocrine/Enzyme (lactose intolerance)
Foods (overfeeding, toxin)
Gut irritation
H3 (HUS, HSP, Hirschsprung) and C3 (Crohn's, Celiac, CF)

Diarrhea (hints for bacterial etiologies)

Bloody stool
Abrupt onset
Cell count increase in stools
Travel abroad
Elevated temperature
Recent antibiotics
Immune deficiency
Anal sex

Domestic violence (management)

Documentation
*
Victim identification
Incidence survey
Options/resources offering
Law enforcement
Evidence collection
Next visit arrangement
Counseling
Environment/safety assurance

Ectopic pregnancy (risk factors)

Endometriosis
Congenital anomaly of tubes
Tubal surgery
Old abdominal scar
PID
In votro fertilization
Contraceptive pills

Endocarditis (Major and minor criteria)

Clinical features and diagnosis include:

Infection (persistent positive cultures) **(M)**
Numerous Echo abnormal findings **(M)**
Foreign materials (m)
Echocardiogram (single) (m)
Culture (single) (m)
Temperature (m)
Immunologic phenomena (Osler's nodes, Roth spots, Rf) (m)
Vascular phenomena (emboli, aneurysm) (m)
Early history of Endocarditis (m)

Endometrial cancer (risk factors)

Estrogen
Nulliparity
Diabetes
Obesity
Menopause after 50
Elevated blood pressure

Fabry Disease

Fleischer vortex dysplasia (corneal clouding)
Angiokeratoma
Brain (CNS)
Renal
Intestinal hyperactivity (diarrhea)
Cardiac
Acroprethesia
Low sweating

Failure to thrive (evaluation)

Family history or genetics (chromosome)
Anemia
Imaging
Lead
Urine
Renal
Endocrine
Skin Test for TB

Fanconi's anemia

Fragile chromosomes
Absent thumb
Nephritic (double or hypoplastic kidneys)
Cutaneous (hyperpigmentation)
Ocular (ptosis, nystagmus)
Neoplastic tendency (leukemia)
IUGR
Short stature

Febrile seizure (clinical features)

Fever as trigger
Early childhood
Brief episode
Recurrence possible
Imaging normal
Lab normal
EEG normal

Fetal alcohol syndrome

Microcephaly
Abnormal facies (short fissures, smooth philtrum)
Thorax (murmur, TOF, coarctation, ribs)
Extremity (joint laxity, palmar creases, clinodactyly)
Retarded growth
Neural-MR
ADHD
Learning disorder

Fetal biophysical profiles
(fetal factors of BPP test)

Fluid (amniotic fluid volume)
Elevated HR
Tone
Activity
Lung (breathing movement)

Fetal Rubella syndrome
(German measles-clinical features)

Mental retardation
Eyes (cataract)
Aortic coarctation or PDA
Skin rash (petechiae)
Liver (hepatitis)
Ears (deafness)
Small for gestational age

Fetal varicella syndrome
(clinical features)

Hypoplastic limbs
Epidermal scars
Retarded (MR)
Prenatal growth deficiency (IUGR)
Eye (retinitis)
Seizure

Fever of unknown origin
(evaluation)
<u>A</u>nalysis of urine
<u>B</u>lood culture
<u>C</u>BC with diff
<u>D</u>ermal Skin Test for TB
<u>E</u>SR

Fever of unknown origin
(common etiologies)
<u>U</u>TI/URI
<u>N</u>eutropenia (cyclic)
<u>K</u>awasaki
<u>N</u>eoplastic (leukemia/Hodgkin)
<u>O</u>steomyelitis
<u>W</u>ound (cat-scratch)
<u>N</u>eurotoxin/drug fever

<u>F</u>actitious
<u>E</u>BV/CMV
<u>V</u>ascular (JRA, SLE, RF)
<u>E</u>ndocarditis
<u>R</u>MSF

FG syndrome
<u>F</u>rontal bossing
<u>G</u>rowth retardation
<u>H</u>ypotonia
<u>I</u>mperforate anus
<u>J</u>oint contracture
<u>K</u>yphoscoliosis
<u>L</u>ow count of dermal ridges
<u>M</u>R

Floating harbor syndrome
<u>H</u>and anomalies
<u>A</u>bnormal speech
<u>R</u>etarded growth
<u>B</u>ulbous nose
<u>O</u>cular/oral anomalies
<u>R</u>ib anomalies

Formula (higher components in kid's formula)
<u>K</u> (vitamin K)
<u>I</u> (Iron)
<u>D</u> (vitamin D)

Fragile X syndrome
<u>F</u>ragile site
<u>R</u>etarded
<u>A</u>utistic/ADHD
<u>G</u>enital anomaly (macro-orchidism)
<u>I</u>ncreased mandible
<u>L</u>anguage problem
<u>E</u>ars (enlarged)

Freeman-Sheldon syndrome
<u>S</u>mall mouth (whistling)
<u>H</u>ypoplastic alae nasi
<u>E</u>xtremity (Talipes Equinovarus)
<u>L</u>ong philtrum
<u>D</u>impled chin ("H" shaped)
<u>O</u>cular (deep-set eyes)
<u>N</u>asal speech

Frequent infections
(evaluation of immune deficiencies)
<u>I</u>mmunization Status
<u>N</u>utritional Hx
<u>F</u>amily Hx
<u>E</u>nzymes (catalase, ADA)
<u>C</u>omplements
<u>T</u>-cells and Subsets
<u>I</u>g-Subsets and Titers To CTMT
<u>O</u>rgans (BM, thymus, etc)
<u>N</u>itroblue Tetrazolium Test
<u>S</u>econdary (HIV, Malignancy, Nephrotic Syndrome)

Gastroesophageal reflux
(complications)
<u>R</u>AD (reactive airway diseases)
<u>E</u>sophagitis
<u>F</u>TT (failure to thrive)
<u>L</u>ung aspiration/infection
<u>U</u>pset stomach
<u>X</u>--SIDS

Gaucher's disease
<u>G</u>lucosidase (beta) deficiency
<u>A</u>utosomal recessive (Accumulation of lipid)
<u>U</u>rologic (renal involvement)
<u>C</u>NS (not for type I)
<u>H</u>ematologic (anemia/bleeding)
<u>E</u>nlarged spleen/liver (hepatosplenomegaly)
<u>R</u>espiratory (lung involvement)
<u>S</u>keletal (osteoporosis/osteopenia)

Goiter (etiologies)

Grave's disease
Oral contraceptives
Infection
Tumors
Environmental
Receptor defects (Resistance to thyroxin)

Heart sounds
  (conditions with increased S2 split)

Septal defect (ASD)
Pulmonary embolus
Left ventricular paced beats
Incomplete pulmonic stenosis
Total right BBB

Henoch-Schönlein Purpura
(HSP) (clinical features)

Hematuria/hematemesis
Skin rashes
Pain of joints/abdomen

Histiocytosis (class II)
  (international criteria for the diagnosis of
  macrophage activation syndrome)

Persistent fever
Hemophagocytosis
Anemia/thrombocytopenia/leukopenia
Glyceride (hypertriglyceridemia)
Enlarged spleen

Histiocytosis (class II)
  (treatment of macrophage activation syndrome)

ATG (antithymocyte antibodies)
BMT (bone marrow transplant)
Cyclosporin (immunosuppressive)
Dexamethasone (steroids)
Etoposide (VP16)

Histoplasmosis
  (clinical features)

Heart
Infiltrate on X-ray
Spleen
Temperature
Ocular
Pneumonitis
Liver
Adenopathy
Skin (erythema nodusa)

Marrow of bone
Amphotericin is choice of treatment

Hypercalcemic crisis (clinical features)

Anorexia
Belly pain
Coma
Delirium
Emesis
Fatigue/weakness

Hyper Ig E syndrome
  (clinical features)

Infection
Growth retardation
Eczema

Hyperkalemia (etiologies)

Kidney
Adrenal dysfunction
Lysis of cells (transfusion, tumors)
Excessive intake
Medications (Digoxin, Heparin, PVK)
Insufficient renin
Acidosis

Hyperkalemia (treatment)

Albuterol (hypokalemia is one of the side
  effects of this drug)
Bicarbonate
Calcium
Dialysis
Exchanger (Kayexalate resin)
Flow of urine (diuretics)
Glucose/insulin
Hyperventilation

Hypokalemia (medication etiologies)

Aminoglycoside
B-amphotericin
Corticosteroids/cisplatin
Diuretics
Epinephrine

Hypertension (causes)

*H*eart (coarctation)
*I*ncreased ICP
*P*heochromocytoma
*E*motional
*R*enal
*T*umors
*E*ndocrine
*N*eurological
*S*teroids (glucocorticoids, minerocorticoids, OCP)
Elicit drugs (cocaine, phencyclidine)
*O*besity
*N*eurofibromatosis

Hypertension (treatment)

*A*CE inhibitors
*B*eta-blockers
*C*alcium channel blockers
*D*iuretics
*E*xercise
*F*ood/fat/sodium adjustment
*G*oal set-up
*H*abit/behavior modification

Intracranial hemorrhage
(etiologies)

*I*nfection (herpes)
*N*ewborn prematurity
*T*rauma
*R*ecent thrombosis (venous sinus)
*A*VM (arterial-venous malformation)
*C*oagulopathy
*R*enal arterial anomalies (hypertension)
*A*neurysm
*N*eoplasm of CNS
*I*nfarction (cerebral)
*A*buse of cocaine
L-Asparaginase

Ig A deficiency (clinical features)

*I*nfection (sinopulmonary)
*G*astrointestinal (IBD, Giardia)
*A*utoimmune diseases (lupus, arthritis)

Iron deficiency (causes)

*I*ncreased growth
*R*educed absorption
*O*vert/occult bleeding
*N*utrition (low iron intake)

Juvenile Rheumatoid Arthritis
(clinical criteria)

*R*heumatoid factors
*H*ands
*E*pidermal (subcutaneous nodules)
*U*nequivocal decalcification on X-ray
*M*orning stiffness
*A*rthritis (symmetric)
*T*hree or more joints involved

Kawasaki disease (clinical features)

*C*onjunctivitis
*O*ral lesions
*W*rist
*A*nkle
*S*kin lesion
*A*denopathy
Key: Temperature > 5 days
*I*VIG is the choice of treatment

Lead poisoning (clinical features)

*L*earning disability
*E*ncephalopathy
*A*nemia
*D*evelopmental delay

Learning disorders (etiologies)

*L*ead Poisoning
*E*pileptic Disorder
*A*DHD
*R*eceptive
*N*eurodegenerative
*I*mpaired Mental Status
*N*utrition
*G*enetics

Legg-Calve-Perthes Disease
(clinical features)

*L*imping
*C*artilage space widening on X-ray
*P*ain
*D*ecreased range of motion by exam

Leprosy (clinical features)

*L*eonine facies
*E*pidermal nodules
*P*eripheral nerves (neuritis)
*R*espiratory mucosa (ulceration)
*O*cular (iritis)

Lyme disease (clinical features)

Tick bite
Impaired memory (meningitis)
Carditis
Knee joint involvement
Skin rashes

Lyme disease

(pathophysiology and treatment)

Skin bite by tick
Pain at bite site
Injection of saliva
Rash is typical (erythema chronicum migrans)
Organ involve via blood
CNS (aseptic meningitis)
Heart (carditis, AV-block)
Extremity (joint pain, arthritis)
Tetracycline is first choice
Erythromycin or Amoxicillin as alternatives

Marden-Walker syndrome

MR
Agenesis of corpus callosum
Retarded growth
Digital and joint anomalies
Emotionless facies
Narrow palpebral fissures

Marfan syndrome

Myopia
Aortic dilatation/insufficiency
Ratio reduction of upper/lower segment
Familial (autosomal dominant)
Arachnodactyly
Narrow face/palate
Stature (thin tall); scoliosis

Marshall syndrome

Myopia/cataract
Anteverted nare of short nose
Robin sequence
Short stature
Hearing loss
Absent frontal sinus
Limb anomalies
Lip thickening

Maternal serum AFP

(elevated MSAFP)

Multiple gestations
Spina bifida (NTDs)
Abdominal wall defects (Omphalocele, gastroschisis)
Fetal death
Placental anomalies

Measles (rubeola) (clinical features)

Rashes
URI
Buccal Koplik's spot
Eye (conjunctivitis, photophobia)
Organomegaly
Lung (pneumonia occurs 6-10%)
Adenopathy

Melanoma and moles

(indication for malignancy)

Margin--irregularity
Odd color
Large diameter
Elevation
Shape--asymmetry

Metabolic acidosis

(with abnormal anion gap)

Alcohol
Non-ketotic coma
Iron/INH
Organic acid
Nephritic (renal) failure
Glycolates
Aspirin
Penicillin/paraldehyde

Metabolic acidosis

(with normal anion gap)

Meds (nephrotoxins)
Extra chloride from TPN
Tubular acidosis
Adrenal insufficiency
Bowel fistula
Ostomy (ureteroenterostomy)
Loose stool (diarrhea)
Intake of chloride
Carbonic anhydrase inhibitors

Mumps (parotitis)(clinical presentation)

Muscular involvement
Up-displaced ears
Malaise
Painful
Swelling

Mumps (parotitis) (complications)

Pancreatitis
Arthritis
Renal (nephritis)
Orchitis/Oophoritis
Thyroiditis
Intracranial (meningitis)
Thrombocytopenia
Intrauterine infection
Sensorineural hearing loss

Myasthenia gravis (clinical presentation)

Growth retardation
Rapid fatigue of muscles
Amblyopia/ptosis
Ventilatory insufficiency
Inability of sucking/swallowing
Seizure

Myasthenia gravis (treatment)

Glucocorticoids
Removal of auto-antibody (plasmapheresis)
Anticholinesterase (Prostigmin)
Ventilation support
IVIG
Surgery (thymectomy)

Myocardial Infarction (management)

Tissue plasminogen activator
Heparin
Rest in bed
Oxygen
Morphine
Beta-blocker
Urinokinase/streptokinase
Salicylate (aspirin)

Near drowning (complication)

ARDS (acute respiratory distress syndrome)
Brain damages
C-spine injuries
DIC
Electrolytes (acidosis)

Necrotizing enterocolitis

(management)
Antibiotics
Bowel resting
Culture/CBC
Decompression (NG tube)
Electrolyte monitoring
Fluid managing

Nephrotic syndrome (clinical features)

Nail whitening
Edema
Proteinuria
Hyperlipidemia
Reduction of albumin
Organomegaly
Thrombosis
Infection (peritonitis)
Calcium loss

Nephrotic syndrome (management)

Corticosteroids
Cyclosporin
Cyclophosphamide
Chlorthiazine/lasix
Cooking with low salt
Consider albumin PRN

Neuroblastoma (poor prognostic factors)

Amplified N-myc
Bone marrow involved
Chromosome #1 deletion
Dehydrogenase (LDH) increased
Enolase positive
Ferritin increased

Neurofibromatosis type-1

(diagnostic criteria)
Cafe-au-lait spots
Axillary freckling
Fibroma (Neurofibroma)
Eye (Lisch nodules)
Skeletal (scoliosis, bowing legs)
Pedigree (positive family Hx)
Optic
Tumors (optic tumor = optic pathway Glioma)

Niemann-Pick disease

Pulmonary involvement
Increased liver an d spleen
CNS involvement

*K*idney involvement

Obesity (assessment)

*O*nset
*B*ehavior
*E*xercise
*S*ocial
*I*Q (mental, school, psych?)
*T*otal daily intake
*Y*oung or old

Obesity (management)

*A*ctivity
*B*ehavior
*C*alorie intake
*D*rugs
*E*ntire family
*F*ollow-ups
*G*oal set-up

Obesity (complications)

*A*irway (asthma, sleeping apnea)
*B*one (orthopedic — SCFE)
*C*ardiovascular diseases
*D*iabetes
*E*motional/psychosocial dysfunction
*F*atty acid metabolic anomaly (lipid)
*G*all bladder diseases
*H*ypertension

Osteogenesis imperfecta

*G*rowth (short stature)
*E*xtremity (deformity, fracture)
*N*eurosensory deafness
*E*ye (blue sclera)
*S*kin (thin skin, scar)
*I*mperfecta of dentinogenesis
*S*pine (scoliosis)

Oxygen saturation curve

(factors for "right shift")

*R*espiratory disease (COPD-resultant 2,3DPG)
*I*ncreased PCO2
*G*lycerate (increased 2,3DPG)
H+ (acidosis)
*T*emperature (fever)

Pancreatitis

(Ranson's poor prognostic factors)

*A*BG (PO2) < 60

*B*UN increase > 5
*C*alcium < 8
*D*eficit of base > 4
*E*rythrocyte loss (Hct) > 10%
*F*luid accumulation > 6000cc

Pancreatitis

(high risk factors for complication)

*A*ge > 55
*B*lood sugar >200
*C*ell count (WBC) >16,000
*D*ehydrogenase (LDH) >350
*E*nzyme (OT) >250

Pancreatitis (management)

*P*ain control
*A*ntibiotics
*N*PO/NG-tube
*C*oagulopathy (DIC)
*R*enal function (UOP, S-Gravity)
*E*lectrolyte monitoring
*A*irway (O2 for hypoxia)
*S*upport with IVF

Parrot fever (clinical features)

*P*neumonitis
*A*denopathy
*R*ashes
*R*igid neck (meningismus)
*O*rganomegaly
*T*hroat (pharyngitis)

Pelvic inflammatory disease

(diagnostic criteria of at least three)

*D*ischarge, vaginal
*I*dentified GC or Chlamydia
*S*ed Rate increase
*E*levation of temperature
*A*bdominal tenderness (m)
*S*ex organ tenderness, bilateral adnexal (m)
*E*xtreme cervix tenderness (m)

Peptic Ulcer Disease (management)

*P*roton-pump inhibitor (Omeprazole)
*E*nhance mucosa protection (Sucralfate)
*P*rostaglandin (Misoprostol)
*T*reating H. Pylori
*I*nhibitor of H2
*C*aCO3
*S*urgery for perforation

Pfeiffer syndrome

Premature closure of cranial sutures
Frontal bossing
Exophthalmos
Imperforate anus
Feet (broad hallux, delta phalanx)
Fused vertebrae
Extremity anomaly (broad thumb)
Retarded

Pierre Robin sequence

Retrognathia
Ocular anomalies (Stickler syndrome)
Breathing problem
Incomplete palate (cleft)
Neonatal FTT

Pneumothorax (risk factors)

Tall stature
Thin body mass
Twenties of age
Tobacco smoking
Trauma
Tumors

Poisoning (contraindications for charcoal use)

Cyanide
Hydrocarbon
Acid/alkali
Relative small compounds
Charged (iron, heavy metals)
Organophosphate
Alcohol
Lithium

Poland syndrome

Pectoralis muscle defect
Oblige/syn/brachydactyly
Limb anomaly
Agenesis of kidney
Nipple anomaly
Dextrocardia

Polyarteritis nodosa (PAN)

(clinical features)

Abdominal pain
Rashes
Temperature
Extremity (arthralgia)
Renal failure
Intestinal infarction

Tip of fingers (necrosis)
Increased blood pressure
Seizure

Polycystic ovarian syndrome

(clinical features)

Obesity
Virilization
Anovulation
Resistance to insulin (diabetes)
Increased hair
Androgen increase
No period

Polymyositis/Dermatomyositis

(diagnostic criteria)

Myositis
Unidentification of infectious agent
Symmetric muscle weakness
Cutaneous rashes
Level of enzyme increase (CPK, Aldolase)
EMG shows myopathy

Portal hypertension

(emergency management)

Hemostasis (Fluid/RBC/Plt)
Endoscopic sclerotherapy/ligation
Portal-systemic shunting
ADH and Anti-H2 (Zantac)
Tamponade
Insertion of NG-tube (lavage)
Coagulopathy prevention (Vit K, FFP)

Prader-Willi syndrome

Poor tone (hypotonia)
Retarded (MR)
Abnormal genitalia
Dysmorphic face
Eating problem (obesity)
Reduced pigmentation

Preeclampsia (PRE)/eclampsia (E)

(clinical features)

Proteinuria
Rise in blood pressure
Edema
Epileptic activity confirm eclampsia

Pregnancy (physiological compensations)

Alkaline phosphatase
Blood volume
Cardiac output
Dilutional anemia
ESR
Factors 7, 8, 9, 10
GFR
Heart rate
Inspiration (tidal volume)

Premenstrual syndrome
(management)

Progesterone/pyridoxine/Prozac
Estrogen reduction (GnRH)
Regular aerobic exercise
Inflammatory control (NSAIDs)
OCP. Omega 3 fatty acids (fish oil)
Danazol (reduce mastalgia)
Spironolactone (aldosterone antagonist)

Primary adrenal insufficiency
(clinical features)

Amenorrhea
Derma (hairless)
Reduced blood sugar
Electrolyte interference (K/CaßàNa)
Nutrition (weight loss, anorexia)
Arthralgia/myoralgia
Low BP
Skin (hyperpigmentation)

Primary adrenal insufficiency
(etiologies)

Addison's disease
ACTH resistance
Adrenoleukodystrophy
Adrenal hypoplasia

Prolong QT syndrome (clinical
features--first three are the triad of EKG findings):

Asymmetric T waves
Bradycardia
Corrected QT > 0.44 second
Death may occur
Episodes of presyncope

Proteus syndrome
Pigmentation (café-au-lait spots)
Retarded >20%

Overgrowth with asymmetry
Tumor tendency
Extremity anomalies
Unilateral
Spinal anomaly

Prune-belly syndrome (clinical triad)

Abdominal musculature anomaly
Bladder/urinary tract abnormality
Cryptorchidism

Pruritus (differential diagnosis)

Psychologic
Rashes
Urticaria
Renal/Uremia
Irritants/Allergens
Tumor (Leukemia/Hodgkin)
Infection
Cholestasis (TPN/Pregnancy)
Systemic Medications

Pseudo-tumor cerebri
(clinical features)

Papilledema
Severe headache
Emesis
Unsteadiness (ataxia)
Dizziness
Oculomotor paralysis (diplopia)

Pseudo-tumor cerebri (management)

Prednisone
Spinal tap
Eye examination
Uncover underlying causes
Diamox (decrease CSF production)
Operation (shunt, optic nerve sheath fenestration)

Psoriasis (medication triggers)
Steroids
Chloroquine
Aspirin (NSAIDs)
Lithium
Esmolol (beta-blockers)

Psoriasis (clinical features--two phenomena, three triggers and four skin anomalies) include:

Plaque of skin
Scaly skin
Oily skin
Red skin
Isomorphic phenomenon (Koebner)
Auspitz phenomenon
Strep infection as trigger
Injury as trigger
Stress as trigger

Pulmonary embolism (management)

TPA (tissue plasminogen activator)
Heparin
Resection of bolus
Oxygen
Maintaining BP
Bicarbonate for acidosis
Urokinase
Streptokinase

Pulmonary hypertension (etiologies)

Pulmonary vasculitis
Upper airway obstruction
Lung diseases (CF)
Muscular hypoventilation
Occlusion of pulmonary vessel (pulmonary embolism)
Newborn (PPH)
Idiopathic
Cardiac (ASD, VSD, CHF, shunt)

Pyelonephritis
(clinical features in newborn)

Poor feeding
Yellow (Jaundice)
Emesis
Lethargy
Odorous urine

Pyloric stenosis (clinical features)

Projectile vomiting
Young male (younger than 6 months)
Loss of fluid/Cl (hypochloremic dehydration)
Olive-shaped mass
Reduced weight
Ultrasound with hypertrophy
String/Shoulder signs on UGI film

Rabies (clinical data)

RNA rhabdovirus
Animal bite
Black inclusion (nigri bodies)
Involuntary motion
Encephalitis
Serological tool for diagnosis ((FA stain)

Rape (management)

Reporting
Antibiotic prophylaxes
Pregnancy prevention
Immunization (HBV or tetanus PRN)
Support (emotional and psychosocial)
Testing for infection or semen

Reiter's syndrome (reactive inflammation-clinical features)

Rashes
Enteritis
Arthritis
Conjunctivitis
Tract of genitourinary (urethritis)

Renal venous thrombosis
(etiologies)

TOF (cyanotic CHD)
H2O deficit (dehydration)
Renal anomalies (congenital)
Overdose of contrast agent (hyperosmolar)
Maternal diabetes
Blood (hemoconcentration)
Oxygen insufficiency (asphyxia)
Shock
Increased muscle tone (hypertonia)
Sepsis

Retropharyngeal abscess
(management)

Airway
Breathing
Start antibiotics ASAP
CT scan as gold standard
ENT consultation
Supportive (fluid/pain)
Surgery PRN

Reye's syndrome (clinical features)

Respiratory distress
Encephalopathy
Yellow liver (fatty degeneration)
Elevation of mitochondrial enzymes
Salicylates as trigger

Rhabdomyolysis (evaluation)

Myoglobinuria
Urinalysis
Serum potassium
Creatinine
Lysis sign on CBC (hemolysis)
Enzyme (CPK) increase

Rheumatic fever

[major (M) and/or minor (m) criteria]

Rashes (M)
Heart disease (M)
Extensor skin nodules (M)
Unique chorea (Sydenham) (M)
Migrating arthritis (M)
Arthralgia (m)
Temperature (m)
Inflammatory (ESR, CRP) (m)
Cardiac blockage on EKG (m)

Rickets (risk factors)

Rapid growth (premie)
Inadequate intake of D and Ca
Chronic liver disease
Kidney insufficiency (calcitriol)
Enteral loss (IBD)
Tubular dysfunction (loss of Ca or Phos)
Sunlight deficit

Roseola infantum (clinical features)

Rashes
Occipital adenopathy
Seizure
Encephalopathy
Ocular (eyelid) edema
Low platelet
Aseptic meningitis

Rubella (clinical features)

Rash
URI
Birth defects
Eye involvement
Lymphadenopathy

Low grade fever
Arthritis

Rubinstein-Taybi syndrome

Retarded growth
Unsteady/stiff gait
Broad thumbs/toes
IQ impairment
Narrow palate with hypoplastic maxilla
Speech difficulties
Tone (hypotonia)
Eye (heavy eyebrows and long eyelashes)
Infection in infancy
Nose (beaked and prominent)

Russell-Silver syndrome

Retarded growth
Uniparental disomy 7
Small/Triangular face with normal HC
Short arm-span, limb asymmetry
Extremity anomaly (clinodactyly)
Low birth weight
Low blood sugar at birth

Salmonella infection (complications)

Sepsis
Adenopathy
Loss of fluids/electrolytes
Myocarditis
Osteomyelitis
Neurological
Enteritis
Lung involvement
Liver involvement
Arthritis

Sarcoidosis (clinical features)

Granuloma
Rashes
Adenopathy
Noncaseating
Uveitis
Lung infiltration
Organomegaly
Malaise
Arthritis

Scarlet fever (clinical features)

Strawberry tongue"
Circumoral pallor"
Adenopathy
Rashes ("sandpaper")
Line of "Pastia"
Enlarged tonsils
Temperature (fever)

Scleroderma (pathogenesis)

Skin as major target
Collagen glycosylation anomaly
Laminin auto-antibodies
Endothelin anomaly
Raynaud phenomenon
Organ involvement

Scleroderma (skin changes)

Discoloration
Edema
Raynaud phenomenon
Morning stiffness
Atrophy

Scleroderma (organ involvement)

Skin
Cardiac
Lung
Esophagus/enteral/oral
Renal
Ocular
Skeletal
Intracranial nerves
Sicca syndrome with parotitis

Seckel syndrome

Short stature
Enlarged nose
CNS anomaly (MR)
Knee/hip anomalies
Eleven ribs
Low ears/large eyes

Sepsis (risk factors)

Sickle cell disease
Engrafted (BMT) patients
Polynuclear cell dysfunction
Steroids usage
Indwelling catheter
SCIDS

Serum sickness (clinical features)

Splenomegaly
Extremity (joint effusion)
Regional lymphadenopathy
Urticarial/maculopapular rashes
Mental change (CNS vasculitis)

Short stature (evaluation)

Skeletal Age/Sweat
Turner's (Genetics)
Anemia
TSH.T4.T3
UA (UTI.RTA)
Renal/electrolytes
ESR/Endocrine

SIADH (etiology)

Secretary tumors (pancreatic carcinoma)
Infection of brain (meningitis, encephalitis)
Asthma/lung diseases (TB, CF, pneumonia)
Drugs (nicotine, clofibrate)
Head trauma

Slipped capital femoral epiphysis (clinical features)

Chronic-most common
Acute slip superimposed on chronic slip also
   common
Pain as major symptom
Internal rotation decreased
Thickening palpable
Atrophy of thigh
Limping or waddling gait

Smith-Magenis syndrome

Short stature
Mental retardation
Insertion of foreign bodies (Polyembolokoiamania)
Tendon reflex absence (neuropathy?)
Hypoplastic mid-face

Smoking (risks to kids with parental smoking)

SIDS
Meningitis
Otitis media
Killed by fire or cancers
Embryopathy (IUGR)
Respiratory (RAD, URI)

Speech problems (etiologies)

*A*utism/Anatomic Abel
*B*lindness/Brain Injury
*C*hromosome/CNS
*D*eafness/DD
*E*nvironment Depression/Early Birth (Premature)

Speech delay (evaluation)

*S*ocial/family history
*P*arenting history
*E*ars (hearing loss)
*A*utism
*K*aryotyping/chromosomes
*I*nfection
*N*eurological imaging
*G*estation-related (preemie)

Spider bites (management for black widow)

*B*enzodiazepine and muscle relaxant
*L*atrodectus antivenom
*A*nalgesic (morphine)
*C*alcium
*K*eep wound clean

Splenomegaly (etiologies)

*S*ickle Cell Anemia
*P*ortal Hypertension
*L*upus
*E*nzyme Deficiencies (Metabolic)
*E*BV Infection
*N*eoplastic (Leukemia/Lymphoma)

Stevens-Johnson syndrome
(clinical features)

*S*ensitivity disorders
*T*emperature high
*E*rythema multiforme rash and bullae of skin
*U*lceration of mucous membranes
*E*ye (conjunctivitis, uveitis)
*N*ephritis (hematuria)
*S*epsis potential

Stickler syndrome

*S*pine (spondylo-epiphyseal dysplasia
*T*horax (MVP, disk herniation)
*I*Q-normal
*C*left palate
*K*nee/hip anomalies
*L*oss of hearing
*E*ye (myopia)
*R*obin sequence

Stroke (risk factors)

*S*ickle cell disease
*T*obacco
*R*ise in Cholesterol
*O*besity
*K*etone (diabetes)
*E*levated blood pressure

Sturge-Weber syndrome

*S*eizure
*T*rigeminal hemangioma
*U*nilateral eye involvement
*R*etarded (MR)
*G*laucoma
*E*ar anomalies

Sudden infant death syndrome
(risk factors)

*S*leeping position
*I*UGR/Premature
*D*efect of airway
*S*moking

Supraventricular tachycardia
(management)

*A*denosine
*B*eta-blockers
*C*alcium blockers
*D*igoxin
*E*lectrocardioversion

Syncope (pathologic etiologies)

*S*tructural Abnormality of Vessels (AVM)
*Y*oungster's Breath Holding
*N*eurological
*C*ardiac
*O*rthostatic Hypotension
*P*rolonged QT syndrome
*E*ndocrine (adrenal insufficiency)

Systemic lupus erythematosus
(diagnostic criteria)

Renal involvement
Hematological
Epidermal photosensitivity
Ulceration of mucous membranes (oral/nasal
    mucosa)
Mallor rashes
ANA (anti-nuclear antibody)
Thorax (pleural/cardial effusion)
Immunological (Anti-dsDNA)
CNS (encephalopathy, seizure etc)
Arthritis
Lupus (discoid lupus)

Teething (features)

Temperature <101
Eat but low appetite
Erupt site swelling/pain
Tylenol helpful
Hand sucking often occurs
Irritable but consolable
No diarrhea but drooling
Gum-rubbing

Toxic shock syndrome (STSS)
(clinical features)

Staph/strep infection
Temperature >102
Skin rashes
Shock (systolic BP < 90)

Toxoplasmosis (caused by toxoplasma
gondii--clinical features)

Growth (IUGR)
Ocular (retinitis)
Neurological (hydrocephalus)
Deafness
Intracerebral calcification
IQ impaired

Townes-Brocks syndrome

Bony defect of hands, thumb anomaly
Rectal/anal anomaly
Otic anomaly (hearing loss and dysplastic ears)
Cardiac defects
Kidney anomaly
Spadias (hypospadias)

Tracheoesophageal fistula
(complications)

Failure to breathe
Immobility of esophagus
Stomach perforation on PPV
Tracheomalacia
Upper airway irritation (cough)
Lower airway infection (pneumonia)
Achalasia

Treacher-Collins syndrome

Treacle gene mutation
Robin sequence
Eye anomalies (lid coloboma)
Antimongoloid palpebral fissures
Conductive hearing loss
Hypoplastic zygomas/mandible
External ear anomalies
Retrognathia

Trisomy 13

Trisomy 13
Holoprosencephaly
IQ low (MR)
Retarded growth
Thorax/heart (80%VSD)
Eye (microphthalmia)
Eating problem (FTT)
Ninety-five percent die with six months

Trisomy 18

Extra chromosome 18
IQ low (MR)
Growth retardation (IUGR)
Hypertonia
Thorax (small chest/heart defects)
Eye/ear/extremities
Eating problem (always requires NGF)
Ninety percent die within first year

Trisomy 21 (Down syndrome)

Age-advanced maternal age
Brain (MR)
Cardiac (CHD)
Dysmorphic features
Eyes (cataract, strabismus)
Feeding problem
GI anomalies (Hirschsprung)
Hypotonia
Infection
Joint laxity
Karyotype (trisomy or translocation)
Leukemia potential
Microcephaly
Neck (cervical spine)

*O*titis (conductive hearing loss, hearing test)

Tuberculosis (side effects of INH)

*I*rritation of GI tract
*N*europathy
*H*epatitis

Tuberous sclerosis (clinical features)

*S*ubependymal nodules
*C*ortical tubers
*L*ipoma
*E*xtremity (ungual fibroma)
*R*habdomyoma (heart)
*O*cular (astrocytic hamartoma)
*S*kin (shagreen patches, ashleaf, CALS and edenoma sebaceum)
*I*nfantile spasm
*S*eizure of any type

Turner syndrome

*T*horacic aortic stenosis/coarctation
*U*nderdeveloped gonads
*R*esidual lymphedema
*N*eck webbing
*E*ndocrine (GH and TSH deficiency)
*R*enal anomaly
*S*exuality (delayed puberty)

Ulcerative colitis/Crohn disease

(extraintestinal manifestation)

*U*veitis
*L*oss of weight
*C*holangitis
*E*xtremity (arthritis)
*R*ed cell (anemia)
*S*pondylitis

Ulcerative colitis

(indications for surgery)

*C*ancer
*O*bstruction
*L*osing blood
*I*neffective medical management
*T*oxic megacolon
*I*ncapacitating disease
*S*low growth (failure to thrive)

Urticaria (management)

(backward order with importance/urgency)

*A*tarax for **a**nti-H1 receptors

*B*enadryl **b**etter
*C*orticoids for **c**hronic phase
*D*iscontinuation of "**d**rugs/offenders"
*E*pinephrine for **e**mergency

Usher syndrome

Clinical features include:
*U*nder-diagnosed (very common in profound deafness/blindness)
*S*ensorineural
*H*earing loss
*E*ye
*R*etinitis pigmentosa

Viral hepatitis (clinical features)

*H*epatomegaly
*E*ncephalopathy
*P*rodromic fever
*A*scites
*T*hrive failure
*O*bstruction
*C*oagulopathy
*Y*ellow (jaundice)
*T*umor potential
*E*dema
*S*plenomegaly

Volvulus (clinical features)

*M*alrotation as trigger
*I*rritable infant
*D*istended abdomen
*G*I track bleeding
*U*p-drawing of legs
*T*enderness on exam

Von Hippel-Lindau syndrome

*V*ision loss
*O*cular (retinal angioma)
*N*ephritic (renal cell carcinoma)
*H*emangioblastoma of brain (cerebella)
*I*ncreased ICP
*P*heochromocytoma
*P*ancreas cyst
*E*ctopic erythropoietin
*L*iver cyst

Wegener granulomatosis
(clinical features)

Weight loss
Enlarged spleen
Glomerulonephritis
Erythematous rashes
Neuropathy
Eye
Respiratory
Sinuses

Whipple's disease (clinical features)

Weight loss
Heart involvement
Intestinal symptoms
Pulmonary symptoms
Polyarthritis
Lymphadenopathy
Enlarged spleen

Williams syndrome

Wide mouth
Iris (stellate)
Lip prominence
Long philtrum
IUGR
Abnormal voice (hoarse voice)
Mental retardation
Supravalvular aortic stenosis

Wilson disease
(copper metabolic disorder-complications)

Cardiomyopathy
Osteoporosis
Pancreatitis

Puberty delay
Eye (Kayser-Fleischer ring)
Red blood cell (anemia)

Wiskott-Aldrich syndrome
(management)

Waive contact sport
IVIG
Splenectomy
Kill germs (Antibiotics) for acute infection
Oral Abx as prophylaxis in post-splenectomy
Transfusion (platelet)
Transplant (BMT)

(Please send your comments and your mnemonics to
Dr. Zhao at: zmnemonics@yahoo.com)

BIBLIOGRAPHY

BOOKS/ARTICLES:

Aaron CK, Bania TC: Insecticides: Organophosphates and Carbamates. In Goldfranks, LR (ed): Goldfrank's Toxicologic Emergencies. East Norwalk, CT, Appleton and Lange, 1994, pp 1105-1116.

Acad Emerg Med 1997; 4:1025

Advanced Cardiac Life Support. Dallas: American Heart Association, 2001.

Advanced Trauma Life Support. Chicago: American College of Surgeons, 1995.

American Academy of Ophthalmology. Basic and Clinical Science Course. Section 8 (1994-95), Section 9 (1996-97) and Section 12 (1997-98).

Anderson, J.E. Grant's Atlas of Anatomy (19th Ed.). Baltimore: Williams & Wilkins, 1999.

Auerbach, P.S. Management of Wilderness and Environmental Emergencies (4th Ed.). St. Louis: C.V. Mosby Company, 2001.

Bakerman, S. ABCs of Interpretive Laboratory Data (3rd Ed.). Greenville: Interpretive Laboratory Data, Inc., 1994.

Barkin, R.M. Emergency Pediatrics (4th Ed.). St. Louis: C.V. Mosby Company, 2004.

Bartlett, J.G. and Gorbach, S.L., The triple threat of aspiration pneumonia.
Chest . 1975. 68: 4.

Berkow, R. The Merck Manual (17th Ed.). Rahway: Merck Sharp & Dohme Research Laboratories, 1999.

Bork, K. Diagnosis and Treatment of Common Skin Diseases. Philadelphia: W.B. Saunders Company, 1999.

Bryson, P.D. Comprehensive Review in Toxicology (2nd Ed.) Aspen Publishers, Inc., 1989

Cahill, B.C. and Ingbar, D.H., Massive hemoptysis. Clinics in Chest Medicine.
1994. 15: 147.

Cullom, RD Jr. and Chang, B (eds.) The Wills Eye Manual: Office and Emergency Room Diagnosis and Treatment of Eye Disease, Second Edition. JB Lippincott Co., Philadelphia. 1994.

Dambro, M.R. Griffith's 5 Minute Clinical Consult. Williams and Wilkins, 2004.

DeGowin, E.L. Bedside Diagnostic Examination (7th Ed.). New York: Macmillan Publishing Co. Inc., 1999.

Diagnostic and Treatment Guidelines on Domestic Violence, AMA Publication.

Diagnostic and Treatment Guidelines on Sexual Assault, AMA Publication.

Firearm Violence: Community Diagnosis and Treatment, Publication and slide show of Physicians for Social Responsibility

Fitzpatrick, T.B. Color Atlas and Synopsis of Clinical Dermatology. New York: McGraw-Hill Publishing Company, 2000.

Harris, J.H. The Radiology of Emergency Medicine (4th Ed.). Baltimore: Williams and Wilkins, 2000.

Harrison, T.R. Principles of Internal Medicine (15th Ed.). New York: McGraw-Hill Book Company, 2000.

Harwood-Nuss, A. The Clinical Practice of Emergency Medicine. Philadelphia: J.B. Lippincott Company, 2nd. Ed, 1996.

Harwood-Nuss, A. The Clinical Practice of Emergency Medicine. (3rd Ed.) Philadelphia: J.B. Lippincott Company, 2001.

Hoppenfeld, S. Physical Examination of the Spine and Extremities. Norwalk: Appleton-Century-Crofts, 1976.

Kirk M   Smoke Inhalation. In Goldfranks, LR (ed): Goldfrank's Toxicologic Emergencies. East Norwalk, CT, Appleton and Lange, 2002, pp. 1183-1272.

Leaverton, P.E. A Review of Biostatistics (5th Ed.). Boston: Little Brown and Company, 1995.

Marriott, H.J.L. Practical Electrocardiography (10th Ed.). Baltimore: Williams and Wilkins, 2001.

Moore, K.L. Clinically Oriented Anatomy. Baltimore: Williams & Wilkins, 1982.

Nelson, Waldo E. Textbook of Pediatrics. Philadelphia: W.B. Saunders Comany, 2004.

Pepose, JS, Holland, GN, and Wilhelmus, KR. Ocular Infection and Immunity. Mosby, St. Louis. 1995.

Perkins, E.S. An Atlas of Diseases of the Eye (4th Ed.). London: Churchill Livingstone, 1993.

Physicians' Desk Reference (58th Ed.). Oradell: Medical Economics Company Inc., 2004.

Plantz, S.H. Emergency Medicine Pearls of Wisdom. (6th Ed.). McGraw-Hill, 2005.

Plantz, SH. Emergency Medicine PreTest, Self-Assessment and Review, McGraw- Hill, 1990.

Robbins, S.L. Pathologic Basis of Disease (3rd Ed.). Philadelphia: W.B. Saunders Company, 1984.

Rosen, P. Emergency Medicine Concepts and Clinical Practice (5th Ed.). St. Louis: Mosby Year Book, 2000.

Rowe, R.C. The Harriet Lane Handbook (15th Ed.). Chicago: Year Book Medical Publishers, Inc., 2002.

Simon, R.R. Emergency Orthopedics The Extremities (3rd Ed.). Norwalk: Appleton & Lange, 1995.

Simon, R.R. Emergency Procedures and Techniques (3rd Ed.). Baltimore: Williams and Wilkins, 2001.

Slaby, F. Radiographic Anatomy. New York: John Wiley & Sons, 1990.

Squire, L.F. Fundamentals of Radiology (5th Ed.). Cambridge: Harvard University Press, 1997.

Stedman, T.L. Illustrated Stedman's Medical Dictionary (27th Ed.). Baltimore: Williams & Wilkins, 2000.

Stewart, C.E. Environmental Emergencies. Baltimore: Williams and Wilkins, 1990.

Textbook of Pediatric Advanced Life Support. Dallas: American Heart Association, 2002.

The Hand Examination and Diagnosis (2nd Ed.). London: Churchill Livingstone, 1983.

The Hand Primary Care of Common Problems (2nd Ed.). London: Churchill Livingstone, 1990.

The Physician's Guide to Domestic Violence, Salber and Taliaferro, Volcano Press, 1995

Tietjen, P., Kaner, R.J. and Quinn, C.E., Aspiration Emergencies. Clinics in Chest Medicine. 1994. 15: 117.

Tintinalli, J.E. Emergency Medicine A Comprehensive Study Guide (5th Ed.). New York: McGraw-Hill, Inc., 1999.

Tsang T, Demby AM. Penile fracture with urethral injury. The Journal of Urology, 1992;147:466-468.

Weinberg, S. Color Atlas of Pediatric Dermatology (4th Ed.). New York: McGraw-Hill, 2001.

Weiner, H.L. Neurology for the House Officer (6th Ed.). Baltimore: Williams & Wilkins, 2004.

Wilkins, E. W. Emergency Medicine (3rd Ed.). Baltimore: Williams & Wilkins, 1989.

NOTES

NOTES

NOTES

NOTES

NOTES

NOTES

NOTES